Opioids in Pain Control

Basic and Clinical Aspects

This book offers a comprehensive overview of the often controversial and confounding use of opioids in pain control. Serving both scientists and clinicians, it informs scientists about unresolved clinical problems of using opioids for pain relief; and it teaches physicians about the practical implications of such use. Written by an internationally recognized group of contributors, it covers topics ranging from the molecular biology of opioid receptors and the basic pharmacology of endogenous and exogenous opioids to the clinical applications of opioids in acute and chronic pain.

Discoveries such as the cloning of the opioid receptors, the transplantation of opioid-producing cells, the inhibition of opioid-degrading enzymes, anti-opioids, and the peripheral effects in visceral and inflammatory pain are discussed along with the actual and potential clinical implications of these developments. Clinically oriented chapters include the application of opioids in malignant and nonmalignant chronic pain, pre-emptive analgesia, intra- and postoperative pain, and obstetrics.

Dr. Christoph Stein, chairman of the Department of Anesthesiology and Critical Care Medicine at Freie Universität Berlin, recently completed a five-year appointment in the Department of Anesthesiology at Johns Hopkins School of Medicine. A recipient of several honors and awards for his work with opioids and their use in pain control, he has contributed numerous articles to publications including the *New England Journal of Medicine,* the *Lancet,* the *Proceedings of the National Academy of Sciences USA,* the *Journal of Clinical Investigation,* the *Journal of Neuroscience,* and *Anesthesiology.*

Opioids in Pain Control

Basic and Clinical Aspects

Edited by

CHRISTOPH STEIN

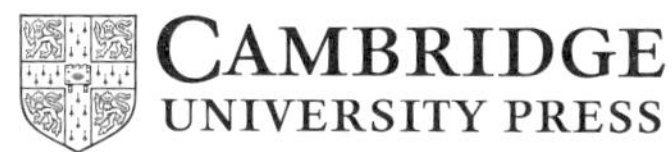

PUBLISHED BY THE PRESS SYNDICATE OF THE UNIVERSITY OF CAMBRIDGE
The Pitt Building, Trumpington Street, Cambridge CB2 1RP, United Kingdom

CAMBRIDGE UNIVERSITY PRESS
The Edinburgh Building, Cambridge CB2 2RU, United Kingdom http: //www.cup.cam.ac.uk
40 West 20th Street, New York, NY 10011–4211, USA http: //www.cup.org
10 Stamford Road, Oakleigh, Melbourne 3166, Australia

First published 1999

Printed in the United States of America

Typeset in 10.5/13.5 Times Roman in QuarkXPress [GH]

A catalogue record for this book is available from the British Library.

Library of Congress Cataloging-in-Publication Data

Opioids in pain control : basic and clinical aspects / edited by Christoph Stein.
p. cm.
ISBN 0-521-62269-7
1. Opioids. 2. Analgesia. 3. Pain. I. Stein, Christoph, 1954–
[DNLM: 1. Narcotics – therapeutic use. 2. Pain – drug therapy.
3. Palliative Care. QV 90 061 1999]
RM328.066 1999
615'.783–dc21
DNLM/DLC 98-19063
CIP

ISBN 0 521 62269 7 hardback

Contents

Contributors

Jean-Jacques Benoliel
Faculté de Médecine
Pitié-Salpêtrière
Paris, France

Christopher M. Bernards
Department of Anesthesiology
University of Washington Medical School
Seattle, Washington

Silvie Bourgoin
Faculté de Médecine
Pitié-Salpêtrière
Paris, France

Lesley Bromley
Division of Anesthesia
University College London Hospital Medical School
Middlesex Hospital
London, United Kingdom

Eduardo Bruera
Division of Palliative Care Medicine
Department of Oncology
University of Alberta
Edmonton, Alberta, Canada

Peter J. Cabot
Department of Anesthesiology and Critical Care Medicine
Johns Hopkins School of Medicine
Baltimore, Maryland

François Cesselin
NeuroPsychoPharmacologie
Moleculaire, Cellulaire et Fonctionnelle
Institut National de la Santé et de la Recherche Médicale
Paris, France

Elisabeth Collin
Faculté de Médecine
Pitié-Salpêtrière
Paris, France

Brian M. Cox
Department of Pharmacology
Uniformed Services University of the Health Sciences
Bethesda, Maryland

Marie-Claude Fournié-Zaluski
Unité de Pharmacochimie Moleculaire et Structurale
Université René Descartes
Paris, France

Claire Gavériaux-Ruff
Ecole Supérieure de Biotechnologie de Strasbourg
Université Louis Pasteur
Illkirch, France

G. F. Gebhart
Department of Pharmacology
University of Iowa College of Medicine
Iowa City, Iowa

Wiebke Gogarten
Klinik und Poliklinik fur Anaesthesiologie und operative Intensivmedizin
Westfälische Wilhelms-Universität
Münster, Germany

Michel Hamon
Faculté de Médecine
Pitié-Salpêtrière
Paris, France

Mary M. Heinricher
Division of Neurosurgery
Department of Physiology and Pharmacology
Oregon Health Sciences University
Portland, Oregon

Carl C. Hug, Jr.
Cardiothoracic Anesthesia
The Emory Clinic
Emory University School of Medicine
Atlanta, Georgia

Brigitte Kieffer
Ecole Supérieure de Biotechnologie de Strasbourg
Université Louis Pasteur
Illkirch, France

Peter Lawlor
Division of Palliative Care Medicine
Department of Oncology
University of Alberta
Edmonton, Alberta, Canada

Klaus A. Lehmann
Klinik für Anaesthesiologie und operative Intensivmedizin
Universität zu Köln
Köln, Germany

Marco A. E. Marcus
Klinik und Poliklinik fur Anaesthesiologie und operative Intensivmedizin
Westfälische Wilhelms-Universität
Münster, Germany

Laurence E. Mather
Department of Anesthesia and Pain Management
University of Sydney at Royal North Shore Hospital
St. Leonard's NSW, Australia

Michael M. Morgan
Department of Psychology
Washington State University
Vancouver, Washington

Dwight E. Moulin
Department of Clinical Neurological Sciences
London Health Sciences Center, Victoria Campus
London, Ontario, Canada

Florence Noble
Unité de Pharmacochimie Moleculaire et Structurale
Université René Descartes
Paris, France

Michel Pohl
Faculté de Médecine
Pitié-Salpêtrière
Paris, France

Narinder Rawal
Department of Anesthesiology and Intensive Care
Orebro Medical Center Hospital
Orebro, Sweden

Bernard P. Roques
Unité de Pharmacochimie Moleculaire et Structurale
Université René Descartes
Paris, France

Jacqueline Sagen
CytoTherapeutics, Inc.
Providence, Rhode Island

Michael Schäfer
Klinik für Anaesthesiologie und operative Intensivmedizin
Universitätsklinikum Benjamin Franklin
Freie Universität Berlin
Berlin, Germany

Jyotirindra N. Sengupta
Department of Pharmacology
University of Iowa College of Medicine
Iowa City, Iowa

Maree T. Smith
School of Pharmacy
University of Queensland
St. Lucia, QLD, Australia

Christoph Stein
Klinik für Anaesthesiologie und operative Intensivmedzin
Universitätsklinikum Benjamin Franklin
Freie Universität Berlin
Berlin, Germany

Xin Su
Department of Pharmacology
University of Iowa College of Medicine
Iowa City, Iowa

Hugo Van Aken
Klinik und Poliklinik fur Anaesthesiologie und operative Intensivmedizin
Westfälische Wilhelms-Universität
Münster, Germany

Paul Walker
Division of Palliative Care Medicine
Department of Oncology
University of Alberta
Edmonton, Alberta, Canada

Zsuzsanna Wiesenfeld-Hallin
Department of Medical Laboratory Sciences
Section of Clinical Neurophysiology, Karolinska Institute
Huddinge University Hospital
Huddinge, Sweden

Clifford Woolf
Division of Anesthesia and Critical Care
Massachusetts General Hospital
Boston, Massachusetts

Xiao-Jun Xu
Department of Medical Laboratory Sciences
Section of Clinical Neurophysiology, Karolinska Institute
Huddinge University Hospital
Huddinge, Sweden

Foreword

In 1680, Sydenham, a famous English physician, wrote, "Among the remedies which it has pleased Almighty God to give to man to relieve his sufferings, none is so universal and so efficacious as opium." Following the isolation of morphine from opium almost 200 years ago and the invention of the hypodermic needle for parenteral application in the middle of the last century, this alkaloid became the remedy of choice for relief of severe pain – although its addictive properties also became more and more apparent. Thus, considerable efforts were undertaken to develop semisynthetic and synthetic derivates that might not be addictive. These attempts, however, were only partially successful.

A new era of opioid research began with the identification of opioid receptors and the detection of endogenous ligands of these receptors 25 years ago. Presently, the occurrence of three opioid receptor types (μ, δ, κ) is well established. They represent the targets of three families of opioid peptides, β-endorphin, enkephalins, and dynorphins. The wide distribution of these opioid receptors and ligands in the central and peripheral nervous systems and other organs points to multiple neuronal and extraneuronal functions. More recently, new opioid peptides and opioid receptor types have been detected, the functional significance of which is so far largely unknown. The recent cloning of opioid receptors will provide new insights into the function of these systems at the molecular level.

In parallel with these fundamental developments in the opioid field, major progress was also made with respect to the neurophysiologic and neurochemical mechanisms of acute and chronic pain. A major role of opioid mechanisms in pain modulatory systems is now well established, and new research has made many contributions to the rational management of acute and chronic pain by a variety of selected opioids. New applications have been found for opioids in various medical disciplines, and most important, new strategies have been developed to minimize the risk of development of addiction.

The first eight chapters of this volume deal with basic aspects of opioid research with respect to pain control. Chapter 1, co-authored by Claire Gavériaux-Ruff and Brigitte Kieffer, who were among the first to clone an opioid receptor, describes recent progress in the molecular biology of opioid receptors and their cDNAs and genes, as well as the pharmacologic and functional properties of cloned μ-, δ-, and κ-opioid receptors. In

Chapter 2, Bernard P. Roques, Florence Noble, and Marie-Claude Fournié-Zaluski deal with the role of endogenous opioid peptides in analgesia and the effects of inhibition of degradation of enkephalins by peptidase inhibitors. Supraspinal mechanisms of pain modulation by opioids and the circuitry involved in supraspinal/spinal interaction are discussed in Chapter 3 by Mary M. Heinricher and Michael M. Morgan. This chapter is complemented by Chapter 4 by François Cesselin, Jean-Jacques Benoliel, Silvie Bourgoin, Elisabeth Collin, Michel Pohl, and Michel Hamon, who examine the interactions between opioids and other neuropeptides. More recent results indicate that besides the brain and the spinal cord, peripheral sites may also participate in opioid modulation of pain. Such peripheral mechanisms of activation of opioid receptors and endogenous ligands under inflammatory conditions as well as their clinical implications are the topic of Chapter 5 by Christoph Stein, the books's editor, Peter J. Cabot, and Michael Schäfer.

Adaptation of the organism to chronic opioid exposure remains an important aspect of pain management. The complicated mechanisms involved in tolerance development are analyzed by Brian M. Cox in Chapter 6, while clinical aspects of prolonged opioid treatment are covered in several subsequent chapters. Modulation of the analgesic effects of opioids by endogenous compounds antagonizing opioid action ("antiopioids") is discussed by Zsuzsanna Wiesenfeld-Hallin and Xiao-Jun Xu in Chapter 7. Chapter 8 by Jacqueline Sagen considers the effects of transplantation of opioid-producing cells – a topic rarely touched to date. Chapter 9 by Christopher M. Bernards summarizes data on the physicochemical properties of clinically relevant opioids and discusses their pharmacokinetic aspects, especially with regard to their topical (spinal) applications.

The second group of chapters, Chapters 10–18, examines the use opioids as analgesics in various clinical disciplines. Chapter 10 by Laurence E. Mather and Maree T. Smith, on the clinical pharmacology of opioid analgesics, focuses on metabolic, pharmacokinetic, and adverse effects. Clifford Woolf and Lesley Bromley describe in Chapter 11 the phenomenon of pre-emptive analgesia, a therapeutic strategy whose clinical usefulness is a topic of much current discussion. Chapter 12, by Carl C. Hug, Jr., discusses the intraoperative use of opioids from the perspective of pharmacokinetics. In Chapter 13, Narinder Rawal deals with the use of opioids in acute pain and the various methods available for their application (in particular, epidural versus intrathecal application). Klaus A. Lehmann in Chapter 14 reviews experience with a large series of opioids in patient-controlled analgesia, a method that seems to be becoming increasingly important with respect to the development of pain-management strategies. Although the extensive use of opioids in cancer pain is presently generally accepted, the same does not apply for the handling of nonmalignant chronic pain. Controversial aspects of opioid use in the latter case, including the development of psychological dependence, are discussed by Dwight E. Moulin in Chapter 15, while aspects of the management of cancer pain are the topic of Chapter 16 by Eduardo Bruera, Paul Walker, and Peter Lawlor. The use of opioids in visceral pain, including experimental data pointing to peripheral sites of κ-opioid receptors, is discussed by G. F. Gebhart,

Jyotirindra N. Segupta, and Xin Su in Chapter 17. Chapter 18, by Marco M. E. Marcus, Wiebke Gogarten, and Hugo Van Aken, provides an overview of the use of opioids in obstetrics.

Summarizing these manifold applications of opioids as potent analgesics in various clinical disciplines leads to the interesting point that, although newer opioids with particular properties (in particular, pharmacokinetics) are widely used in special cases, the genuine opium alkaloid morphine, which binds with high affinity to the μ-opioid receptor, remains the standard analgesic. It is also striking that opioids which bind preferentially to the δ- and κ-opioid receptors and induce analgesia as well have nevertheless not yet been introduced into routine pain therapy, even though some aspects of their pharmacologic actions – for example, with respect to dependence liability – indicate them to be promising therapeutic candidates. Although this book provides an excellent overview of our current understanding of the use of opioids in the clinical management of pain, observations such as the last one indicate that much basic and clinical research remains to be done. In the meantime, this volume will not only assist practicing clinicians to select appropriate treatment modalities and protocols but will also serve as a useful stimulus for future research.

Martinsried
May 1998

Albert Herz
Max-Planck-Institute for Neurobiology

Preface

The impetus to write this book was based on several recent developments in the field of opioid pharmacology, specifically with regard to the pain-relieving effects of these compounds. A careful review of the existing literature revealed that although some volumes deal with opioid pharmacology in general, no recent books focus on the analgesic actions or integrate basic research with clinical applications. The past several years have seen some extremely exciting research developments that have shed new light on mechanisms of opioid analgesia and have stimulated novel approaches to the treatment of acute and chronic pain. Thus, the aim of this book was to gather a group of internationally renowned experts in basic and clinical aspects of opioid actions in pain control. I am extremely grateful to all the contributors who have made extraordinary efforts to write these overviews of their respective fields. Also, I extend my thanks to the publisher, in particular to Jo-Ann Strangis and to my colleagues in the Department of Anesthesiology at Freie Universität Berlin for their invaluable help. In the end, the spirit for this collaborative effort was fueled by my mentor and one of the most prominent investigators in the field, Albert Herz.

CHAPTER ONE

Opioid Receptors: Gene Structure and Function

CLAIRE GAVERIAUX-RUFF AND BRIGITTE KIEFFER

Introduction

Opiates, the prototype of which is morphine, are potent analgesic and addictive drugs that act through opioid receptors (Barnard, 1993; Browstein, 1993). The opioid system plays a major role in pain-controlling systems (Dickenson, 1991) and affective behavior, including motivation and reward (Di Chiara and North, 1992; Koob 1992). It also modulates locomotor activity, learning and memory, neuroendocrine physiology, and autonomic and immune functions (Olson et al., 1996). Three classes of opioid receptors, μ, δ, and κ, have been identified by pharmacologic approaches (Goldstein and Naidu, 1989). Their endogenous ligands are the opioid peptides (enkephalins, endorphins, and dynorphins), which share a common N-terminal sequence (NH_2-Tyr-Gly-Gly-Phe-Met/Leu-COOH), and are encoded by three different genes known as preproopiomelanocortin, preproenkephalin, and prodynorphin (Day et al., 1993; Rossier, 1993; Young et al., 1993). A new class of highly μ-selective endogenous peptides has been discovered recently (Zadina et al., 1997). These short tetrapeptides, called endomorphines, are structurally distinct from opioid peptides (NH_2-Tyr-Pro-Trp/Phe-Phe-$CONH_2$), and their genes still need to be isolated. The understanding of pain control or drug addiction, and the development of novel classes of analgesic compounds, require a detailed knowledge of the molecular properties of opioid receptors. Although opioid binding sites have been extensively characterized in the last two decades on the basis of opioid ligand pharmacology, the molecular characterization of the receptors has been initiated only recently (Evans et al., 1992; Kieffer et al., 1992). The first identification of an opioid receptor, cDNA, has opened the way to the identification of the opioid receptor gene family and provided molecular tools to study opioid receptor diversity and function both in vitro and in vivo.

This chapter briefly summarizes the identification of the opioid receptor cDNA and genes, together with the pharmacologic and functional properties of the cloned μ, δ, and κ receptors in vitro. These issues have been reviewed in detail elsewhere (Kieffer, 1995, 1997; Knapp et al., 1995; Reisine, 1995; Satoh and Minami, 1995). We then will emphasize our present knowledge about the organization and splicing

Christoph Stein, ed., *Opioids in Pain Control: Basic and Clinical Aspects*. Printed in the United States of America.

of opioid receptor genes and their function in vivo. Studies using antisense or knock-out strategies have just begun. These approaches are paving the way toward the understanding of opioid neurotransmission at the molecular level.

Molecular Characterization of Opioid Receptors

cDNA Cloning of Opioid Receptors

The first cDNA encoding an opioid receptor was isolated simultaneously by two laboratories in 1992. This cDNA was identified by expression cloning in mammalian cells (Evans et al., 1992; Kieffer et al., 1992) and encodes a mouse δ receptor (mDOR). Sequence analysis of the mDOR protein 372 aminoacid residues in length indicates that the cloned receptor belongs to the family of seven transmembrane G-protein–coupled receptors (Kenakin, 1996). Homology cloning strategies led to the identification of DOR from other mammalian species, as well as cDNAs encoding μ and κ opioid receptors (MOR and KOR respectively; for reviews, see Kieffer, 1995, 1997). Using a PCR-based technology, Li and colleagues identified MOR- and DOR-like DNA sequences in other vertebrate species including chick, frog, bass, and shark (Li et al., 1996a, 1996b). These DNA stretches, encoding short conserved regions of the receptors, display 96–98% homology with the corresponding deduced protein sequences in rodent or human receptors. This suggests that multiple members of the opioid receptor family may exist in lower vertebrates and that the opioid receptor gene family has been conserved during vertebrate evolution.

Another opioid receptor-related cDNA, with high-sequence homology to the three cloned opioid receptors, was isolated from rat, mouse, and human brain cDNA libraries (reviewed in Kieffer, 1997). Attempts to measure specific opioid binding to the recombinant receptor expressed in COS cells was unsuccessful, and this cDNA was named opioidlike orphan receptor (ORL-1). Recently, two groups have reported the isolation of an endogenous ligand for this receptor (Meunier et al., 1995; Reinscheid et al., 1995). This heptadecapeptide, called orphaninFQ or nociceptin, displays structural similarities to opioid peptides but does not act at opioid receptors. This new ligand-receptor system may play a role in pain perception (Meunier et al., 1995; Reinscheid et al., 1995; Grisel et al., 1996; Mogil et al., 1996; Rossi et al., 1996; Xu et al., 1996) and locomotion (Reinscheid et al., 1995; Devine et al., 1996; Florin et al., 1996; Noble and Roques, 1997).

Binding and Functional Properties of the Cloned MOR, DOR, and KOR Receptors

Cell lines expressing cloned receptors allow us to study the binding properties of each receptor type independently. The recombinant receptors have been produced in mammalian cells, and affinities of a large number of opioid ligands have been determined (reviewed in Kieffer, 1995, 1997). From these studies it is clear that DOR, MOR, and KOR encode μ, δ, and κ receptor sites, respectively. Unlimited sources of human recombinant receptors are now available. They represent highly valuable screening tools in drug design programs and in the search for novel therapeutic agents.

The concept of multiple receptor subtypes within each μ, δ, and κ receptor class has emerged from accumulating pharmacologic data. Indeed, δ1, δ2, μ1, μ2, μ3, κ1, κ2, and κ3 subtypes have been proposed (reviewed in Millan, 1990; Pasternak, 1993; Traynor and Elliot, 1993; Makman, 1994), whereas only three opioid receptor genes have been characterized (DOR, MOR, and KOR). Hence, the issue of opioid receptor diversity remains a major matter of debate. Several molecular mechanisms may be responsible for creating the largely documented opioid receptor diversity (see comments in Zaki et al., 1996). These include: (1) the implication of yet uncloned opioid receptor genes; (2) the generation of receptor isoforms by alternative splicing from the known DOR, MOR, and KOR genes; and (3) versatile properties of the MOR-, DOR-, and KOR-encoded proteins, depending on ligand-induced receptor conformational changes, post-translational modifications, association with distinct sets of G-proteins or other proteins, and cellular compartmentalization. The possible existence of a gene different from the described DOR, MOR, and KOR genes was suggested following the isolation of a putative δ receptor-encoding cDNA from lymphocytes (Heagy et al., 1996). Also, the possibility that diversity arises from variable activation mechanisms of the known receptor proteins by distinct agonists is now gaining support from several studies (see comments in Befort and Kieffer, 1997).

Functional expression of DOR, MOR, and KOR receptors in several mammalian host cells suggests that cloned opioid receptors are able to interact with a number of G-protein α subunits. Recombinant opioid receptors may couple to Gi2α, Gi3α, Go2α, and Gz and to an unknown G-protein subunit (Henry et al., 1994, 1995; Prather et al., 1994, 1995; Chakrabarti et al., 1995; Lai et al., 1995; Tsu et al., 1995; Ueda et al., 1995a, 1995b). Several studies using heterologous expression systems showed that receptor-agonist interaction induces the simultaneous activation of multiple G-proteins (Prather et al., 1994, 1995; Chakrabarti et al., 1995; Mullaney et al., 1996). It is of note that a recent report from Wu and colleagues demonstrated the conversion of DOR from inhibitory to excitatory in the presence of GM1 ganglioside, presumably by facilitating the interaction of DOR with Gs (Wu et al., 1997). This confirms a role for lipid environment in the modulation of opioid receptor activity.

The demonstration that cloned opioid receptors are negatively coupled to adenylate cyclase and voltage-gated Ca^{2+} channels or positively coupled to inwardly rectifying K^+ channels and phosphatidyl inositol turnover is well documented (reviewed in Kieffer, 1997). These data have confirmed previous studies conducted on endogenous receptor preparations from nervous tissues (Cox, 1993; North, 1993). Recent studies using heterologous expression systems have found evidence for other possible mechanisms of opioid-mediated cellular response. An implication of G-protein β and γ subunits was suggested for the opioid-induced modulation of hormone release in MOR- and DOR-transfected GH3 cells (Piros et al., 1996). Another finding was the discovery of MOR, DOR, and KOR coupling to mitogen activated protein kinase (MAPK) and phospholipase A2 in stable CHO transfectants (Fukuda et al., 1996). A possible crosstalk with growth factor signaling pathways was described by Law and colleagues, who showed that activation of DOR, but not MOR, potentiates tyrosine-kinase receptor-mediated cell proliferation (Law et al., 1997). MOR can also couple to cystic fibrosis transmembrane conductance regulator (CFTR), as demonstrated by Cl^- currents produced by the μ agonist DAMGO when MOR and the CFTR channel are coexpressed in *Xenopus* oocytes (Wotta et al., 1997).

Opioid tolerance may be partly due to loss of opioid receptor function under sustained exposure to an agonist. Receptor desensitization is now extensively studied using the cloned receptors, and rapid desensitization has been reported for MOR or DOR expressed in heterologous host cells. One mechanism involves receptor phosphorylation (Arden et al., 1995; Pei et al., 1995; Zhang et al., 1996). The implication of nonspecific protein kinases (PKC or unknown kinase) or G-protein–coupled receptor kinases seems to rely on the receptor-expressing cell (reviewed for DOR in Befort and Kieffer, 1997), indicating that multiple receptor sites may be phosphorylated, depending on the cellular context. Rapid receptor sequestration represents another desensitization mechanism. Both MOR and DOR were shown to internalize within a few minutes following agonist treatment in transfected cell lines (Keith et al., 1996) as well as in vivo (Sternini et al., 1996). Interestingly, these studies show that opioid peptides, but not morphine, induce receptor sequestration, indicating that desensitization may be ligand dependent. This phenomenon adds another level of diversity in opioid responses at the cellular level. Finally, the observation of unchanged DOR mRNA levels in DOR-expressing CHO cells following chronic DADLE treatment suggests that long-term receptor down-regulation does not occur at the transcriptional level but rather results from protein degradation (Law et al., 1994).

Altogether these data indicate that opioid receptor activation and functional coupling are complex and highly dependent on the agonist involved, the lipid membrane environment, the G-protein content, and the presence of regulatory proteins in the host cell under study. These observations are critical with regard to our understanding of opioid receptor function in the central nervous system. It is likely that specific properties of neurons, which are found in distinct areas of opioid pathways, are determinant in defining responses to opiates. Accordingly, diverse cellular events may be generated by opiate treatment depending on the neurons involved, and this contributes to the complexity of opioid pharmacology in vivo.

Structural Features of the Cloned Opioid Receptors

Sequence comparison between members of the opioid receptor family (Fig. 1.1) shows high similarity in some protein regions. Putative transmembrane domains (TM), in particular TM 2, 3, 5, 6, and 7; the three intracellular loops; and a short

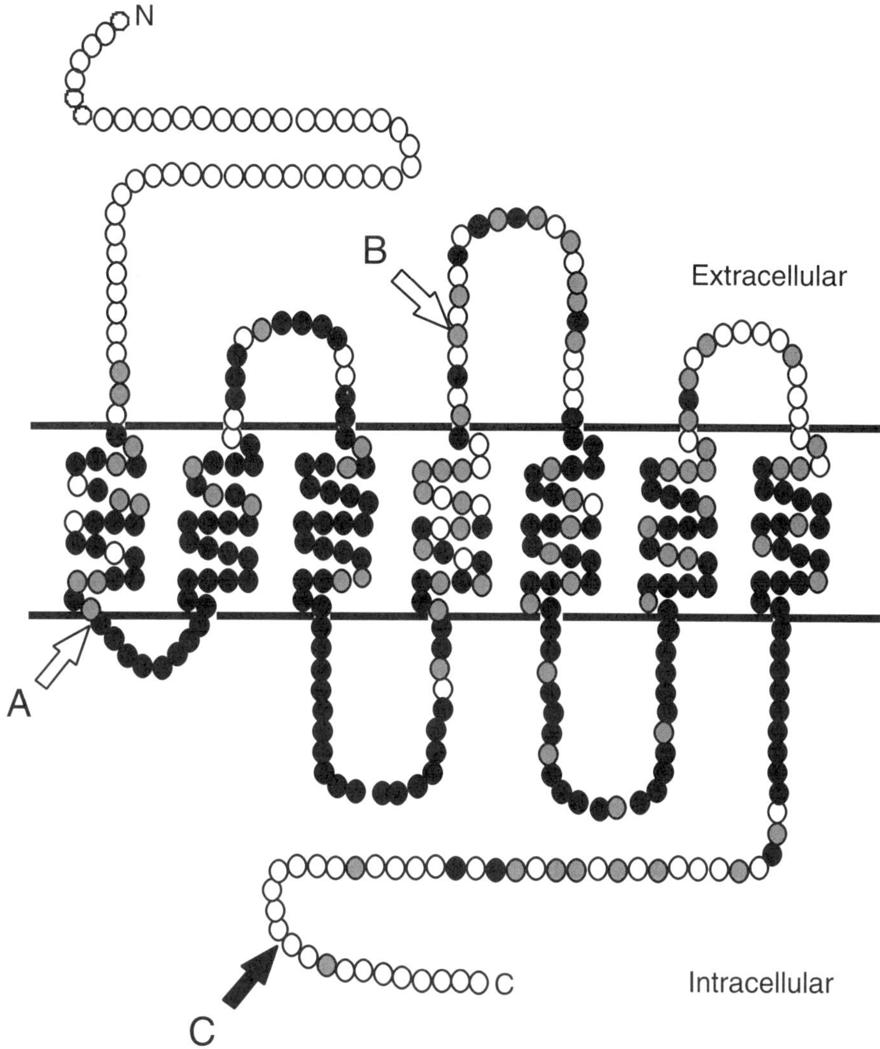

Figure 1.1. Homology between μ, δ, and κ opioid receptors and the localization of splice sites. Putative transmembrane topology of hDOR is illustrated. Each amino acid residue is shown as a circle. White circles indicate amino acid residues that differ between hDOR, hMOR, and hKOR. Gray circles show amino acids that are conserved in two of three receptors, and black circles represent amino acid residues identical in all three receptors. White arrows show splice sites found at equivalent positions in all three genes (A and B), and the black arrow indicates a splice site specific to the MOR gene (C). Alternative splicing was reported at site A for DOR, site B for KOR, and site C for MOR.

region of the C-terminal tail proximal to the membrane are almost identical across subtypes and species. In contrast, little or no homology is found in the extracellular loops or in the N- and C-terminal tails. From this and from our knowledge of structure-function relationships in other cloned G-protein–coupled receptors (Strader et al., 1994), we may predict structural motives that are important for ligand binding and subtype specificity within transmembrane and extracellular domains. We may also anticipate that coupling properties are similar for all three receptor types, whereas the regulation of their activity may differ widely.

Three-dimensional computer modeling and analysis of the binding properties of chimeric or point-mutated opioid receptors have confirmed structural determinants involved in ligand recognition. The general picture that emerges from these studies has been reviewed for MOR by Traynor (1996) and for DOR by Befort and Kieffer (1997). The seven-helical bundle forms an opioid-binding pocket, highly similar across opioid receptor types, in which hydrophilic and aromatic residues from TM II to VII seem to participate in ligand binding. Noteworthy is the demonstrated diversity of interaction modes between DOR and a wide set of opioid ligands (Befort et al., 1996), suggesting the existence of multiple forms of ligand-receptor complexes. Extracellular loops, which differ in sequence between opioid receptor types, play a role in discriminating μ, δ, and κ opioid ligands. Metzger and Ferguson (1995) have suggested that these ectodomains act as a gate that allows binding for some ligands while excluding others.

Intracellular domains of the receptors are implicated in receptor signaling and regulation. The third intracellular loop and the juxtamembraneous part of the C-terminus are involved in coupling to G-proteins. This was shown by the ability of synthetic peptides, which mimic intracellular portions of the receptor, to interfere with G-protein activation following δ-agonist stimulation (Merkouris et al., 1996). The C-terminal portion of DOR, comprising the last 37 aminoacid residues, was shown to be important for receptor desensitization, with distinct parts of the intracellular tail involved in receptor trafficking (Trapaidze et al., 1996) or down-regulation (Cvejic et al., 1996).

Deduced protein sequences of human opioid receptors present 85–90% identity to their rodent counterparts. Regions that are weakly conserved between subtypes, particularly N- and C-terminal domains, also exhibit high variability across species. A striking interspecies divergence was noticed for the KOR sequence, where the first 21 aminoacids are conserved in rat, mouse, and human receptors, but are totally different in the guinea pig receptor (Xie et al., 1994). One should note that no species-specific binding properties of the receptors have been reported to date. Thus, differences in sequences across species do not seem to lead to distinct receptor pharmacologic properties.

Overproduction of Opioid Receptor Proteins for Structural Studies

Computer modeling and the study of mutant recombinant opioid receptors expressed in mammalian cells have permitted establishment of structure-function relationships. Although these data provide useful information about dynamic molecular properties of the receptors, they do not allow delineation of receptor organization at an atomic resolution. This knowledge should come from the determination of 2D- or 3D-crystal structures, a highly challenging goal under present circumstances. One major limitation stems from the requirement of large protein amounts; also, overexpression of recombinant receptors has to be improved. Nonmammalian heterologous expression systems are attractive because they allow low-cost mass production. Recently, opioid receptors have been successfully expressed in *E. coli* (L. Stanisala, personal communication), in the yeast *Pichia pastoris* (Talmont et al., 1996), and in baculovirus-infected insect cells (Obermeier et al., 1996; Massotte et al., 1997). Affinities of agonists for opioid receptors expressed in these organisms are generally lower than in mammalian cells, although binding affinities of antagonist compounds are preserved. This is likely due to the lack *(E. coli)* or inappropriate (yeast, insect cells) expression of G-proteins that may associate with these receptors. At the moment, expression levels (maximum 2 pmol receptor/mg membrane protein) do not exceed those obtained in mammalian cells hosts, as is the case for other GPRs (Grisshammer and Tate, 1995). Large-scale production of these host cells needs to be undertaken, or, alternatively, novel expression systems need to be developed in order to obtain protein amounts sufficient to allow detailed structural studies of the receptors.

Opioid Receptor Genes

General Organization of the Genes

Opioid receptor gene organization has been studied most extensively in the mouse, and chromosomal assignments have been determined in both the mouse and human (for a review, see Kieffer, 1997). Opioid receptor genes share a similar exon/intron organization of their coding regions. These are distributed over three exons, and their splice sites are found at homologous positions after the first and fourth putative TM (see Fig. 1.1). The MOR gene differs from the DOR and KOR genes at the level of exon 3. This exon terminates before the stop codon, the 12 C-terminal aminoacids being encoded by a fourth exon.

Initiation of Transcription and Promoter Regions

Transcription initiation sites have been proposed for all three opioid receptor genes on the basis of RNAse protection and primer extension experiments. Within the MOR gene, two transcriptional start sites have been identified upstream from the ATG translation initiation codon. These are located at positions –793 and between –291 and –269 for the mouse gene (Min et al., 1994; Liang et al., 1995) or at positions –880 and –230 for the rat gene (Kraus et al., 1995). Transcriptonal promoter activity of these regions has been measured in the human SHSY-5Y or SK-N-SH neuroblastoma cell lines known to express μ and δ receptors using a reporter gene assay. In the mouse, a promoter region was identified within a 210 bp portion upstream from the –793 nt transcription start site. In the rat, promoter activity was found to lie within a region spanning 1,198 to 229 bp upstream from the ATG start codon. These regions lack consensus

TATA or CAAT boxes, but contain putative AP1 and AP2 sites. The mouse DOR gene also displays multiple putative transcription initiation sites, including two strong sites located at positions –142 and –324 upstream from the ATG codon (Augustin et al., 1995). In the rat KOR gene, Yakovlev and colleagues identified two clusters of transcription initiation sites upstream from the translational start codon in regions –932 to –907 and –569 to –565, preceded by two TATA boxes and a CAAT box, respectively (Yakovlev et al., 1995). The 5′ region of the mouse KOR gene differs from the rat gene. Three major transcription start sites have been located – 334, 340, and 711 bp upstream from the translation start codon – but no TATA or CAAT boxes could be identified within upstream 1,000 bp (Liu et al., 1995). To our knowledge, no transcriptional activity has been reported for these 5′ regions of the DOR and KOR genes.

Alternative Splicing

The existence of alternative splicing mechanisms was evidenced by analysis of cDNA clones and from RT-PCR experiments. Splice variants have been identified for MOR, DOR, and KOR mRNAs. MOR mRNA isoforms with distinct C-terminal sequences have been described in the rat and human (MOR 1B and MOR 1A; see Fig. 1.2A). MOR 1B derives from alternative splicing at the donor site of exon 3, which is unique to the MOR gene (Zimprich et al., 1995). Analysis of the MOR gene shows the presence of two alternative coding exons downstream from exon 3 (exons 4 and 5) (Mayer et al., 1996). The classically described transcript (MOR) contains exon 5, whereas the rat MOR variant (rMOR 1B) described by Zimprich et al. displays exon 4 instead of 5 at its 3′ end (Fig. 1.2A). The receptor protein encoded by the MOR 1B mRNA was expressed in mammalian cells and was shown to exhibit desensitization properties different from those of the classically described MOR receptor (Zimprich et al., 1995). Recently, the respective anatomic distributions of MOR and MOR 1B were compared by immunocytochemistry. MOR represents the major isoform throughout the brain,

---

Opposite

Figure 1.2. Exon/intron structure and alternative splicing in the coding regions of MOR, DOR, and KOR genes. The organization of the genes is shown for MOR (A), KOR (B), and DOR (C). Transcribed regions are shown by boxes. White boxes represent the classically described exons. Alternative exons, or portion of exons, are shown as filled boxes with various motives. Stars represent the first stop codon for each transcript. (A). MOR mRNA corresponds to the transcript classically isolated from brain. MOR1 B and MOR1 A splice variants have been isolated from rat brain and from the SK-N-SH neuroblastoma cell line and human brain, respectively (see text). (B). The KOR gene displays a 5′ untranslated exon, not described in MOR and DOR genes (exon 1). Exons 2, 3, and 4 in the KOR gene are therefore homologous to exons 1, 2, and 3 in MOR and DOR genes. KOR mRNAs with distinct 5′ untranslated regions have been isolated from mouse and rat. A KOR transcript arising from an alternative splicing mechanism between exon 3 and 4 was reported in human immune cell lines. (C). The classically described DOR mRNA is presented below the gene structure. An mDOR variant has been isolated by RT-PCR from mouse brain. Analysis of this variant suggests the existence of an alternative exon located between exon 1 and 2 (exon 1′).

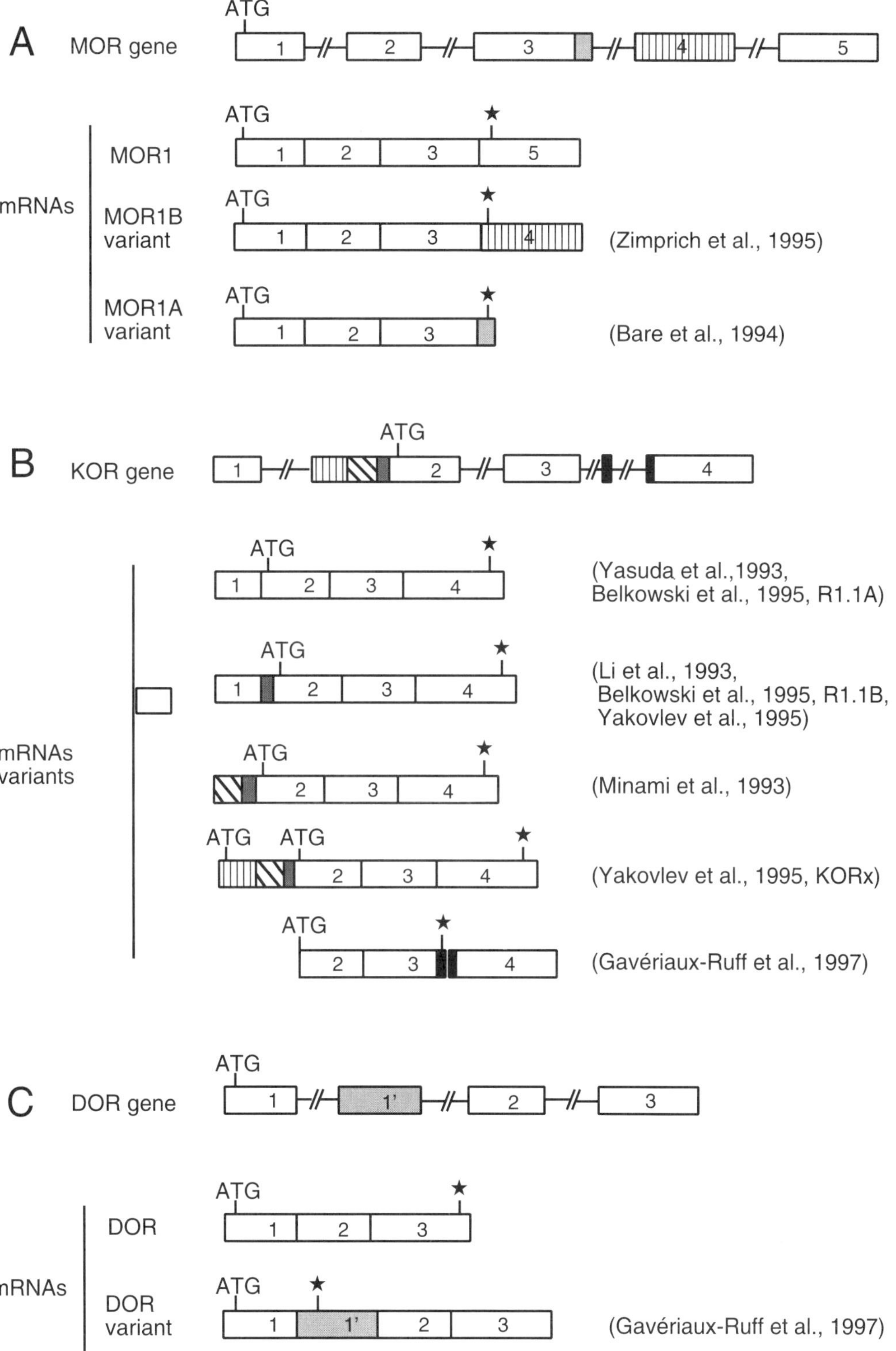
A
MOR gene
ATG
1
2
3
4
5
mRNAs
MOR1
MOR1B
variant
MOR1A
variant
(Zimprich et al., 1995)
(Bare et al., 1994)
B
KOR gene
mRNAs
variants
(Yasuda et al.,1993,
Belkowski et al., 1995, R1.1A)
(Li et al., 1993,
Belkowski et al., 1995, R1.1B,
Yakovlev et al., 1995)
(Minami et al., 1993)
(Yakovlev et al., 1995, KORx)
(Gavériaux-Ruff et al., 1997)
C
DOR gene
1'
DOR
DOR
variant
(Gavériaux-Ruff et al., 1997)

whereas expression of the MOR 1B protein seems to be restricted to the olfactory bulb, suggesting a specific role for the MOR 1B-encoded receptor (Schulz et al., 1997). The human transcript isoform described by Bare and colleagues (MOR 1A; see Fig. 1.2A) differs from MOR and MOR 1B in that the intronic sequence located 3′ of exon 3 has not been spliced out (Bare et al., 1994). An in-frame termination codon is found 12 nucleotides downstream from the consensus splice site. Thus, the receptor protein encoded by this mRNA isoform displays a C-terminal sequence distinct from those of MOR and MOR 1B. When expressed in CHO cells, this variant seems to display pharmacologic and transduction properties identical to the MOR protein (Bare et al., 1994).

In the KOR gene, the existence of a 5′ non-coding exon has been demonstrated by two groups (Liu et al., 1995; Yakovlev et al., 1995). In Figure 1.2B, this exon is therefore referred to as exon 1, whereas the three coding exons have been renamed 2, 3, and 4 despite their strong homology to exons 1, 2, and 3 in the MOR and DOR genes. Further, various transcripts have been shown to arise by alternative splicing occurring in the 5′ untranslated region of exon 2, in both rodents and humans (Fig. 1.2B). Two populations of KOR mRNAs were detected in the R1.1 mouse thymoma cell line (Belkowski et al., 1995). One presents an exon 1/exon 2 junction identical to the previously published transcript reported by Yasuda et al. (1993). Another R1.1B mRNA displays a 30-nucleotide insertion located 15 bases upstream from the start codon (Belkowski et al., 1995). This insertion may not be specific to immune cells because it was also detected in the rat brain (Li et al., 1993; Yakovlev et al., 1995). In the rat KOR cDNA sequence reported by Minami et al., the alternative 30-nucleotide DNA stretch is also present, with an additional 5′ 63-nucleotide sequence (Minami et al., 1993). Exon 1 was not found in this cDNA. Finally, another transcript was identified in the rat brain (KORx; see Yakovlev et al., 1995). This mRNA would arise from alternative splicing at a site located 284 bp upstream from the ATG start codon. This extended 5′ portion contains an in-frame ATG codon upstream from the classically described translation start site. Whether this mRNA encodes a protein with a longer N-terminal tail is not known. In conclusion, a 5′ noncoding exon has been identified in the KOR gene, and three alternative splice acceptor sites seem to be used in the first coding exon. These features have not been described for the MOR and the DOR genes.

RT-PCR was used to detect unusual transcripts that may arise from alternative splicing within the coding regions of opioid receptor mRNAs. This approach allowed identification of novel DOR and KOR mRNA forms in the mouse brain and human lymphocytic cell lines, respectively (Gavériaux-Ruff et al., 1997). The alternative DOR transcript displays an additional sequence inserted at the level of the junction between the first and second coding exons. This portion of DNA defines a novel exon that is localized 9 kb upstream from exon 2 within the mDOR gene (Fig. 1.2C). The KOR mRNA variant presents a deletion at the 3′ end of exon 3, followed by a DNA insertion. The latter was found in the KOR gene within the intron joining exon 3 to exon 4 (Fig. 1.2B). In both isoforms, an in-frame stop codon is present in the additional sequences, potentially leading to expression of truncated receptor proteins.

The search for alternative transcripts essentially provides a description of unusual mRNA isoforms. The existence of encoded protein in nervous tissues was reported for the MOR 1B variant only. Noticeably, detailed study of this receptor protein produced in heterologous host cells did not permit the demonstration of altered binding properties that may account for the existence of μ opioid receptor subtypes. Therefore μ opioid receptor heterogeneity probably involves other mechanisms.

Opioid Peptide and Receptor Gene Function in Vivo

The contribution of each receptor to opioid function in vivo may now be assessed by genetic approaches. The role of each receptor type was analyzed by altering receptor expression using administration of antisense oligodeoxynucleotides or gene disruption in mice. Also, the role of endogenous peptides was investigated by gene targeting.

Antisense Strategies

When injected in vitro or in vivo antisense oligodeoxynucleotides interfere with gene expression processes by hybridizing to complementary sequences in the target gene or its messenger RNA, thereby leading to reduced protein levels. Antisense studies applied to opioid receptors have confirmed the implication of DOR (reviewed by Zaki et al., 1996) and MOR (reviewed by Traynor, 1996) in opioid-induced analgesia. Also, an antisense oligonucleotide based on conserved opioid receptor regions (DOR residues 82–88, TM2) diminished the antinociceptive action of μ, δ, and κ agonists (Bilsky et al., 1996). Noticeably, spinal administration of DOR antisense oligodeoxynucleotides suppressed the antinociception induced by DPDPE (δ1) and deltorphin II (δ2), whereas supraspinal administration prevented deltorphin II but not DPDPE analgesia (Bilsky et al., 1994; Lai et al., 1994; Standifer et al., 1994), suggesting that DOR may give rise to the δ2 receptor subtype in defined regions of the central nervous system. The antisense approach was also used to demonstrate the implication of DOR in tolerance and physical dependence on morphine in mice (Kest et al., 1996). A role of μ and κ receptors in the regulation of body temperature was shown by the ability of MOR- and KOR-specific antisense oligodeoxynucleotides to abolish μ agonist-induced hyperthermia and κ agonist-induced hypothermia, respectively (Chen et al., 1995).

Knock-Out Mice

The generation of mice deficient in several components of the opioid system has now been described. Genes encoding MOR, DOR, KOR, β-endorphin, and preproenkephalin have been disrupted in mice by homologous recombination. The five mutant animal strains are fertile, grow normally, and present no apparent developmental abnormality. In the MOR knock-out animals there is no detectable alteration in the expression of other opioid receptors or endogenous opioid peptides, whereas mice deficient in the preproenkephalin gene display upregulation of μ and δ receptor sites in specific brain areas (Brady et al., 1996). This suggests that the absence of μ receptor does not alter the expression of other components of the opioid system, whereas the levels of endogenous ligand regulate opioid transmission. Brain mapping or binding studies performed in the MOR-deficient mice have yielded an interesting clue to the issue of opioid receptor diversity. The data indicate a total loss of DAMGO binding sites in those mice, suggesting that both reported μ1 and μ2 subsites arise from the MOR gene (Matthes et al., 1996). Since alternative splicing mechanisms do not seem to account for these subtypes (see "Alternative Splicing," p. 8), it is likely that μ opioid receptor diversity arises from distinct conformational states of the protein itself.

Behavioral studies of mice lacking opioid peptide or receptor genes have addressed spontaneous behavior, pain perception, and stress response, as well as responses to drugs, in particular, morphine. The results are summarized in Table 1.1.

Horizontal locomotor activity was found reduced in both μ receptor and preproenkephalin-deficient animals. The measurement of nociceptive thresholds by the tail-flick and hot-plate tests in MOR knock-out mice showed that endogenous activation of MOR receptors is not essential (Matthes et al., 1996), but may contribute (Sora et al., 1997) to the control of thermal nociceptive perception. In mice lacking the preproenkephalin gene, pain perception was found dramatically modified in the hot-plate but not in the tail-flick test, suggesting that enkephalins are involved in the modulation of supraspinal, but not spinal, pain responses. Also, an altered behavioral response was observed to formalin-induced inflammatory pain in those mice (König et al., 1996). Although the mouse phenotypes overlap only partially, it is likely that MOR and preproenkephalin gene products act as partners to modulate locomotor activity and pain sensitivity. Stress response was investigated in mice lacking endogenous peptides. Unexpectedly, cold-swim stress experiments showed that enkephalins are not critically implicated in stress-induced analgesia (König et al., 1996). Yet, β-endorphin–deficient mice exhibited alterations in responses to the cold-water-swim stress and an absence of mild-swim stress-induced analgesia (opioid mediated), demonstrating the implication of β-endorphin in stress-mediated responses (Rubinstein et al., 1996). Finally, mice lacking preproenkephalin exhibited increased anxiety and aggressive behavior (König et al., 1996), a phenotype that has not been described for the three other mutant mouse strains.

The lack of MOR protein abolished the antinociceptive action of morphine when the drug was administred at classical analgesic doses (up to 10 mg/kg; Matthes et al., 1996; Sora et al., 1997). Also, morphine-induced place-preference activity was absent in those mice (Matthes et al., 1996). Finally, the absence of μ receptor prevented the development of physical dependence, as indicated by the lack of naloxone-induced withdrawal symptoms following the chronic administration of escalating morphine doses (up to 100 mg/kg; Matthes et al., 1996). These data demonstrate that the μ receptor represents the molecular target of morphine in vivo and mediates

Table 1.1. ***Effect of Gene Disruption in Mice by Homologous Recombination***

Disrupted gene	μ-opioid receptor (1, 2, 3, 8)	δ-opioid receptor (4)	κ-opioid receptor (5)	Preproenkephalin (6)	β-endorphin (7)
Locomotion	No change *R* (2), *H* (2), *V* (3) Weak reduction (20%) *H* (1) Strong reduction (>50%) *H* (3)	NR	No change *H*	Weak reduction (20%) *OF*	No change *H, V*
Nociceptive threshold	No change *TF* (1), *HP* (1) Reduction *TF* (2), *HP* (2)	NR	No change *TF, HP* Reduction *W*	No change *TF* Reduction *HP* Increase/altered behavior *F*	No change
Stress-induced analgesia	NR	NR	NR	No change *TF*	Abolished *HP, W*
Drug response	Abolishment of morphine effects • locomotor response (3) • analgesia *TF, HP* (1, 2) • reward *PP* (1) • physical dependence*WS* (1) • immunosuppression (8)	No modification of morphine analgesia *TF* Abolishment of DPDPE analgesia *TF*	Abolishment of U50,488H effects • locomotor response • analgesia *TF, HP* • aversion Morphine effects: • no modification of analgesia *TF, HP* • no modification of reward *PP* • reduction of physical dependence *WS*	NR	No modification of morphine analgesia *W, HP*
Other	Increased proliferative activity of hematopoietic cells (3) Reduced sexual functions in males (3)	NR	NR	Increased anxiety *OF, OM* Increased aggressive behavior *RI*	NR

Behavioral tests are indicated in italics. Locomotion is assessed by actimetry (horizontal activity, or *H*), measurement of rearing behavior (vertical activity, or *V*), using the rotarod (*R*) or the open-field (*OF*). Painful stimuli used to evaluate nociceptive thresholds, analgesia, or stress-induced analgesia are of thermal (tail flick, or *TF*), chemical (writhing test, or *W*) or inflammatory (formalin test, or *F*) type. The tail-flick test involves spinal responses, whereas the hot-plate test reflects supraspinal mechanisms. Stress-induced analgesia refers to the opioid component of stress response in the cold-swim stress. Morphine reward is evaluated using the place-preference paradigm (*PP*), and physical dependence is based on the observation of somatic and vegetative withdrawal symptoms (*WS*) following naloxone administration. Anxiety is observed in the open-field (*OF*) and the O-maze (*OM*). Aggressive behavior is revealed using the resident-intruder test (*RI*). NR: not reported. References are from Matthes et al., 1996 (1), Sora et al., 1997 (2), Tian et al., 1997 (3), Zhu et al., 1997 (4), Simonin et al., 1998 (5), König et al., 1996 (6), Rubinstein et al., 1996 (7), and Gavériaux-Ruff et al., 1998 (8).

the major biologic actions of the drug. In mice lacking the δ receptor (Zhu et al., 1997) and the κ receptor (Simonin et al., 1998), morphine analgesia was preserved, further strengthening the previous conclusion. Interestingly, morphine abstinence was attenuated in KOR-deficient mice, suggesting that although the μ receptor is necessary to mediate morphine dependence, the κ receptor contributes to this phenomenon.

Other biologic functions were investigated in MOR-deficient mice. The mutant animals displayed altered hematopoiesis, with increased in vitro proliferation of both bone marrow and spleen progenitor cells of the granulocyte-macrophage, erythroid, and mutlipotential lineages (Tian et al., 1997). Also, the μ-receptor gene may be involved in sexual functions of males. Tian et al. (1997) described decreased mating activity, sperm count, and motility in their mutant mice, suggesting reduced reproductive performance. Impaired fertility was not reported for other mutant mice lacking the μ-receptor gene (Matthes et al., 1996; Sora et al., 1997), perhaps because of their different genetic backgrounds. No altered reproductive function was noticed in mutant mice lacking enkephalins or β-endorphin.

Summary

Gene cloning has led to the molecular characterization of three receptor proteins and opened new avenues toward the understanding of opioid receptor function. The study of recombinant receptors in vitro has shed light on structural requirements for ligand recognition and receptor coupling. Further investigations will undoubtedly delineate molecular mechanisms of transduction and desensitization at the receptor level. The isolation of genes encoding all components of the opioid system and the advent of antisense and knock-out strategies now allow the investigation of the implication of each peptide and receptor in opioid function in vivo. In the future, careful comparative analysis of mice lacking proenkephalin, β-endorphin, prodynorphin, and MOR, DOR, and KOR receptors will provide detailed information about ligand-receptor partnerships and homeostasis mechanisms that regulate opioid transmission in response to threatening stimuli. These mouse strains also represent unique tools to redefine the specific mode of action of opiate drugs. Finally, triple mutant mice lacking the three opioid receptor genes should definitely confirm or rule out the possible existence of yet uncloned opioid receptor genes, providing a clue about opioid receptor heterogeneity. Altogether, these data should help the development of novel therapeutic strategies for the treatment of pain and drug addiction.

REFERENCES

Arden, J.R., Segredo, V., Wang, Z., Lameh, J., and Sadée, W. (1995). Phosphorylation and agonist specific intracellular trafficking of an epitope-tagged μ-opioid receptor expressed in HEK 293 cells. *J. Neurochem.* **65,** 1636–1645.

Augustin, L.B., Flesheim, R.F., Min, B.H., Fuchs, S.M., Fuchs, J.A., and Loh, H.H. (1995).

Genomic structure of the mouse delta opioid receptor gene. *Biochem. Biophys. Res. Comm.* **207,** 111–119.

Bare, L.A., Mansson, E., and Yang, D.M. (1994). Expression of two variants of the human mu opioid receptor mRNA in SK-N-SH cells and human brain. *FEBS Lett.* **354,** 213–216.

Barnard, E. A. (1993). Pipe dreams realized. *Curr. Biol.* **3,** 211–214.

Befort, K., and Kieffer, B.L. (1997). Structure-activity relationships in the δ-opioid receptor. *Pain reviews.* London: Arnold.

Befort, K., Tabbara, L., Kling, D., Maigret, B., and Kieffer, B.L. (1996). Structure-activity relationships in the δ-opioid receptor. *J. Biol. Chem.* **271,** 10161–10168.

Belkowski, S.M., Zhu, J., Liu-Chen, L.-Y., Eisenstein, T.K., Adler, M.W., and Rogers, T.J. (1995). Sequence of κ-opioid cDNA in the R1.1 thymoma cell line. *J. Neuroimmunol.* **62,** 113–117.

Bilsky, E.J., Bernstein, R.N., Hruby, V.J., Rothman, R.B., Lai, J., and Porreca, F. (1996). Characterisation of antinociception to opioid receptor selective agonists following antisense oligodeoxynucleotide-mediated "knock-down" of opioid receptors in vivo. *J. Pharmacol. Exp. Ther.* **277,** 491–501.

Bilsky, E.J., Bernstein, R.N., Pasternak, G.W., Hruby, V.J., Patel, D., Porrecca, F., and Lai, J. (1994). Selective inhibition of [D-Ala2, Glu4] deltorphin antinociception by supraspinal, but not spinal, administration of an antisense oligodeoxynucleotide to an opioid delta receptor. *Life Sci.* **55,** 37–43.

Brady, L.S., Herkenham, M., Rothman, R.B., Partilla, J.S., König, M., Zimmer, A.M., and Zimmer, A. (1996). Regionally specific up-regulation of mu and delta opioid receptor binding in enkephalin knock-out mice. *Society for Neuroscience.* Washington, DC, 380.2.

Browstein, M. (1993). A brief history of opiates, opioid peptides and opioid receptors. *Proc. Natl. Acad. Sci. U.S.A.* **90,** 5391–5393.

Chakrabarti, S., Prather, P.L., Yu, L., Law, P.-Y., and Loh, H.H. (1995). Expression of the μ-opioid receptor in CHO cells: Ability of μ-opioid ligands to promote α-Azidoanilido[^{32}P]GTP labeling of multiple G protein α subunits. *J. Neurochem.* **64,** 2534–2543.

Chen, X.-H., Geller, E.B., Kim de Riel, J., Liu-Chen, L.-Y., and Adler, M.W. (1995). Antisense oligodeoxynucleotides against μ- or κ-opioid receptors block agonist-induced body temperature changes in rat. *Brain Res.* **688,** 237–241.

Cox, B.M. (1993). Opioid receptor-G proteins interactions: Acute and chronic effects of opioids. *Opioids I: Handbook of experimental pharmacology.* Berlin: Springer-Verlag, 145–180.

Cvejic, S., Trapaidze, N., Cyr, C., and Devi, L.A. (1996). Thr353, located within the COOH-terminal tail of the δ opiate receptor, is involved in receptor down-regulation. *J. Biol. Chem.* **271,** 4073–4076.

Day, R., Trujillo, K.A., and Akil, A. (1993). Prodynorphin biosynthesis and posttranslational processing. In Herz, A. (ed.), *Opioids I: Handbook of experimental pharmacology.* Berlin: Springer-Verlag, 449–463.

Devine, D.P., Taylor, L., Reinscheid, R.K., Monsma, F.J., Civelli, O., and Akil, H. (1996). Rats rapidly develop tolerance to the locomotor-inhibiting effects of the novel neuropeptide orphanin FQ. *Neurochem. Res.* **21**(11), 1387–1396.

Di Chiara, G., and North, A. (1992). Neurobiology of opiate abuse. *Trends Pharmacol. Sci.* **13,** 185–193.

Dickenson, A.H. (1991). Mechanisms of the analgesic action of opiates and opioids. *Br. Med. Bull.* **47,** 690–702.

Evans, C.J., Keith, D.E., Morrison, H., Magendzo, K., and Edwards, R.H. (1992). Cloning of a delta opioid receptor by functional expression. *Science.* **258,** 1952–1955.

Florin, S., Suaudeau, C., Meunier, J.C., and Costentin, J. (1996). Nociceptin stimulates locomotion and exploratory behaviour in mice. *Eur. J. Pharmacol.* **317,** 9–13.

Fukuda, K., Kato, S., Morikawa, H., Shoda, T., and Mori, K. (1996). Functional coupling of the δ-, μ-, and κ-opioid receptors to mitogen-activated protein kinase and arachidonate release in chinese hamster ovary cells. *J. Neurochem.* **67,** 1309–1316.

Gavériaux-Ruff, C., Matthes, H.W.D., Peluso, J., and Kieffer, B.L. (in press). Abolition of morphine-immunosuppression in mice lacking the m-opioid receptor gene. *Proc. Natl. Acad. Sci. U.S.A.*

Gavériaux-Ruff, C., Peluso, J., Befort, K., Simonin, F., Zilliox, C., and Kieffer, B. (1997). Detection of opioid receptor mRNA by RT-PCR reveals alternative splicing for the δ- and κ-opioid receptors. *Mol. Brain Res.* **48,** 298–304.

Goldstein, A., and Naidu, A. (1989). Multiple opioid receptors: Ligand selectivity profiles and binding site signatures. *Mol. Pharmacol.* **36,** 265–272.

Grisel, J.E., Mogil, J.S., Belknap, J.K., and Grandy, D.K. (1996). Orphanin FQ acts as a supraspinal, but not a spinal, anti-opioid peptide. *Neuroreport.* **7,** 2125–2129.

Grisshammer, R., and Tate, C.G. (1995). Overexpression of membrane proteins for structural studies. *Quarterly Rev. Biophysics.* **28,** 315–422.

Heagy, W., Finberg, R., Teng, E., McAllen, K., and Sharp, B. (1996). Opioid receptors and signalling in lymphocytes. *J. Neuroimmunol.* **69,** 5–7.

Henry, D.J., Kovoor, A., and Chavkin, C. (1994). Effects of treatment with kinase activators and inhibitors on mu and delta opioid receptor coupling to G-protein gated K+ channels in Xenopus oocytes. *Regul. Pept.* **54,** 157–158.

Keith, D.E., Murray, S.R., Zaki, P.A., Chu, P.C., Lissin, D.V., Kang, L., Evans, C.J., and Von Zastrow, M. (1996). Morphine activates opioid receptors without causing their rapid internalization. *J. Biol. Chem.* **277,** 19021–19024.

Kenakin, T. (1996). The classification of seven transmembrane receptors in recombinant expression systems. *Pharmacol. Rev.* **48,** 413–463.

Kest, B., Lee, C.E., McLemore, G.L., and Inturrisi, C.E. (1996). An antisense oligodeoxynucleotide to the delta opioid receptor (DOR-1) inhibits morphine tolerance and acute dependence in mice. *Brain Res. Bull.* **39,** 185–188.

Kieffer, B.L. (1995). Recent advances in molecular recognition and signal transduction of active peptides: Receptors for opioid peptides. *Cell. Mol. Neurobiol.* **15,** 615–635.

Kieffer, B.L. (1997). Molecular aspects of opioid receptors. *Pain: Handbook of experimental pharmacology.* Berlin: Springer-Verlag.

Kieffer, B.L., Befort, K., Gavériaux-Ruff, C., and Hirth, C.G. (1992). The δ-opioid receptor: Isolation of a cDNA by expression cloning and pharmacological characterization. *Proc. Natl. Acad. Sci. U.S.A.* **89,** 12048–12052.

Knapp, R.J., Malatynska, E., Collins, N., Fang, L., Wang, J.Y., Hruby, V.J., Roeske, W.R., and I, Y.H. (1995). Molecular biology and pharmacology of cloned opioid receptors. *FASEB J.* **9,** 516–525.

König, M., Zimmer, A.M., Steiner, H., Holmes, P.V., Crawley, J.N., Brownstein, M.J., and Zimmer, A. (1996). Pain responses, anxiety and aggression in mice deficient in preproenkephalin. *Nature.* **383,** 535–538.

Koob, G.F. (1992). Drug of abuse: Anatomy, pharmacology and function of reward pathways. *TiPS.* **13,** 177–184.

Kraus, J., Horn, G., Zimprich, A., Simon, T., Mayer, P., and Höllt, V. (1995). Molecular cloning and functional analysis of the rat μ opioid receptor gene promoter. *Biochem. Biophys. Res. Commun.* **215,** 591–597.

Lai, H.W.L., Minami, M., Satoh, M., and Wong, Y.H. (1995). Gz coupling to the rat kappa opioid receptor. *FEBS Lett.* **360,** 97–99.

Lai, J., Blisky, E.J., Rothman, R.B., and Porreca, F. (1994). Treatment with oligodeoxynucleotide to the opioid δ receptor selectively inhibits δ_2-agonist antinociception. *Neuroreport.* **5,** 1049–1052.

Law, P.Y., McGinn, T.M., Campbell, K.M., Erickson, L.E., and Loh, H.H. (1997). Agonist activation of δ-opioid receptor but not m-opioid receptor potentiates fetal calf serum or tyrosine kinase receptor-mediated cell proliferation in a cell-line-specific manner. *Mol. Pharmacol.* **51,** 152–160.

Law, P.Y., McGinn, M.J., Erikson, L.J., and Loh, H.H. (1994). Analysis of delta-opioid receptor activities stably expressed in CHO cell lines: Function of receptor density? *J. Pharmacol. Exp. Ther.* **271,** 1686–1694.

Li, S., Zhu, J., Chen, C., Chen, Y.-W., Deriel, J.K., Ashby, B., and Lui-Chen, L.-Y. (1993). Molecular cloning and expression of a rat κ opioid receptor. *Biochem. J.* **295,** 629–633.

Li, X., Keith, D.E., and Evans, C.J. (1996a). Mu opioid receptor-like sequences are present throughout vertebrate evolution. *J. Mol. Evol.* **43,** 179–184.

Li, X., Keith, D.E., and Evans, C.J. (1996b). Multiple opioid receptor-like genes are identified in diverse vertebrate phyla. *FEBS Lett.* **397:** 25–29.

Liang, Y., Mestek, A., Yu, L., and Carr, L.G. (1995). Cloning and characterization of the promoter region of the mouse μ-opioid receptor gene. *Brain Res.* **679,** 82–88.

Liu, H.-C., Lu, S., Augustin, L.B., Felsheim, R.F., Chen, H.-C., Loh, H.H., and Wei, L.-N. (1995). Cloning and promoter mapping of mouse κ-opioid receptor gene. *Biochem. Biophys. Res. Comm.* **209,** 639–647.

Makman, M.H. (1994). Morphine receptors in immunocytes and neurons. *Advan. Neuroimmunol.* **4,** 69–82.

Massotte, D., Baroche, L., Simonin, F., Yu, L., Kieffer, B., and Pattus, F. (1997). Characterization of δ, κ, and μ human opioid receptors overexpressed in baculovirus-infected insect cells. *J. Biol. Chem.* **272,** 1998–1992.

Matthes, H.W.D., Maldonado, R., Simonin, F., Valverde, O., Slowe, S., Kitchen, I., Befort, K., Dierich, A., Le Meur, M., Dollé, P., Tzavara, E., Hanoune, J., Roques, B.P., and Kieffer, B.L. (1996). Loss of morphine-induced analgesia, reward effect and withdrawal symptoms in mice lacking the μ-opioid-receptor gene. *Nature.* **383,** 819–823.

Mayer, P., Schulzeck, S., Kraus, J., Zimprich, A., and Höllt, V. (1996). Promoter region and alternatively spliced exons of the rat μ-opioid receptor gene. *J. Neurochem.* **66,** 2272–2278.

Merkouris, M., Dragatsis, I., Megaritis, G., Konidakis, G., Zioudrou, C., Milligan, G., and Georgoussi, Z. (1996). Identification of the critical domains of the δ-opioid receptor involved in G protein coupling using site-specific synthetic peptides. *Mol. Pharmacol.* **50,** 985–993.

Metzger, T.G., and Ferguson, D.M. (1995). On the role of extracellular loops of opioid receptors in conferring ligand selectivity. *FEBS Lett.* **375,** 1–4.

Meunier, J.-C., Mollereau, C., Toll, L., Suaudeau, C., Moisand, C., Alvinerie, P., Butour, J.-L., Guillemot, J.-C., Ferrara, P., Monsrrat, B., Mazarguil, H., Vassart, G., Parmentier, M., and Costentin, J. (1995). Isolation and structure of the endogenous agonist of opioid receptor-like ORL_1 receptor. *Nature.* **377,** 532–535.

Millan, M.J. (1990). κ-opioid receptors and analgesia. *TiPS.* **11,** 70–76.

Min, B.H., Augustin, L.B., Felsheim, R.F., Fuchs, J.A., and Loh, H.H. (1994). Genomic structure and analysis of promoter sequence of a mouse mu opioid receptor gene. *Proc. Natl. Acad. Sci. U.S.A.* **91,** 9081–9085.

Minami, M., Toya, T., Katao, Y., Maekawa, K., Nakumura, S., Onogi, T., Kaneko, S., and Satoh, M. (1993). Cloning and expression of a cDNA for the rat κ-opioid receptor. *FEBS Lett.* **329,** 291–295.

Mogil, J.S., Grisel, J.E., Reinscheid, R.K., Civelli, O., Belknap, J.K., and Grandy, D.K. (1996). Orphanin FQ is a functional anti-opioid peptide. *Neuroscience.* **75,** 333–337.

Mullaney, I., Carr, I.C., and Milligan, G. (1996). Analysis of inverse agonism at the δ opioid receptor after expression in Rat-1 fibroblasts. *Biochem. J.* **315,** 227–234.

Noble, F., and Roques, B.P. (1997). Association of aminopeptidase N and endopeptidase 24.15 inhibitors potentiate behavioral effects mediated by nociceptin/orphanin FQ in mice. *FEBS Lett.* **401,** 227–229.

North, R.A. (1993). Opioid action on membrane ion channels. *Opioids I: Handbook of experimental pharmacology.* Berlin: Springer-Verlag, 773–793.

Obermeier, H., Wehmeyer, A., and Schulz, R. (1996). Expression of μ-, δ-, and κ-opioid receptors in baculovirus-infected insect cells. *Eur. J. Pharmacol.* **318,** 161–166.

Olson, G.A., Olson, R.D., and Kastin, A.J. (1996). Endogenous opiates: 1995. *Peptides.* **17,** 1421–1466.

Pasternak, G.W. (1993). Pharmacological mechanisms of opioid analgesics. *Clin. Pharmacol.* **16,** 1–18.

Pei, G., Kieffer, B.L., Lefkowitz, R.J., and Freedman, N.J. (1995). Agonist-dependent phosphorylation of the mouse delta-opioid receptor: Involvement of G protein-coupled receptor kinases but not protein kinase C. *Mol. Pharmacol.* **48,** 173–177.

Piros, E.T., Hales, T.G., and Evans, C.J. (1996). Functional analysis of cloned opioid receptors in transfected cell lines. *Neurochem. Res.* **21,** 1277–1285.

Prather, P.L., McGinn, T.M., Claude, P.A., Liu-Chen, L.Y., Loh, H.H., and Law, P.Y. (1995). Properties of a κ-opioid receptor expressed in CHO cells: Interaction with multiple G-proteins is not specific for any individual Ga subunit and is similar to that of other opioid receptors. *Mol. Brain Res.* **29,** 336–346.

Prather, P.L., McGinn, T.M., Erickson, L.J., Evans, C.J., Loh, H.H., and Law, P.Y. (1994). Ability of delta-opioid receptors to interact with multiple G-proteins is independent of receptor density. *J. Biol. Chem.* **269,** 21293–21302.

Reinscheid, R.K., Nothacker, H.-P., Bourson, A., Ardati, A., Henningsen, R.A., Bunzow, J.R., Grandy, D.K., Langen, H., Monsma, F.J., and Civelli, O. (1995). Orphanin FQ: A neuropeptide that activates an opioid-like G protein-coupled receptor. *Science.* **270,** 792–794.

Reisine, T. (1995). Opiate receptors. *Neuropharmacology.* **34**(5), 463–472.

Rossi, G.C., Leventhal, L., and Pasternak, G.W. (1996). Naloxone sensitive orphanin FQ-induced analgesia in mice. *Eur. J. Pharmacol.* **311,** R7–R8.

Rossier, J. (1993). Biosynthesis of enkephalins and proenkephalin-derived peptides. *Opioids I: Handbook of experimental pharmacology.* 104/1, Berlin: Springer-Verlag.

Rubinstein, M., Mogil, J.S., Japòn, M., Chan, E.C., Allen, R.G., and Low, M.J. (1996). Absence of opioid stress-induced analgesia in mice lacking β-endorphin by site-directed mutagenesis. *Proc. Natl. Acad. Sci. U.S.A.* **93,** 3995–4000.

Satoh, M., and Minami, M. (1995). Molecular pharmacology of the opioid receptors. *Pharmacol. Ther.* **68,** 343–364.

Schulz, S., Schreff, M., Koch, T., Zimprich, A., Elde, R., and Höllt, V. (in press). Immunolocalization of two mu opioid receptor isoforms (MOR1 and MOR1B) in the rat central nervous system. *Neuroscience.*

Simonin, F., Valverde, O., Smadja, C., Slowe, S., Kitchen, I., Dierich, A., Le Meur, M., Roques, B.P., Maldonado, R., and Kieffer, B.L. (1998). Disruption of the k-opioid receptor gene in mice enhances sensitivity to chemical visceral pain, impairs pharmacological actions of the selective k-agonist U-50,488H and attenuates morphine withdrawal. *EMBO J.* **17,** 886–897.

Sora, I., Takahashi, N., Funada, M., Ujike, H., Revay, R.S., Donovan, D.M., Miner, L.L., and Uhl, G.R. (1997). Opiate receptor knockout mice define μ receptor roles in endogenous nociceptive responses and morphine-induced analgesia. *Proc. Natl. Acad. Sci. U.S.A.* **94,** 1544–1549.

Standifer, K.M., and Al, E. (1994). Selective loss of δ opioid analgesia and binding by antisense oligodeoxynucleotides to a δ opioid receptor. *Neuron.* **12,** 805–810.

Sternini, C., Spann, M., Anton, B., Keith, D.E., Bunnett, N.W., Von Zastrow, M., Evans, C.J., and Brecha, N.C. (1996). Agonist-selective endocytosis of m opioid receptor by neurons in vitro. *Proc. Natl. Acad. Sci. U.S.A.* **93,** 9241–9246.

Strader, C.D., Fong, T.M., Tota, M.R., and Underwood, D. (1994). Structure and function of G protein-coupled receptors. *Ann. Review Biochem.* **63,** 101–132.

Talmont, F., Sidobre, S., Demange, P., Milon, A., and Emorine, L.J. (1996). Expression and pharmacological characterization of the human μ-opioid receptor in the methylotropic yeast *Pichia pastoris. FEBS Lett.* **394,** 268–272.

Tian, M., Broxmeyer, H.E., Fan, Y., Lai, Z., Zhang, S., Aronica, S., Cooper, S., Bigsby, R.M., Steinmetz, R., Engle, S.J., Mestek, A., Pollock, J.D., Lehman, M.N., Jansen, H.T., Ying, M., Stambrook, P.J., Tischfield, J.A., and Yu, L. (1997). Altered hematopoiesis, behavior, and sexual function in μ opioid receptor-deficient mice. *J. Exp. Med.* **185,** 1517–1522.

Trapaidze, N., Keith, D.E., Cvejic, S., Evans, C.J., and Devi, L.A. (1996). Sequestration of the δ opioid receptor: Role of the C terminus in agonist-mediated internalization. *J. Biol. Chem.* **271,** 29279–29285.

Traynor, J.R. (1996). The μ-opioid receptor. *Pain Rev.* **3,** 221–248.

Traynor, J.R., and Elliot J. (1993). δ-opioid receptor subtypes and cross talk with μ-receptors. *Trends Pharmacol. Sci.* **14,** 84–85.

Tsu, R.C., Chan, J.S.C., and Wong, Y.H. (1995). Regulation of multiple effectors by the cloned δ-opioid receptor: Stimulation of phospholipase C and type II adenylyl cyclase. *J. Neurochem.* **64,** 2700–2707.

Ueda, H., Miyamae, T., Fukushima, N., Takeshima, H., Fukuda, K., Sasaki, Y., and Misu, Y. (1995). Opioid μ- and κ-opioid receptors mediate phospholipase C activation through Gi1 in *Xenopus* oocytes. *Mol. Brain Res.* **32,** 166–170.

Ueda, H., Miyamae, T., Hayashi, C., Watanabe, S., Fukushima, N., Sasaki, Y., Iwamura, T., and Misu, Y. (1995). Protein kinase C involvement in homologous desensitization of δ-opioid receptor coupled to Gi1-phospholipase C activation in *Xenopus oocytes. J. Neurosci.* **15,** 7485–7499.

Wotta, D.R., Birnbaum, A.K., Wilcox, G.L., Elde, R., and Law, P.-Y. (1997). μ-opioid receptor regulates CFTR coexpressed in *Xenopus* oocytes in a cAMP independent manner. *Mol. Brain Res.* **44,** 55–65.

Wu, G., Lu, Z.-H., and Ledeen, R.W. (1997). Interaction of the δ-opioid receptor with GM1 ganglioside: Conversion from inhibitory to excitatory mode. *Mol. Brain Res.* **44,** 341–346.

Xie, G.X., Meng, F., Mansour, A., Thompson, R.C., Hoversten, M.T., Goldstein, A., Watson, S.J., and Akil, H. (1994). Primary structure and functional expression of a guinea pig kappa opioid (dynorphin) receptor. *Proc. Natl. Acad. Sci. U.S.A.* **91,** 3779–3783.

Xu, X.J., Hao, J.X., and Weisenfel-Hallin, Z. (1996). Nociceptin or antinociceptin: Potent spinal antinociceptive effect of orphanin FQ/nociceptin in the rat. *Neuroreport.* **7,** 2092–2094.

Yakovlev, A.G., Krueger, K.E., and Faden, A.I. (1995). Structure and expression of a rat κ opioid receptor gene. *J. Biol. Chem.* **270,** 6421–6424.

Yasuda, K., Raynor, K., Kong, H., Breder, C.D., Takeda, J., Reisine, T., and Bell, G.I. (1993). Cloning and functional comparision of κ and δ opioid receptors from mouse brain. *Proc. Natl. Acad. Sci. U.S.A.* **90,** 6736–6740.

Young, E., Bronstein, D., and Akil, H. (eds.) (1993). *Proopiomelanocortin biosynthesis, processing and secretion: Functional implications.* 104/1. Berlin: Springer-Verlag.

Zadina, J.E., Hackler, L., Ge, L.-J., and Kastin, A.J. (1997). A potent and selective endogenous agonist for the μ-opiate receptor. *Nature.* **386,** 499–502.

Zaki, P.A., Bilsky, E.J., Vanderah, T.W., Lai, J., Evans, C.J., and Porreca, F. (1996). Opioid receptor types and subtypes: The δ receptor as a model. *Ann. Rev. Pharmacol. Toxicol.* **36,** 379–401.

Zhang, L., Yu, Y., Mackin, S., Weight, F.F., Uhl, G.R., and Wang, J.B. (1996). Differential μ opiate receptor phosphorylation and desensitization induced by agonists and phorbol esters. *J. Biol. Chem.* **271,** 11449–11454.

Zhu, Y., King, M., Schuller, A., Unterwald, E., Pasternak, G., and Pintar, J.E. (1997). Genetic disruption of the mouse delta opioid gene. *Eur. Opioid Conf.* Guildford, UK, 6.

Zimprich, A., Simon, T., and Höllt, V. (1995). Cloning and expression of an isoform of the rat mu opioid receptor (rMOR1B) which differs in agonist-induced desensitization from rMOR1. *FEBS Lett.* **359,** 142–146.

CHAPTER TWO

Endogenous Opioid Peptides and Analgesia

BERNARD P. ROQUES, FLORENCE NOBLE,
AND MARIE-CLAUDE FOURNIE-ZALUSKI

Introduction

The pain-suppressive effect of morphine is related to the interaction of this alkaloid with binding sites located in the central nervous system (CNS) and more precisely within structures known for their involvement in the regulation of nociceptive stimuli. Moreover, the wide distribution of opioid receptors in the brain accounts for the multiplicity of pharmacologic responses elicited by morphine administration. Psychic dependence and respiratory depression, which are among the major side effects of narcotics, are related to overstimulation of brain receptors, respectively, in behavioral and bulbar respiratory controls. The reduction in intestinal transit is another drawback frequently associated with chronic morphine treatment. Thus, despite the considerable interest in morphine and surrogates for treatment of severe pain, there is a crucial need for new analgesics to fill the gap between opioid analgesics and antalgics, such as aspirin and paracetamol. Such compounds may be of major interest for the treatment of various pain syndromes (postoperative, neurogenic, osteoarthritic) and more easily used in children, the elderly, and patients with respiratory problems.

Although many factors seem to be involved in pain control, the prevailing role of the opioid μ receptor type in analgesia has hampered the discovery of analgesics devoid of the severe morphine side effects, which were proposed to result from the stimulation of μ receptors. This hypothesis has recently been firmly established using transgenic mice with a deletion of the μ-receptor gene (Matthes et al., 1996). This does not preclude an interest in δ agonists, since these compounds were shown to elicit potent antinociceptive responses, especially against inflammatory-related painful stimuli, and to remain active in animals tolerant to morphine (Desmeules et al., 1993). Nevertheless, chronic administration of these selective agonists was also reported to induce side effects (Maldonado et al., 1990). Another extensively used approach consists in developing antagonists for receptors of hyperalgesic endogenous effectors such as SP, bradykinin, excitatory aminoacids, and cholecystokinin (Besson and Chaouch, 1987). However, the analgesic effects of these compounds were found to be closer to those of anti-inflammatory drugs than to opiates (Seguin et al., 1995). A new, attractive approach has been offered by the discovery of several

Christoph Stein, ed., *Opioids in Pain Control: Basic and Clinical Aspects*. Printed in the United States of America.

endogenous peptides endowed with high affinities for various opioid receptors and thus acting as natural opioid substances. However, it has been rapidly demonstrated that the use of these endogenous peptides is hindered by their brief half-life in vivo and their low bioavailability. Moreover, an enkephalin analog with favorable pharmacokinetic properties and μ selectivity was shown to generate the same side effects as morphine (Roemer et al., 1977). However, the discovery that the interruption of the physiologic action of the endogenous enkephalins is ensured by ectopeptidases located at the proximity of the opioid receptors has given rise to a novel strategy inherent in the design of the inhibitors of these peptidases. These compounds seem capable of filling the gap between antalgics and analgesics. This observation was recently reinforced by a study showing that enkephalins modulate responses to painful stimuli in transgenic mice deficient in preproenkephalin (König et al., 1996).

Endogenous Opioid Peptides

Mammalian opioid peptides are encoded by three different genes that are widely distributed throughout the central and peripheral nervous systems: pro-opiomelanocortin (POMC), proenkephalin, and prodynorphin (see review in Cesselin, 1995). These large precursors are maturated by cleavage at the level of pair basic residues to generate final active peptides acting at specific receptors (μ, δ, and κ) also largely distributed centrally and peripherally. At least 20 peptides are known, all of which have the amino-terminal amino-acid sequence Tyr-Gly-Gly-Phe-Met or Tyr-Gly-Gly-Phe-Leu (Table 2.1). These pentapeptide sequences are by themselves the two shortest opioids – that is, Met- and Leu-enkephalin.

The POMC gene is mainly expressed in the anterior pituitary and the CNS. As indicated by its name, POMC is the precursor of opioid (β-endorphin), melanotropic, and corticotropic peptides. POMC is synthesized by neurons located in the hypothalamus and brain stem. Hypothalamic POMC neurons have very diffuse projections in the brain. Several structures involved in nociception (such as the thalamus, the periaqueductal gray [PAG], and the reticular formation) contain POMC terminals.

Proenkephalin is mainly synthesized in the adrenal medulla and the CNS. Each molecule of proenkephalin contains seven sequences of opioids. The major ones are Met- and Leu-enkephalin, an heptadecapeptide Met-enkephalin-Arg^6-Phe^7, and an octapeptide Met-enkephalin-Arg^6-Gly^7-Leu^8. Proenkephalin-synthesizing neurons are numerous and largely distributed. They are found essentially in the striatum, cerebral cortex, olfactory tubercle, hippocampus, septum, thalamus, PAG, and dorsal horn of the spinal cord. They are mainly interneurons, although some send long projections. Enkephalins are also present in peripheral neurons, notably in some primary afferent fibers that innervate the pelvic viscera.

Each molecule of prodynorphin contains three Leu-enkephalin sequences. However, the main products of prodynorphin are longer peptides – that is, neoendorphins

Table 2.1. *Peptide Products of the Proenkephalin, Pro-opiomelanocortin, and Prodynorphin Precursors*

Peptides derived from proenkephalin	
Met-enkephalin	Tyr-Gly-Gly-Phe-Met
Leu-enkephalin	Tyr-Gly-Gly-Phe-Leu
Met-enkephalin-8	Tyr-Gly-Gly-Phe-Met-Arg-Gly-Leu
Met-enkephalin-Arg^6-Phe^7	Tyr-Gly-Gly-Phe-Met-Arg-Phe
Peptides derived from prodynorphin	
α-neo-endorphin	Tyr-Gly-Gly-Phe-Leu-Arg-Lys-Tyr-Pro-Lys
β-neo-endorphin	Tyr-Gly-Gly-Phe-Leu-Arg-Lys-Tyr-Pro
Dynorphin A-(1–8)	Tyr-Gly-Gly-Phe-Leu-Arg-Arg-Ile
Dynorphin A-(1–17)	Tyr-Gly-Gly-Phe-Leu-Arg-Arg-Ile-Arg-Pro-Lys-Leu-Trp-Asp-Asn-Gln
Dynorphin B-(1–13)	Tyr-Gly-Gly-Phe-Leu-Arg-Arg-Gln-Phe-Lys-Val-Val-Thr
Peptides derived from POMC (Pro-opiomelanocortin)	
β-endorphin	Tyr-Gly-Gly-Phe-Met-Thr-Ser-Glu-Lys-Ser-Gln-Thr-Pro-Leu-Val-Thr-Leu-Phe-Lys-Asn-Ala-Ala-Ile-Val-Lys-Asn-Ala-His-Lys-Lys-Gly-Gln

and dynorphins A and B. In the CNS, the distribution of neurons synthesizing prodynorphin is as large as that of proenkephalin neurons.

Endorphins, enkephalins, and dynorphins bind with low to moderate specificity to the three opioid receptors. β-endorphin binds to the μ and δ receptors with comparable affinity, but because of their selectivity, Met- and Leu-enkephalin are considered the endogenous ligands for the δ receptor, although they also recognize μ receptors. Dynorphins bind to the κ receptor. Recently, two peptides have been characterized (Tyr-Pro-Phe-Phe-NH_2 and Tyr-Pro-Trp-Phe-NH_2) that have the highest specificity and affinity for the μ receptor of any endogenous substance so far described (Zadina et al., 1997).

However, the ORL_1 receptor, which structurally resembles opioid receptors, has recently been described; it does not bind to any of the known opiate ligands with high affinity. A heptadecapeptide (nociceptin/orphanin FQ) was identified as an endogenous ligand for ORL_1 (Meunier et al., 1995; Reinscheid et al., 1995). Numerous studies have investigated the pharmacologic effects of this peptide following central administration. Nevertheless, the physiologic role of this peptide remain to be determined.

Enkephalin-Degrading Enzymes

Early studies with enkephalins showed that they had a very short half-life both in vitro and in vivo conditions. These results accounted for the weak and transient

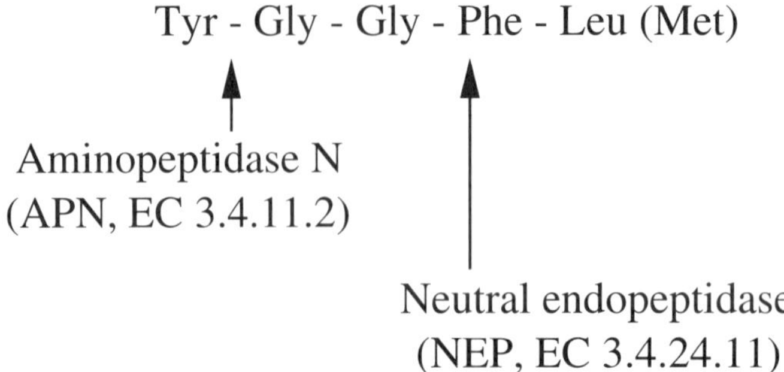

Figure 2.1. Sites of enzymatic cleavage of enkephalins.

analgesia obtained only for high doses of ICV-administered enkephalins (Belluzi et al., 1976) and for the higher potency of enkephalin analogs protected from peptidases releasing Tyr (Pert et al., 1976) and Tyr-Gly-Gly (Fournié-Zaluski et al., 1979; Guyon et al., 1979) (Fig. 2.1). These results supported the occurrence of peptidase activities on the cell surface, acting therefore as ectoenzymes (see review by Roques et al., 1993). A Tyr-Gly-Gly–releasing enzyme was detected in rat striatal membranes (Craves et al., 1978; Malfroy et al., 1978). The physiologic relevance of the enzyme designated enkephalinase in enkephalin catabolism was firmly established by the naloxone-reversible antinociceptive properties elicited by its first synthetic inhibitor, thiorphan (Roques et al., 1980). This enzyme was then shown to be neutral endopeptidase 24.11 (NEP, EC 3.4.24.11) (Relton et al., 1983), an already well-described Zn metallopeptidase present in large quantities in the brush border cells of the proximal tubules of the kidney (Kerr and Kenny, 1974).

The aminopeptidase selectively involved in the physiologic cleavage of the Tyr-Gly bond of enkephalins (Meek et al., 1977; Guyon et al., 1979) was shown to be aminopeptidase N (APN, EC 3.4.11.2), thanks to the increased analgesic potency of selective inhibitors of this membrane-bound enzyme (Waksman et al., 1985).

Localization of Neutral Endopeptidase 24.11, Enkephalins, and Opioid Receptors

The first precise localization of NEP in the CNS was obtained by autoradiography using the tritiated inhibitor [^{3}H]HACBO-Gly (Waksman et al., 1986). A good correspondence was found between the distribution of the enzyme, the endogenous enkephalins, and the opioid receptors (Waksman et al, 1986, and references cited therein). Thus, in the caudate putamen, [^{3}H]HACBO-Gly binding overlapped both patchy μ sites and diffusely labeled δ receptors. High concentrations of both NEP (Fig. 2.2) and μ receptors were found in the periaqueductal gray matter and the substantia gelatinosa of the spinal cord, areas that are implicated in pain perception and

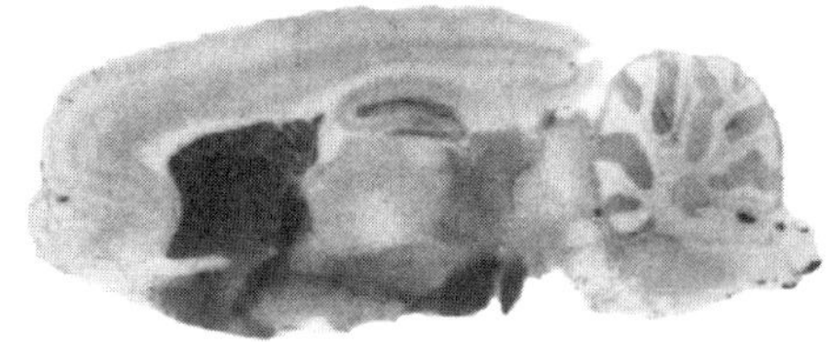

Figure 2.2. Autoradiogram showing the distribution of NEP at different levels of the rat brain. Tissue section was incubated with [^{125}I] RB 104.

analgesia. The substantia gelatinosa contains high levels of δ- and μ-opioid binding sites, a finding in agreement with the involvement of both opioid receptors in spinal analgesia (Dickenson et al., 1986, 1987). At this level, most of the opioid receptors are located on primary afferent terminals, whereas NEP is located on interneurons (Besse et al., 1990).

Rational Design of Peptidase Inhibitors

Development of Selective NEP or APN Inhibitors

Although the sequence of NEP shows only a weak homology with those of other Zn metallopeptidases, some of the most important amino acids in the active site of thermolysin (TLN), which has been crystallized alone and with a variety of inhibitors, appear to have been conserved. Several of these residues are included in consensus sequences VxxHExxH and ExxxD, which have been found in numerous other Zn endopeptidases (see review in Roques et al., 1993). The design of NEP inhibitors has been based on active site models derived from structural data on TLN, whose active site appears to be very similar to that of NEP, as confirmed by site-directed mutagenesis (Beaumont et al., 1997, and references cited therein). The specificity of NEP is essentially ensured by the S'_1 subsite, which interacts preferentially with aromatic or large hydrophobic moieties, whereas the S'_2 subsite has a poor specificity (Fournié-Zaluski et al., 1979, 1984; Llorens et al., 1980). These observations were used to design thiorphan HS-CH_2-CH(CH_2Φ)-CONH-CH_2-COOH (Roques et al., 1980) and retrothiorphan HS-CH_2-CH(CH_2Φ)-NHCO-CH_2-COOH (Roques et al., 1983), which were the first potent synthetic NEP inhibitors described, the latter being unable to recognize ACE, which is involved in the control of blood pressure. Protection of the thiol and carboxyl groups of thiorphan led to acetorphan, a compound able to cross the blood-brain barrier after systemic administration. In addition to acetorphan, other active NEP inhibitors containing a thiol group such as SQ 29,072 [HS-CH_2-CH(CH_2Φ)-CONH-$(CH_2)_6$-COOH] (Seymour et al., 1989) or RU 44,004 [(R,S)HS-CH_2-CH(CH_2Φ)-CONH-NC_4H_8O]; a carboxyl group such as SCH 39,370 [Φ-CH_2-CH_2-CH(COOH)-NH-CH(CH_2Φ)-CONH-CH_2-CH(OH)-COOH] (Sybertz et al., 1990) or UK 69,758, candoxatril [CH_3O-CH_2-CH_2-OCH_2-CH(COOH)-CH_2-X-CONH-Y, where *X* is cyclopentyl and *Y* is *p*-carbonyl cyclohexyl] (Northridge et al., 1989); hydroxamate in bidentate inhibitors such as HACBO-Gly [N-[(2R,S)-4-(hydroxy amino)-1,4-dioxo-2-(phenylmethyl)-butyl]-glycine] (Fournié-Zaluski et al., 1985; Xie et al., 1989) have been developed (see review in Roques et al., 1993). The replacement of Gly in retro-HACBO-Gly by a highly hydrophobic aromatic moiety led to the inhibitor RB 104 [2-[(3-iodo-4-hydroxy)-phenylmethyl]-4-N-[3-hydroxyamino-3-oxo-1-(phenylmethyl)propyl]amino-4-oxobutanoic acid]. [^{125}I]RB 104 is the most potent NEP inhibitor that has been described so far (K_I = 0.03 nM), a property that has been used to directly visualize NEP in crude membrane fractions after gel electrophoresis (Fournié-Zaluski, Soleilhac et al., 1992). Another interesting series of inhibitors are the phosphorus-containing dipeptides (Elliot et al., 1985), among which is the natural competitive inhibitor of NEP, phosphoramidon. Numerous NEP inhibitors were synthesized in the pharmaceutical industry when NEP was demonstrated to be involved in the physiologic inactivation, mostly in the kidney, of the atrial natriuretic peptide ANP (Stephenson and Kenny, 1987).

Various natural aminopeptidase inhibitors have been isolated. These include puromycin, bestatin, amastatin, and derivatives. However, these molecules have little selectivity for aminopeptidase N. Simple molecules that recognize only the S_1 subsite and interact with the Zn atom were found to be highly potent APN inhibitors (see review in Roques et al., 1993). The bioavailability of phenylalanine-thiol (K_I = 20 nM) was improved by introducing a hydrophobic carbamate group on the thiol function (Gros et al., 1988).

Development of Mixed Inhibitors of NEP/APN

The concept of mixed inhibitors was developed to take into account the previously mentioned inactivation of endogenous enkephalins by two Zn-metallopeptidases, NEP and APN (Fournié-Zaluski et al., 1984). This was first achieved using hydroxamate-containing inhibitors. The loss of binding affinity arising from a relative inability of the lateral chains of a single inhibitor to fit adequately the respective S_1, S_1', S_2' subsites of the two different enzymes was expected to be counterbalanced by the strength of the coordination to the Zn atom. This was indeed obtained with bidentate-containing inhibitors such as kelatorphan [(R,S)(HONH-CO-CH_2-CH($CH_2\Phi$)-CONH-CH(CH_3)-COOH], which strongly inhibits NEP (IC_{50} = 1.8 nM) and APN (IC_{50} = 380 nM) (Fournié-Zaluski et al., 1984). A large number of analogs have been synthesized using this new concept, all having a pseudodipeptide structure. RB 38A [(R,S)(HONH-CO-CH_2-CH($CH_2\Phi$)-CONH-CH($CH_2\Phi$)-COOH] is as active as kelatorphan on NEP, but is a more potent inhibitor of APN (IC_{50} = 120 nM) (Schmidt et al., 1991). However, although these molecules gave promising results in numerous pharmacologic tests (see review in Roques et al., 1993), they are too hydrophilic to cross the blood-brain barrier, precluding peripheral administration. Another strategy was therefore employed that consisted of linking highly potent thiol-containing APN and NEP inhibitors by a disul-

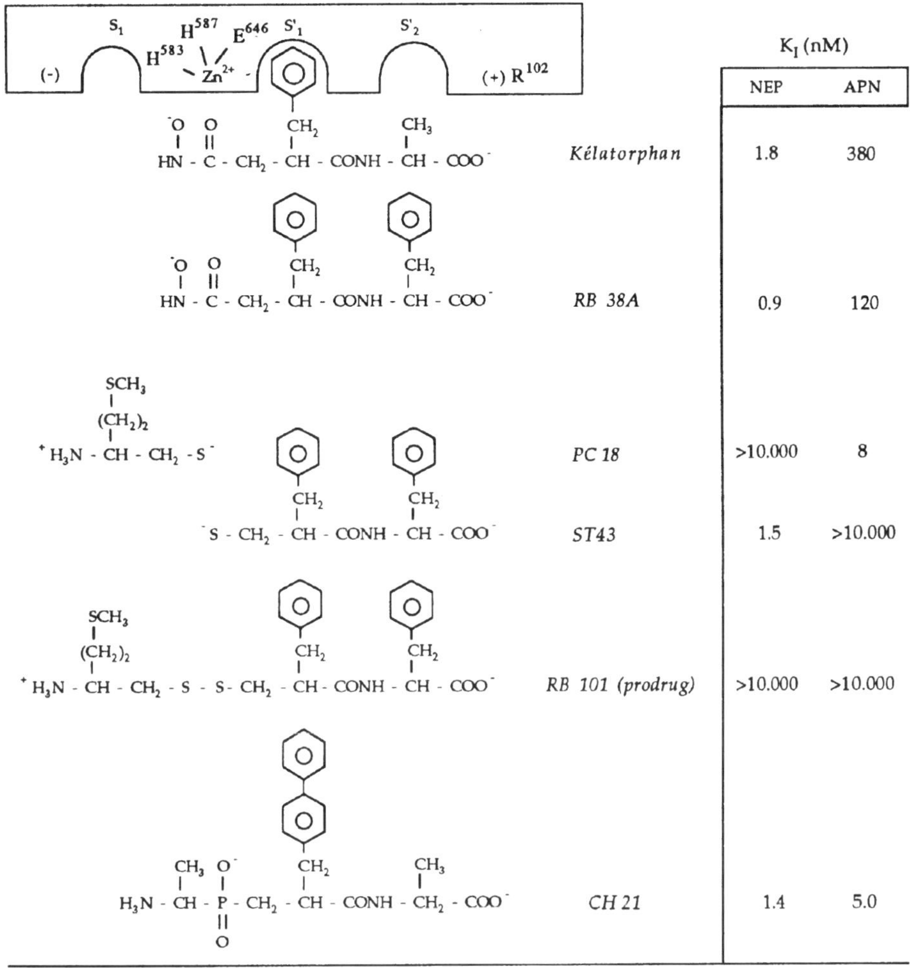

Figure 2.3. Mixed inhibitors of NEP/APN.

phide bond, which led to the synthesis of RB 101 and RB 120. In addition to the easy modulation of their hydrophobicity, one of the main advantages of these mixed inhibitor prodrugs is the stability of the disulphide bond in plasma, in contrast with its relatively rapid breakdown in brain by a biologically dependent process to release the selective APN and NEP inhibitors (Fig. 2.3) (Fournié-Zaluski, Coric et al., 1992). However, the first dual inhibitors able to recognize the S_1, S_1' and S_2' subsites of both APN and NEP have only recently been developed after numerous unfavorable assays. These phosphinic acid derivatives (M.C. Fournié-Zaluski, H. Chen, and B.P. Roques, French Patent 96.13082), exemplified by CH 21 (Fig. 2.3), exhibit nanomolar affinities for both enzymes and could be endowed with improved pharmacokinetic properties as compared to RB 101 and derivatives.

In Vitro and in Vivo Studies of Enkephalin Degradation by NEP and APN

The protection of exogenous or endogenous opioid peptides has been studied using slices of brain (Patey et al., 1981; Waksman et al., 1985; Bourgoin et al., 1986) from which the enkephalins can be released by depolarization and the metabolites measured in the superfusion medium. Under these conditions, the NEP inhibitor thiorphan was found to reduce the formation of Tyr-Gly-Gly but enhance Tyr levels formed by APN action. However, the opposite effect was observed with the APN inhibitor bestatin, showing that a blockade of both enzymes by a mixed NEP/APN inhibitor such as kelatorphan is required to obtain a major increase in the extracellular level of enkephalins (Waksman et al., 1985; Bourgoin et al., 1986).

A demonstration of the increase in levels of enkephalins following enkephalin-degrading enzyme inhibitors was also indirectly obtained by in vivo binding experiments performed under the conditions commonly used for pharmacologic studies (Meucci et al., 1989; Ruiz-Gayo et al., 1992a). Thus, an increase in "synaptic" levels of enkephalins was shown by in vivo inhibition (15%) of [^{3}H]diprenorphine binding to brain opioid receptors in normal mice and about 32% in stressed animals after IV administration of RB 101 (Ruiz-Gayo et al., 1992a). The increase of endogenous enkephalins released from neurons by kelatorphan was also evidenced by the radioligand displacement assay proposed by Chavkin and collaborators (Wagner et al., 1990), which constitues a sensitive measure of transmitter release under physiologically relevant conditions – that is, after focal electrical stimulation of the preparation.

A more direct demonstration of the increase in "synaptic" levels of enkephalins following peptidase inhibitor administration was obtained by microdialysis, which enabled the evaluation of the in vivo functioning of peptidergic pathways in awake and freely moving rats and the quantification of the peptides in the extracellular space released under basal or stimulated conditions. Using this method, Daugé et al. (1996) have shown that RB 101, which easily crosses the blood-brain barrier, as shown by the complete inhibition of cerebral NEP following IV injection in mice (Noble, Soleilhac et al., 1992), induced a dose-dependent and long-lasting increase in the extracellular levels of Met-enkephalin-like material in the nucleus accumbens of freely moving rats after IP administration (Fig. 2.4).

Various nociceptive stimuli have been shown to enhance Met-enkephalin levels in the spinal cord (Yaksh and Elde, 1981; Cesselin et al., 1982). Kelatorphan almost completely prevented the spinal degradation of exogenous [^{3}H]Met-enkephalin in superfusions of halothane-anesthetized rats (Bourgoin et al., 1986). In contrast, in the same in vivo model, thiorphan or bestatin alone were inactive and, when co-administered, were only half as active as kelatorphan. Moreover, when the spontaneous outflow of endogenous Met-enkephalin was measured there was a twofold better recovery in the presence of kelatorphan and a fivefold enhancement during noxious stimulation (muzzle pinching), with no apparent change in the release

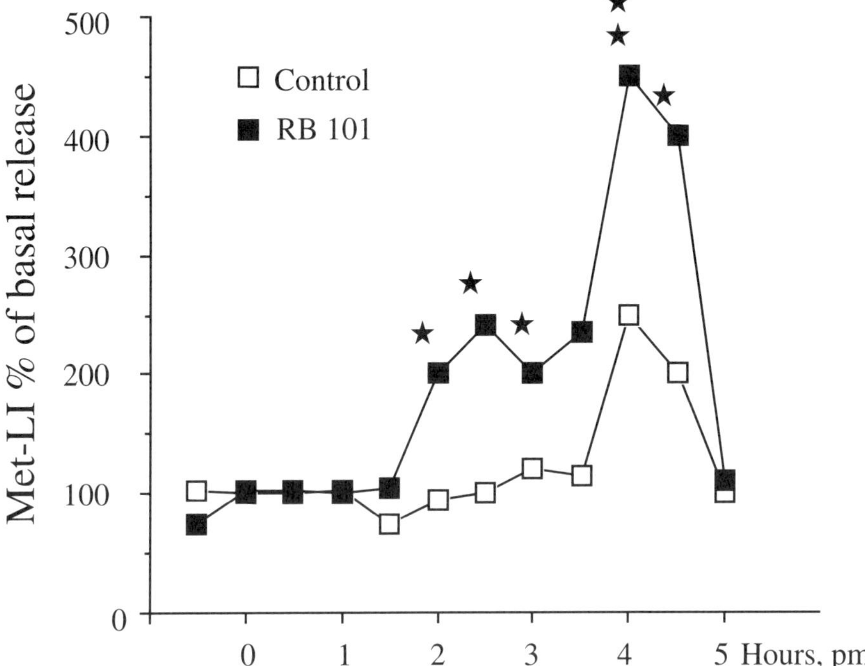

Figure 2.4. Long-lasting effect of RB 101 on the extracellular efflux of Met-enkephalin-like material (Met-LI) in the nucleus accumbens of rats using microdialysis in awake and freely moving rats. The rats were perfused beginning at 9 A.M. for 2 hours, and samples were then collected until 5 P.M. RB 101 was IP injected at 1 P.M. at a dose of 80 mg/kg. Samples were collected every 30 minutes. Results are expressed as the percentage change in basal levels of Met-LI. ★ $P < 0.05$ and ★★ $P < 0.01$ as compared to the control group.

process itself (Bourgoin et al., 1986). This latter result shows that protection of extracellularly released enkephalin has no significant effect on the secretion of the opioid peptides, indicating that mixed inhibitors can be used to investigate the existence of tonically or phasically active enkephalinergic pathways (Dickenson et al., 1986; Williams et al., 1987; Roques, 1991; Daugé et al., 1992).

Analgesic Responses Induced by Enkephalin-Degrading Enzyme Inhibitors

Inhibitor-Induced Central Analgesia

Owing to the complementary roles of NEP and APN in enkephalin inactivation, selective inhibition of only one of the peptidases gives weak antinociceptive effects, whereas mixed inhibitors or co-administered APN and NEP inhibitors are much more effective (Fig. 2.5). Thus, kelatorphan was shown to decrease the ICV dose of Met-enkephalin required to obtain 50% analgesia (ED_{50}) by a factor of 50,000 (Fournié-

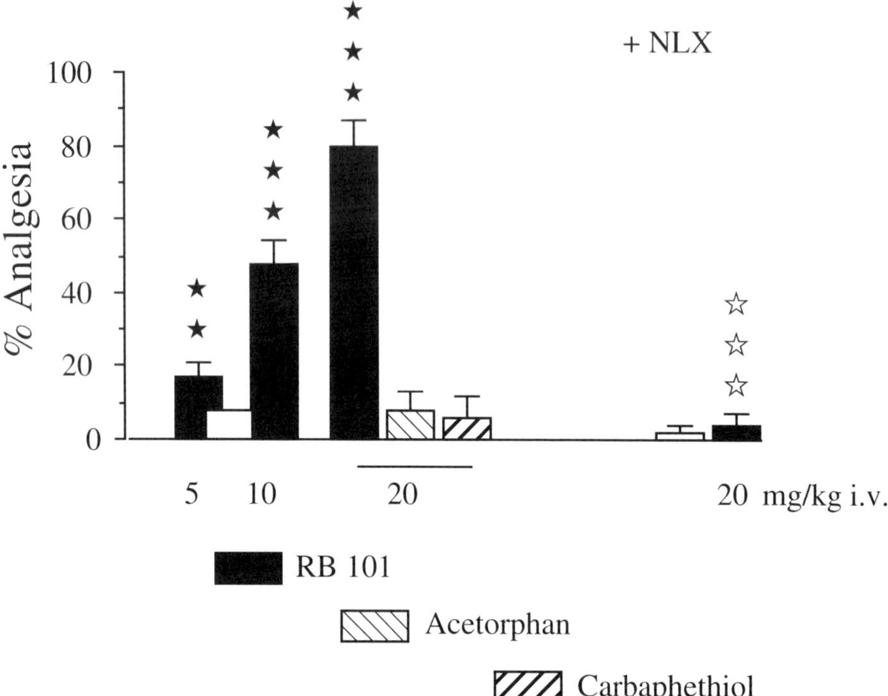

Figure 2.5. Comparison of analgesic potencies (hot-plate test) of selective and mixed inhibitors of enkephalin-degrading enzymes. Acetorphan (NEP inhibitor) and carbaphethiol (APN inhibitor) were administered IV for 15 minutes, and RB 101 for 10 minutes, before testing, that is, at the time corresponding to their maximum effects. Naloxone was injected SC for 20 minutes before testing. The analgesic responses were expressed as percentages of analgesia using the following equation: % analgesia = (test latency – control latency)/(cut-off time – control latency) × 100 (cut-off time = 240 seconds). ★★★ $P < 0.011$ as compared to control group; ☆☆☆ $P < 0.01$ as compared to the same dose of RB 101 without antagonist.

Zaluski et al., 1984), leading to an ED_{50} value of Met-enkephalin not very different from that of the μ agonist DAMGO, in agreement with the similar in vitro affinities of both compounds for the opioid receptors. Various types of stress, such as foot shock in rats, immobilization in mice, warm water in mice (see review in Chipkin, 1986), and transcranial electrostimulation analgesia (Malin et al., 1989) increase the release of enkephalins in regions involved in pain control and thus improve the antinociceptive effects of the catabolizing enzyme inhibitors. The complete inhibition of enkephalin metabolism by ICV RB 38A, IV RB 101, or PO RB 120 (Table 2.2) induced naloxone-antagonized antinociceptive responses in all the various assays commonly used to select analgesics, not only in tests in which naloxone produces pronociceptive effects as initially thought (Schwartz, 1983) but more generally in morphine-sensitive assays (Schmidt et al., 1991; Noble, Soleilhac et al., 1992; Noble et al., 1997). Given their comparable affinities for opioid-binding sites, similar analgesic responses could theoretically be obtained with morphine and endogenous

Table 2.2. *Antinociceptive Effects Induced by PO Administration of RB 120 on Various Animal Models of Pain*

	Animal Models	Antinociceptive Responses	
Severe	Hot plate (mice)		ED_{50} = 410 mg/kg (325–516)
	Tail electric stimulation (rat)	Motor response	active from 200 mg/kg
		Vocalization	active from 200 mg/kg
		Vocalization postdischarge	active from 150 mg/kg
Inflammatory	Formalin (mice)	Early phase	ED_{50} = 73 mg/kg (27–193)
		Late phase	active from 60 mg/kg
	Paw pressure (inflamed paw) (rat)		active from 62 mg/kg
Visceral	Writhing (mice)		ED_{50} = 53 mg/kg (3–960)

enkephalins if identical opioid receptor occupancy could be achieved (Roques and Fournié-Zaluski, 1986).

However, even at very high concentrations, at which they have been shown to completely inhibit enkephalin degradation, mixed inhibitors were unable to produce the maximum analgesic effect induced by morphine in animal models of severe pain, for example, 80% in the hot-plate and 40% in the tail-flick tests (Schmidt et al., 1991; Noble, Soleilhac et al., 1992). These results indicate that the local increase in enkephalin levels is too low to saturate opioid-binding sites, in agreement with in vivo binding experiments (Ruiz-Gayo et al., 1992a), thus eliminating, or at least minimizing, receptor overstimulation, which is thought to be responsible for the major side effects of morphine.

The endogenous enkephalins protected from degrading enzymes were shown to induce supraspinal antinociceptive responses through a preferential involvement of μ receptors, at least regarding thermal nociceptive stimuli (Michael-Titus et al., 1989; Baamonde et al., 1991; Noble, Soleilhac et al., 1992).

Inhibitor-Induced Spinal Antinociception

The enkephalins are found at high levels in the spinal cord, especially in the substantia gelatinosa, a region also enriched in μ and δ opioid receptors and in NEP (Waksman et al., 1986). The antinociceptive properties of kelatorphan, locally infused onto the spinal cord, were inhibited by the selective δ-opioid antagonist ICI 174,864 (Dickenson et al., 1986) and are shown to be additive with those of the μ-selective agonist DAMGO, but not with those of the selective δ agonist DSTBULET (Dickenson et al., 1988), confirming that endogenous enkephalins and δ-selective agonists act on a common binding site to produce spinal antinociception. Given that there are pharmacologically discernible μ– and δ-receptor populations in the spinal cord that independently modulate noxious transmission, mixed inhibitors such as kelatorphan and/or selective δ agonists may be of clinical interest in patients insensitive to or tolerant of morphine. These drugs may also be useful as a means of eliminating unwanted side effects mediated by stimulation of μ receptors. This novel approach to analgesia has provided promising preliminary clinical results after intrathecal administration of kelatorphan.

The expression of immediate early genes can be used to investigate spinal neuronal activity in an attempt to differentiate the pain modulatory effects of exogenously administered opioids from those induced by tonically released endogenous opioid peptides. When administered IV before heat stimulation, both morphine and to a lesser extent kelatorphan and RB 101 reduce the induction of immediate early genes, such as c-fos, in the superficial dorsal horn and the deep dorsal horn of rats (Abbadie et al., 1994; Tölle et al., 1994) (Fig. 2.6). However, the decrease of immediate early gene expression by kelatorphan and its increase by naloxone supports the existence of a tonically active opioidergic gating system in the dorsal horn. Accordingly, electrophoretic administration of kelatorphan in the substantia gelatinosa of the cat spinal cord leads to naloxone-reversible inhibition of nociceptive responses and marked potentiation of co-administered Met-enkephalin (Morton et al., 1987).

Yet, a reduction of the C-fiber reflex elicited by electrical stimulation of the receptive field of the sural nerve in the ipsilateral biceps femoris muscle was obtained following IV administration of RB 101 (Keime et al., 1996; Xu et al., 1997). This effect was observed in decerebrate, spinalized, unanesthetized rats (Xu et al., 1997), demonstrating that the depression observed involves spinal mechanisms.

Peptidase Inhibitors in Chronic Pain

Using a centrally integrated test (the vocalization threshold to paw pressure), researchers have established that the mixed inhibitors kelatorphan and PC 12, a derivative of RB 101 (Fournié-Zaluski, Coric et al., 1992), when administered systemically produce a potent antinociceptive effect in arthritic rats (Kayser et al., 1989; Perrot et al., 1993). Given the very weak passage of kelatorphan into the brain and the lack of changes in the level of NEP or μ– and δ-opioid receptors in the arthritic rats (Delay-Goyet et al., 1989), the strong antinociceptive effects of kelatorphan in inflammatory pain raise the question of a possible action at the level of peripheral nociceptors, where all opioid targets, including NEP, seem to be present (Stein et al., 1989, 1993). Moreover, on a model of unilateral inflammatory "pain" (intraplantar injection of Freund's complete adjuvant), the elevation of paw pressure threshold in inflamed paws induced by systemic administration of RB 38A or RB 101 was blocked by SC quaternary naltrexone, administered at doses shown to act exclusively at a peripheral level, suggesting a peripheral site of action of enkephalin-like peptides in this model. Nevertheless, in this study, a reduction of the RB 101–induced antinociceptive response was also

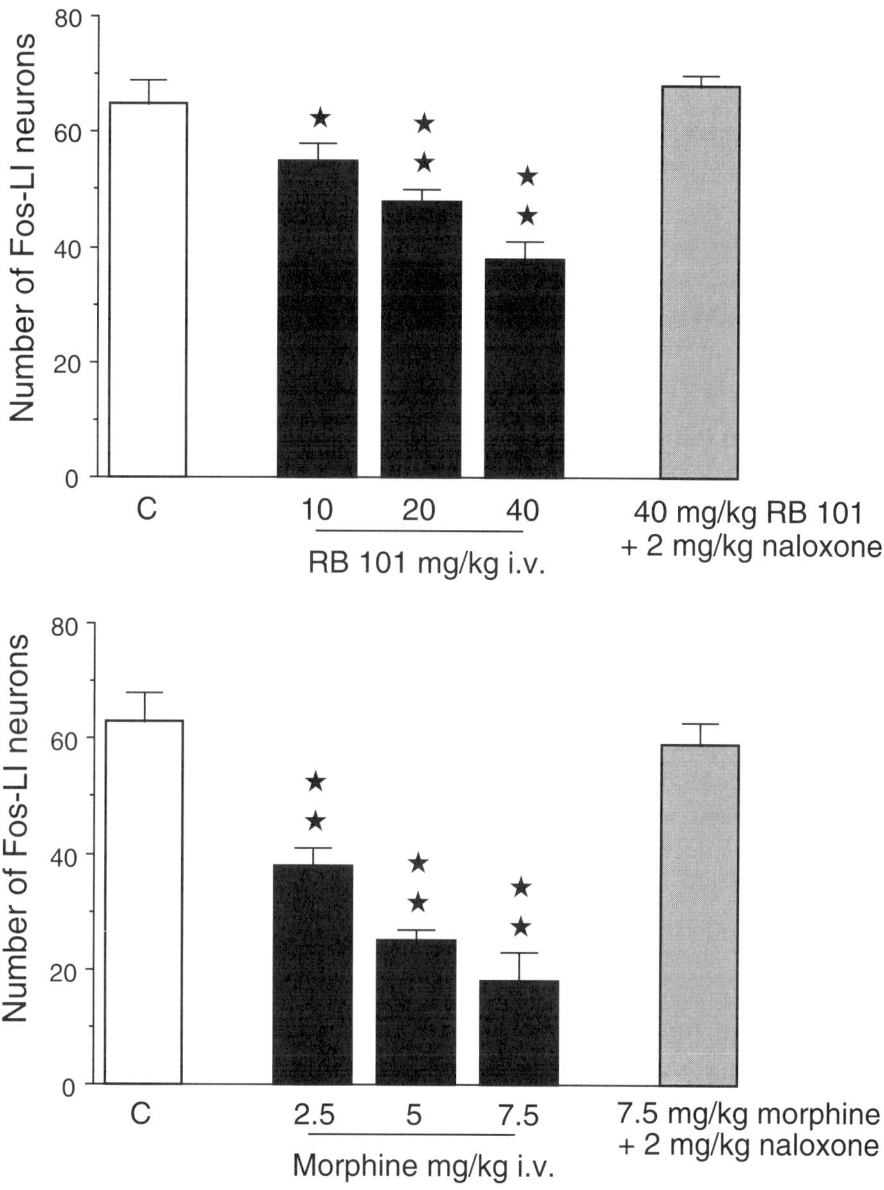

Figure 2.6. Effects of RB 101 and morphine on Fos-like (Fos-LI) immunoreactivity in the superficial dorsal horn and the deep dorsal horn 2 hours after heat stimulation (52° C for 15 seconds) applied to the rat's right foot and reversion by naloxone (2 mg/kg SC). Rats were treated 10 minutes prior to stimulation. ★ $P < 0.05$, ★★ $P < 0.01$ as compared to control.

observed after central administration of methylnaloxonium, suggesting an additional action at the supraspinal level of the mixed inhibitor (Maldonado et al., 1994).

The formalin test measures the response to a long-lasting nociceptive stimulus and thus is often considered to have similarity with clinical pain, such as postoperative pain. Intraperitoneal injection of RB 101 (50 mg/kg) induces antinociceptive responses during early (0–5 minutes postformalin) and late (20–30 minutes postformalin) observation phases (Noble et al., 1995). RB 120 was also capable of inducing strong antinociceptive effects in the inflammatory paw test and in the formalin test in rats and mice, respectively, after oral administration.

Kelatorphan was found to be highly active in rats with pain-related disorders as a result of peripheral mononeuropathy (Attal et al., 1991), although many clinical observations have stated that neuropathic pain is resistant to opioids. However, recent reports showed that patients with neuropathy can benefit from opioid treatment and that the consequences of deafferentation can be reduced by opioids (Foley, 1993).

Tolerance, Dependence, and Possible Side Effects of Enkephalin-Degrading Enzyme Inhibitors

A major side effect of opiate analgesia is a central respiratory depression, which is mainly due to the inhibition of bulbar respiratory neurons. Activation of μ and δ receptors decreases the firing of these neurons with a subsequent diminution in respiratory rhythm and tidal volume (Morin-Surun et al., 1984). After injection of kelatorphan into the nucleus ambiguous of cats or IV injection of RB 101 in anesthetized rats at concentrations that give analgesic responses there was a weak effect on respiratory frequency (Morin-Surun et al., 1992; Keime et al., 1996). Furthermore, no signs of withdrawal were observed after administration of naloxone in animals chronically treated with RB 101 (Noble, Coric et al., 1992). Moreover, chronic administration of the mixed inhibitor prodrug did not induce tolerance or cross tolerance with morphine (Noble, Turcaud et al., 1992) and unlike morphine did not induce psychic dependence (Noble, Fournié-Zaluski et al., 1993) (Fig. 2.7).

Side effects following chronic treatment with opiates are probably due to multiple cellular events involving several components of the cyclic AMP signal transduction cascade (Nestler, 1992; Matsuoka et al., 1994) such as CREB (Maldonado et al., 1996). The main advantage of modifying the concentration of endogenous peptides by use of peptidase inhibitors is that pharmacologic effects are induced only at receptors tonically or phasically stimulated by the natural effectors. Moreover, in contrast to exogenous agonists or antagonists, chronic administration of mixed enkephalin-degrading enzyme inhibitors does not induce changes in the synthesis of the enzymes and the opioid receptors or in that of the enkephalin precursor and in the secretion of the active peptides (Delay-Goyet et al., 1989). The moderate degree or the lack of tolerance and the physical or psychic dependence observed with the mixed inhibitors could be explained by a weaker but more specific stimulation of the opioid-binding sites by the tonically or phasically released endogenous opioids, minimizing receptor desensitization or down-regulation, which usually occurs after the ubiquitous stimulation of opioid receptors by exogenously administered agonists. This assumed limited opioid receptor occupation by the endogenous enkephalins is

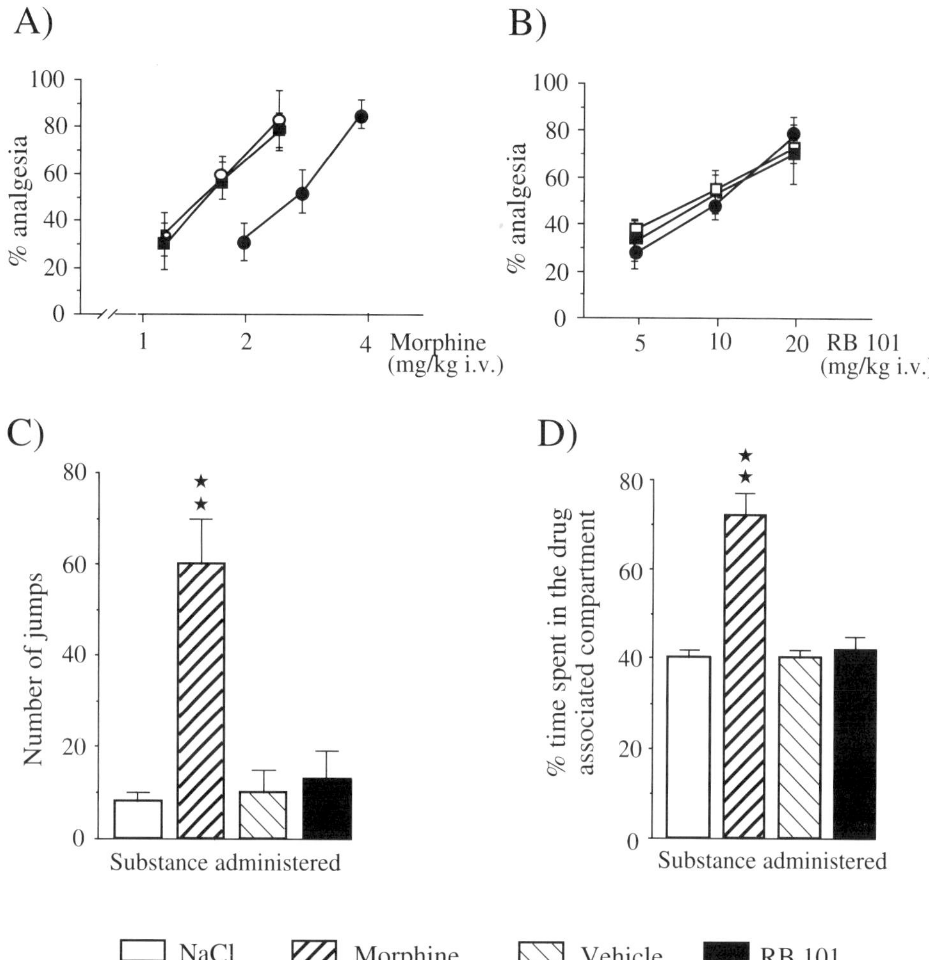

Figure 2.7. (A) Antinociceptive dose-response curves recorded in the hot-plate test 10 minutes after IV administration of morphine to mice chronically pretreated with saline (○), RB 101 (■, 80 mg/kg) or morphine (□, 3 mg/kg) IP twice daily for 4 days. (B) Antinociceptive dose-response curves recorded in the hot-plate test 10 minutes after IV administration of RB 101 to mice chronically pretreated with vehicle (□), RB 101 (■, 80 mg/kg), or morphine (●, 3 mg/kg) IP twice daily for 4 days. (C) Comparison of the withdrawal symptoms induced by naloxone after chronic treatment with morphine (6 mg/kg) or RB 101 (160 mg/kg) injected IP twice daily for 5 days. (D) Comparison of the psychic dependence induced by chronic morphine (6 mg/kg) or RB 101 (160 mg/kg) injected IP in the place-preference test.

in agreement with in vivo binding studies (see review in Roques et al., 1993). Although the locus coeruleus has been clearly demonstrated to be a critical structure implicated in the development of physical dependence and withdrawal syndrome, it has been shown that there is little or no tonic endogenous opioid action in this structure (Williams et al., 1987). This is probably one of the major reasons no significant withdrawal syndrome was observed after chronic treatment by peptidase inhibitors as compared to exogenous opioids (Noble, Soleilhac et al., 1992; Nobel, Turcaud et al., 1992).

The biochemical mechanisms involved in the rewarding effects of morphine are unknown, but several studies have shown that dopaminergic neurons, particularly those that project from the ventral tegmental area (VTA) to the nucleus accumbens, may play a major role in the euphorogenic properties of opiates. The importance of the dopaminergic mesolimbic system in opioid-induced psychic dependence was recently confirmed by the loss of these effects in transgenic mice lacking D_2 receptors (Maldonado et al., 1997). The failure of mixed inhibitors to establish a psychic dependence probably results from a lower recruitment of opioid receptors, as discussed in more detail earlier, and the relatively poor capability of endogenous enkephalins to modulate the dopaminergic transmission in the nucleus accumbens. This hypothesis is supported by the minimal changes in dopamine release in the nucleus accumbens after local administration of kelatorphan into the VTA (Daugé et al., 1992).

Other side effects should have been expected from the blockade of NEP in peripheral tissues where the enzyme has been shown to be involved in the physiologic metabolism of regulatory peptides such as APN, bradykinin, and SP (see review in Roques et al., 1993). However, no side effect resulting from the protection of the degradation of these peptides has been observed after treatment of a great number of patients with Tiorfan, a prodrug of thiorphan that entered the market as a new antidiarrheal, antisecretory agent protecting the enkephalin activity on the δ receptors in the intestine wall (see review in Roques et al., 1993).

Interactions between the Cholecystokinin and Enkephalin Systems in the Control of Pain

The overlapping distribution of the neuropeptides enkephalin and cholecystokinin (CCK) and their respective receptors in pain-processing regions of the brain and spinal cord (Gall et al., 1987; Pohl et al., 1990) has focused attention on the role of CCK in nociception. It has been suggested that CCK_8 has an antiopioid activity. Thus, Faris et al. (1983) found that CCK reduced the antinociceptive effects produced by the stress-induced release of endogenous opioids and did not modify nonopiate responses induced by hind paw foot shock. In addition, numerous studies have shown that peripherally administered CCK antagonists or active immunization against CCK potentiate exogenous opiate-produced antinociception (Faris et al., 1984; Baber et al., 1989).

However, few studies have been performed on the possible physiologic interactions between endogenous CCK and endogenous opioid systems. Recently, the existence of regulatory mechanisms between CCK and enkephalin systems in the control of pain have been proposed. Activation of CCK-A receptors by ICV administration of a CCK_8 derivative, BDNL, potentiates the analgesic effects of RB 101, whereas

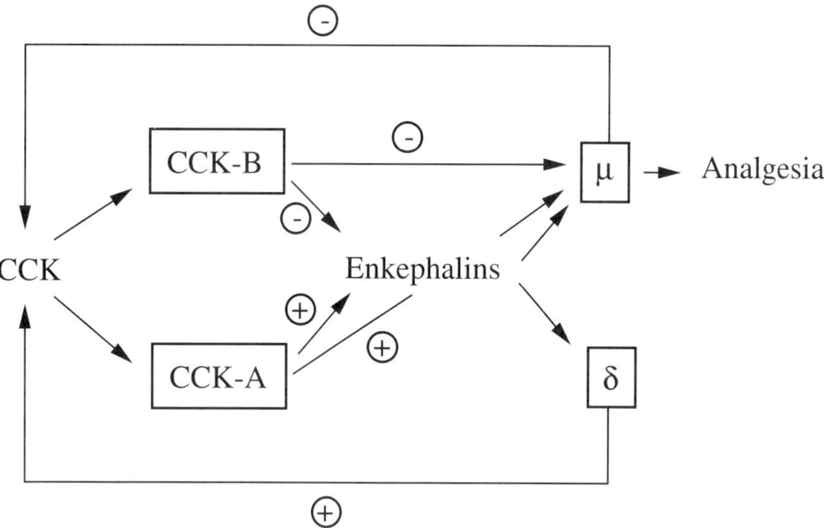

Figure 2.8. Hypothetical model of the interactions between CCK, via CCK-A and CCK-B receptors, and the opioid system via δ-opioid and μ-opioid receptors. CCK agonists, endogenous and/or exogenous, stimulate the CCK-B and/or the CCK-A receptors, which can modulate the opioidergic systems either directly (via binding of opioid agonists or via C-fiber–evoked activity) or indirectly (via the release of endogenous enkephalins). In addition, activation of μ-opioid receptors, which leads to antinociceptive responses, could negatively modulate the release of endogenous CCK, whereas δ-opioid receptors may enhance it.

activation of CCK-B receptors by ICV injection of the selective agonist BC 264 reduce them (Derrien et al., 1993; Noble, Derrien et al., 1993). Taken together these results suggest the existence of a regulatory mechanism between CCK and enkephalin systems in the control of pain. Schematically, stimulation of CCK-A receptors could enhance opioid release and/or directly improve the efficacy of transduction processes occurring at the μ sites, which might be allosterically evoked by CCK-A site occupation (Magnuson et al., 1990). In contrast, CCK-B receptor activation could negatively modulate the opioidergic system (Fig. 2.8). This is supported by the blockade of CCK-B binding sites by selective antagonists, which strongly increase the antinociceptive responses induced by RB 101 in the rat tail-flick test and the mouse hot-plate test (Maldonado et al., 1993; Valverde et al., 1994) and reduce the carrageenin-evoked spinal c-fos expression (Honoré et al., 1997). Furthermore, if stimulation of CCK sites is capable of modulating the opioid system, this system could in turn regulate the release of CCK peptides. Thus, it has been shown that the stimulation of δ-opioid receptors, through RB 101–induced protection of enkephalin enhances the release of endogenous CCK (Ruiz-Gayo et al., 1992b).

Peripheral nerve injury induces complex changes in the level of neuropeptides in primary sensory neurons and in the spinal cord (Hökfelt et al., 1994). Thus, an increase in primary sensory neurons of endogenous CCK was observed after peripheral axotomy in the rat (Verge et al., 1993; Stanfa et al., 1994). It could be suggested that a possible increased release of CCK from terminals of primary afferents will antagonize the actions of opioid analgesics either released endogenously or applied exogenously, resulting in the development of neuropathic pain syndrome and the relative ineffectiveness of opioids (Xu et al., 1993). Thus, it has been demonstrated that a combination of opioids and selective CCK-B antagonists enhanced morphine antiallodynic efficacy (Nichols et al., 1995) and suppressed the development of autotomy behavior in a model of neuropathic pain in the rat (Xu et al., 1993; Xu, Hökfelt et al., 1994) and effectively relieved the allodynia-like symptoms in spinally injured rats (Xu, Hao et al., 1994). As expected, RB 101 was also shown to produce similar effects (Xu et al., 1997).

Summary

Numerous neuromediators are involved in both the control and transmission of nociceptive messages. Several lines of research have been developed to obtain new analgesics to fill the existing gap between opioid analgesics (morphine and surrogates) and antalgics (aspirin, paracetamol, NSAIDs). Recent investigations with transgenic mice have clearly shown that μ agonists are not suitable, and the clinical interest in potent and selective δ agonists remains to be demonstrated. As discussed in this chapter, the inhibitors of enkephalin degradation produce their physiologic effects by increasing the extracellular levels of endogenous opioid peptides, the main advantage being that their pharmacologic effects are induced only at receptors tonically or phasically stimulated by the natural effectors. The putative side effects of inhibitors appear to be strongly reduced by the existence of selective inactivation pathways for most of the important neuropeptides (enkephalin, neurotensin, CCK_8, galanin, nociceptin, angiotensin II, SP), a finding that was initially not expected owing to the low specificity of ectopeptidases measured in vitro. The goal of discovering orally active analgesics endowed with a potency similar to that of morphine, but devoid of major side effects, seems to have been reached with the mixed NEP/APN inhibitors. Based on results obtained in animal models of pain, the clinical trials now under way with one of these compounds are believed to give more insight into the potentiality of these compounds in analgesia.

In addition, results obtained in rodents suggest that orally active mixed inhibitors could be used in the treatment of drug abuse (see review in Roques and Noble, 1995). They could represent more efficient compounds than methadone in the treatment of opioid addiction because they do not seem to induce dependence, a problem generated by the long-lasting agonist methadone. The complete inhibitors could be administered alone or in combination with the selective CCK-B antagonists to increase the endogenous opioid peptide levels, thus reducing the discomfort of the short-term withdrawal syndrome (Ruiz et al., 1996). The protracted abstinence syndrome could also be improved owing to the antidepressant-like properties of the mixed inhibitors (Baamonde et al., 1992; Smadja et al., 1995), thus minimizing relapse, the most important problem in the management of opioid addiction.

REFERENCES

Abbadie, C., Honoré, P., Fournié-Zaluski, M.C., Roques, B.P., and Besson, J.M. (1994). Effects of opioids and nonopioids on c-Fos-like immunoreactivity induced in rat lumbar spinal cord neurons by noxious heat stimulation. *Eur. J. Pharmacol.* **258,** 215–227.

Attal, N., Desmeules, J., Kayser, V., Jazat, F., and Guilbaud, G. (1991). Effects of opioids in a rat model of peripheral mononeuropathy. In *Lesions of primary afferent fibers as a tool for the study of clinical pain,* ed. J.M. Besson and G. Guilbaud. Amsterdam: Elsevier Science Publishers, pp. 245–258.

Baamonde, A., Daugé, V., Gacel, G., and Roques, B.P. (1991). Systemic administration of (Tyr-D-Ser(O-Tert-Butyl)-Gly-Phe-Leu-Thr(O-Tert-Butyl), a highly selective delta opioid agonist, induces mu receptor-mediated analgesia in mice. *J. Pharmacol. Exp. Ther.* **257,** 767–773.

Baamonde, A., Daugé, V., Ruiz-Gayo, M., Fulga, I.G., Turcaud, S., Fournié-Zaluski, M.C., and Roques, B.P. (1992). Antidepressant-type effects of endogenous enkephalins protected by systemic RB 101 are mediated by opioid δ and dopamine D_1 receptor stimulation. *Eur. J. Pharmacol.* **216,** 157–166.

Baber, N.S., Dourish, C.T., and Hill, D.R. (1989). The role of CCK, caerulein, and CCK antagonists in nociception. *Pain.* **39,** 307–328.

Beaumont, A., Fournié-Zaluski, M.C., Noble, F., Maldonado, R., and Roques, B.P. (1997). The chemistry and pharmacology of cell-surface peptidase inhibitors. In *Cell-suface peptidases in health and disease,* ed. J. Kenny and C.M. Boustead. Oxford: BIOS Scientific Publishers, 5, pp. 59–78.

Belluzi, J.D., Grant, N., Garsky, V., Sarantakis, D., Wise, C.D., and Stein, D. (1976). Analgesia induced in vivo by central administration of enkephalin in rat. *Nature (Lond.).* **260,** 625–626.

Besse, D., Lombard, M.C., Zajac, J.M., and Roques, B.P. (1990). Pre- and post-synaptic distribution of μ, δ and κ opioid receptors in the superficial layers of the cervical dorsal horn of the rat spinal cord. *Brain Res.* **521,** 15–22.

Besson, J.M., and Chaouch, A. (1987). Peripheral and spinal mechanisms of nociception. *Physiol. Rev.* **67,** 67–186.

Bourgoin, S., Le Bars, D., Artaud, F., Clot, A.M., Bouboutou, R., Fournié-Zaluski, M.C., Roques, B.P., Hamon, M., and Cesselin, F. (1986). Effects of kelatorphan and other peptidase inhibitors on the in vitro and in vivo release of Met-enkephalin-like material from the rat spinal cord. *J. Pharmacol. Exp. Ther.* **238,** 360–366.

Cesselin, F. (1995). Opioid and anti-opioid peptides. *Fundam. Clin. Pharmacol.* **9,** 109–433.

Cesselin, F., Oliveras, J.L., Bourgoin, S., Sierralta, F., Michelot, R., Besson, J.M., and Hamon, M. (1982). Increased levels of Met-enkephalin-like material in the CSF of anesthetized cats after tooth pulp stimulation. *Brain Res.* **237,** 325–338.

Chipkin, R.E. (1986). Inhibitors of enkephalinase: The next generation of analgesics. *Drugs Future.* **11,** 593–606.

Craves, F.B., Law, P.Y., Hunt, C.A., and Loh, H.H. (1978). The metabolic disposition of radiolabeled enkephalins in vitro and in situ. *J. Pharmacol. Exp. Ther.* **206,** 492–506.

Daugé, V., Kalivas, P.W., Duffy, T., and Roques, B.P. (1992). Effect of inhibiting enkephalin catabolism in the VTA on motor activity and extracellular dopamine. *Brain Res.* **599,** 209–214.

Daugé, V., Mauborgne, A., Cesselin, F., Fournié-Zaluski, M.C., and Roques, B.P. (1996). The dual peptidase inhibitor RB 101 induces a long-lasting increase in the extracellular level of Met-enkephalin in the nucleus accumbens of freely moving rats. *J. Neurochem.* **67,** 1301–1308.

Delay-Goyet, P., Zajac, J.M., and Roques, B.P. (1989). Effects of repeated treatment with haloperidol on rat striatal neutral endopeptidase EC 3.4.24.11, and on μ and δ opioid binding sites: Comparison with chronic morphine and chronic kelatorphan. *Neurosci. Lett.* **103,** 197–202.

Derrien, M., Noble, F., Maldonado, R., and Roques, B.P. (1993). Cholecystokinin-A but not cholecystokinin-B receptor stimulation induces endogenous opioid-dependent antinociceptive effects in the hot plate test in mice. *Neurosci. Lett.* **160,** 193–196.

Desmeules, J.A., Kayser, V., Gacel, G., Guilbaud, G., and Roques, B.P. (1993). The highly selective delta agonist BUBU induces an analgesic effect in normal and arthritic rat and this action is not affected by repeated administration of low doses of morphine. *Brain Res.* **611,** 243–248.

Dickenson, A.H., Sullivan, A., Feeney, C., Fournié-Zaluski, M.C., and Roques, B.P. (1986). Evidence that endogenous enkephalins produce δ-opiate receptor mediated neuronal inhibitions in rat dorsal horn. *Neurosci. Lett.* **72,** 179–182.

Dickenson, A.H., Sullivan, A.F., Fournié-Zaluski, M.C., and Roques, B.P. (1987). Prevention of degradation of endogenous enkephalins produces inhibition of nociceptive neurones in rat spinal cord. *Brain Res.* **408,** 36–44.

Dickenson, A.H., Sullivan, A.F., and Roques, B.P. (1988). Evidence that endogenous enkephalins and a δ opioid receptor agonist have a common site of action in spinal antinociception. *Eur. J. Pharmacol.* **148,** 437–439.

Elliot, R.L., Marks, N., Berg, M.J., and Portoghese, P.S. (1985). Synthesis and biological evaluation of phosphonomidate peptide inhibitors of enkephalinase and angiotensin converting enzyme. *J. Med. Chem.* **28,** 1208–1216.

Faris, P.L., Komisaruk, B.R., Watkins, L.R., and Mayer, D.J. (1983). Evidence for the neuropeptide cholecystokinin as an antagonist of opiate analgesia. *Science.* **219,** 310–312.

Faris, P.L., McLaughlin, C.L., Baile, C.A., Olney, J.W., and Komisaruk, B.R. (1984). Morphine analgesia potentiated but tolerance not affected by active immunization against cholecystokinin. *Science.* **226,** 1215–1217.

Foley, K.M. (1993). Opioid analgesics in clinical pain management. In *Opioids II: Handbook of experimental pharmacology,* ed. A. Herz, H. Akil, and E.J. Simon. Berlin, Heidelberg: Springer-Verlag, pp. 697–743.

Fournié-Zaluski, M.C., Chaillet, P., Bouboutou, R., Coulaud, A., Chérot, P., Waksman, G., Costentin, J., and Roques, B.P. (1984). Analgesic effects of kelatorphan, a new highly potent inhibitor of multiple enkephalin degrading enzymes. *Eur. J. Pharmacol.* **102,** 525–528.

Fournié-Zaluski, M.C., Coric, P., Turcaud, S., Lucas, E., Noble, F., Maldonado, R., and Roques, B.P. (1992). Mixed-inhibitor prodrug as a new approach towards systemically active inhibitors of enkephalin degrading enzymes. *J. Med. Chem.* **35,** 2474–2481.

Fournié-Zaluski, M.C., Coulaud, A., Bouboutou, R., Chaillet, P., Devin, J., Waksman, G., Costentin, J., and Roques, B.P. (1985). New bidentates as full inhibitors of enkephalin degrading enzymes: Synthesis and analgesic properties. *J. Med. Chem.* **28,** 1158–1169.

Fournié-Zaluski, M.C., Perdrisot, R., Gacel, G., Swerts, J.P., Roques, B.P., and Schwartz, J.C. (1979). Inhibitory potency of various peptides on enkephalinase activity from mouse striatum. *Biochem. Biophys. Res. Comm.* **91,** 130–135.

Fournié-Zaluski, M.C., Soleilhac, J.M., Turcaud, S., Lai-Kuen, R., Crine, P., Beaumont, A., and Roques, B.P. (1992). Development of [^{125}I]RB104, a new potent inhibitor of neutral endopeptidase-24,11 and its use in detecting nanogram quantities of the enzymes by "Inhibitor Gel Electrophoresis." *Proc. Natl. Acad. Sci. U.S.A.* **89,** 6388–6392.

Gall, C., Lauterborn, J., Burks, D., and Seroogy, K. (1987). Co-localization of enkephalins and cholecystokinin in discrete areas of rat brain. *Brain Res.* **403,** 403–408.

Gros, C., Giros, B., Schwartz, J.C., Vlaiculescu, A., Costentin, J., and Lecomte, J.M. (1988). Potent inhibition of cerebral aminopeptidases by carbaphethiol, a parenterally active compound. *Neuropeptides.* **12,** 111–118.

Guyon, A., Roques, B.P., Guyon, F., Foucault, A., Perdrisot, R., Swerts, J.P., and Schwartz, J.C. (1979). Enkephalin degradation in mouse brain studied by a new H.P.L.C. method: Further evidence for the involvement of carboxydipeptidase. *Life Sci.* **25,** 1605–1612.

Hökfelt, T., Xu, Z., Verge, V., Villar, M., Elde, R., Xu, X.J., and Wiesenfeld-Hallin, Z. (1994). Messenger plasticity in primary sensory neurons. In *Neuropeptides, nociception, and pain,* ed. T. Hökfelt, H.G. Schaible, and R.F. Schmidt. Weinheim: Chapman and Hall, pp. 71–84 .

Honoré, P., Buritova, J., Fournié-Zaluski, M.C., Roques, B.P., and Besson, J.M. (1997). Antinociceptive effects of RB 101, a complete inhibitor of enkephalin-catabolizing enzymes, are enhanced by a CCK-B receptor antagonist as revealed by noxiously-evoked spinal c-fos expression in the rat. *J. Pharmacol. Exp. Ther.* **281,** 208–217.

Kayser, V., Fournié-Zaluski, M.C., Guilbaud, G., and Roques, B.P. (1989). Potent antinociceptive effects of kelatorphan (a highly efficient inhibitor of multiple enkephalin degrading enzymes) systemically administered in normal and arthritic rats. *Brain Res.* **497,** 94–101.

Keime, F., Strimbu, M., Le Bars, D., Roth, V., Noble, F., Roques, B.P., and Willer, J.C. (1996). Effects of intravenous enkephalin-metabolizing enzymes inhibitor, RB 101, on a C-fiber reflex in the rat. *Proc. Eur. Neurosci. Ass.* (Abstract). Strasbourg, France, European Neuroscience Association.

Kerr, M.A., and Kenny, A.J. (1974). The purification and specificity of a neutral endopeptidase from rabbit kidney brush border. *Biochem. J.* **137,** 477–488.

König, M., Zimmer, A.M., Steiner, H., Holmes, P.V., Crawley, J.N., Brownstein, M.J., and Zimmer, A. (1996). Pain responses, anxiety and aggression in mice deficient in pre-proenkephalin. *Nature.* **383,** 535–538.

Llorens, C., Gacel, G., Swerts, J.P., Perdrisot, R., Fournié-Zaluski, M.C., Schwartz, J.C., and Roques, B.P. (1980). Rational design of enkephalinase inhibitors: Substrate specificity of enkephalinase studied from inhibitory potency of various peptides. *Biochem. Biophys. Res. Commun.* **96,** 1710–1715.

Magnuson, D.S.K., Sullivan, A.F., Simonnet, G., Roques, B.P., and Dickenson, A.H. (1990). Differential interactions of cholecystokinin and FLFQPQRF-NH_2 with μ and δ opioid antinociception in the rat spinal cord. *Neuropeptides.* **16,** 213–218.

Maldonado, R., Blendy, J.A., Tzavara, E., Gass, P., Roques, B.P., Hanoune, J., and Schütz, G. (1996). Reduction of morphine abstinence in mice with a mutation in the gene encoding CREB. *Science.* **273,** 657–659.

Maldonado, R., Derrien, M., Noble, F., and Roques, B.P. (1993). Association of the peptidase inhibitor RB 101 and a CCK-B antagonist strongly enhances antinociceptive responses. *Neuroreport.* **4,** 947–950.

Maldonado, R., Féger, J., Fournié-Zaluski, M.C., and Roques, B.P. (1990). Differences in physical dependence induced by selective μ or δ opioid agonists and by endogenous enkephalins protected by peptidase inhibitors. *Brain Res.* **520,** 247–254.

Maldonado, R., Saiardi, A., Valverde, O., Samad, T.A., Roques, B.P., and Borreli, E. (1997). Absence of opiate rewarding effects in mice lacking dopamine D_2 receptors. *Nature (Lond.).* **388,** 586–589.

Maldonado, R., Valverde, O., Turcaud, S., Fournié-Zaluski, M.C., and Roques, B.P. (1994). Antinociceptive response induced by mixed inhibitors of enkephalin catabolism in peripheral inflammation. *Pain.* **58,** 77–83.

Malfroy, B., Swerts, J.P., Guyon, A., Roques, B.P., and Schwartz, J.C. (1978). High-affinity enkephalin-degrading peptidase in mouse brain and its enhanced activity following morphine. *Nature (Lond.).* **276,** 523–526.

Malin, D.H., Lake, J.R., Hamilton, R.F., and Skolnick, M.H. (1989). Augmentated analgesic effects of enkephalinase inhibitors combined with transcranial electrostimulation. *Life Sci.* **44,** 1371–1376.

Matsuoka, I., Maldonado, R., Defer, N., Noël, F., Hanoune, J., and Roques, B.P. (1994). Chronic morphine administration causes region-specific increase of brain type VIII adenylyl cyclase mRNA. *Eur. J. Pharmacol. (Mol. Pharm. Sec.).* **268,** 215–221.

Matthes, H.W., Maldonado, R., Simonin, F., Valverde, O., Slowe, S., Kitchen, I., Befort, K., Dierich, A., Le Meur, M., Dollé, P., Tzavara, E., Hanoune, J., Roques, B.P., and Kieffer, B.L. (1996). Loss of morphine-induced analgesia, reward effect and withdrawal symptoms in mice lacking the μ-opioid-receptor gene. *Nature (Lond.).* **383,** 819–823.

Meek, J.L., Yang, H.Y.T., and Costa, E. (1977). Enkephalin catabolism in vitro and in vivo. *Neuropharmacology.* **16,** 151–154.

Meucci, E., Delay-Goyet, P., Roques, B.P., and Zajac, J.M. (1989). Binding in vivo of selective μ and δ opioid agonists: Opioid receptor occupancy by endogenous enkephalins. *Eur. J. Pharmacol.* **171,** 167–178.

Meunier, J.C., Mollereau, C., Toll, L., Suaudeau, C., Moisand, C., Alvinerie, P., Butour, J.L., Guillemot, J.C., Ferrara, P., Monsarrat, B., Mazarguil, H., Vassart, G., Parmentier, M., and Costentin, J. (1995). Isolation and structure of the endogenous agonist of opioid receptor-like ORL1 receptor. *Nature (Lond.).* **377,** 532–535.

Michael-Titus, A., Dourmap, N., Caline, H., Costentin, J., and Schwartz, J.C. (1989). Role of endogenous enkephalins in locomotion and nociception studied with peptidase inhibitors in two inbred strains of mice. *Neuropharmacology.* **28,** 117–122.

Morin-Surun, M.P., Boudinot, E., Fournié-Zaluski, M.C., Champagnat, B.P., Roques, B.P., and Denavit-Saubié, M. (1992). Control of breathing by endogenous opioid peptides: Possible involvement in sudden infant death syndrome. *Neurochem. Int.* **20,** 103–107.

Morin-Surun, M.P., Boudinot, E., Gacel, G., Champagnat, J., Roques, B.P., and Denavit-Saubié, M. (1984). Different effects of delta and mu opiate agonists on respiration. *Eur. J. Pharmacol.* **98,** 235–240.

Morton, C.R., Zhao, Z.Q., and Duggan, A.W. (1987). Kelatorphan potentiates the effect of Met^5-enkephalin in the substantia gelatinosa of the cat spinal cord. *Eur. J. Pharmacol.* **140,** 195–201.

Nestler, E.J. (1992). Molecular mechanisms of drug addiction. *J. Neurosci.* **12,** 2439–2450.

Nichols, M.L., Bian, D., Ossipov, M.H., Lai, J., and Porreca, F. (1995). Regulation of morphine antiallodynic efficacy by cholecystokinin in a model of neuropathic pain in rats. *J. Pharmacol. Exp. Ther.* **275,** 1339–1345.

Noble, F., Blommaert, A., Fournié-Zaluski, M.C., and Roques, B.P. (1995). A selective CCK-B receptor antagonist potentiates μ- but not δ-opioid receptor-mediated antinociception in the formalin test. *Eur. J. Pharmacol.* **273,** 145–151.

Noble, F., Coric, P., Fournié-Zaluski, M.C., and Roques, B.P. (1992). Lack of physical dependence in mice after repeated systemic administration of the mixed inhibitor prodrug of enkephalin-degrading enzymes, RB 101. *Eur. J. Pharmacol.* **223,** 91–96.

Noble, F., Derrien, M., and Roques, B.P. (1993). Modulation of opioid analgesia by CCK at the supraspinal level: Evidence of regulatory mechanisms between CCK and enkephalin systems in the control of pain. *Br. J. Pharmcol.* **109,** 1064–1070.

Noble, F., Fournié-Zaluski, M.C., and Roques, B.P. (1993). Unlike morphine, the endogenous enkephalins protected by RB 101 are unable to establish a conditioned place preference in mice. *Eur. J. Pharmacol.* **230,** 139–149.

Noble, F., and Roques, B.P. (1995). Assessment of endogenous enkephalin's efficacy in the hot plate test in mice: Comparative study with morphine. *Neurosci. Lett.* **185,** 75–78.

Noble, F., Smadja, C., Valverde, O., Maldonado, R., Coric, C., Turcaud, S., Fournié-Zaluski, M.C., and Roques, B.P. (1997). Pain-suppressive effects on various nociceptive stimuli (thermal, chemical, electrical and inflammatory) of the first orally active enkephalin-metabolizing enzyme inhibitor RB 120. *Pain.* **73,** 381–391.

Noble, F., Soleilhac, J.M., Soroca-Lucas, E., Turcaud, S., Fournié-Zaluski, M.C., and Roques, B.P. (1992). Inhibition of the enkephalin-metabolizing enzymes by the first systemically active mixed inhibitor prodrug RB 101 induces potent analgesic responses in mice and rats. *J. Pharmacol. Exp. Ther.* **261,** 181–190.

Noble, F., Turcaud, S., Fournié-Zaluski, M.C., and Roques, B.P. (1992). Repeated systemic administration of the mixed inhibitor of enkephalin degrading enzymes, RB 101, does not induce either antinociceptive tolerance or cross-tolerance with morphine. *Eur. J. Pharmacol.* **223,** 83–89.

Northridge, D.B., Alabaster, C.T., Connell, J.M.C., Dilly, S.G., Lever, A.F., Jardine, A.G., Barclay, P.L., Dargie, H.J., Findlay, I.N., and Samuels, G.M.R. (1989). Effects of UK 69578: A novel atriopeptidase inhibitor. *Lancet,* **2,** 591–593.

Patey, G., De La Baume, S., Schwartz, J.C., Gros, C., Fournié-Zaluski, M.C., Lucas-Soroca, E., and Roques, B.P. (1981). Selective protection of methionine enkephaline released from brain slices by thiorphan, a potent enkephalinase inhibitor. *Science.* **212,** 1153–1155.

Perrot, S., Kayser, V., Fournié-Zaluski, M.C., Roques, B.P., and Guilbaud, G. (1993). Antinociceptive effect of systemic PC 12, a prodrug mixed inhibitor of enkephalin-degrading enzymes in normal and arthritic rats. *Eur. J. Pharmacol.* **214,** 129–133.

Pert, C., Pert, A., Chang, J.K., and Fong, B.T.W. (1976). [D-Ala^2]-Met-enkephalinamide: A potent, long-lasting synthetic pentapeptide analgesic. *Science.* **194,** 330–332.

Pohl, M., Benoliel, J.J., Bourgoin, S., Lombard, M.C., Mauborgne, A., Taquet, H., Carayon, A., Besson, J.M., Cesselin, F., and Hamon, M. (1990). Regional distribution of calcitonin gene-related peptide-, substance P-, cholecystokinin-, Met^5-enkephalin-, and dynorphin A (1–8)-like materials in the spinal cord and dorsal root ganglia of adult rats: Effects of dorsal rhizotomy and neonatal capsaicin. *J. Neurochem.* **55,** 1122–1130.

Reinscheid, R.K., Nothacker, H.P., Bourson, A., Ardati, A., Henningsen, R.A., Bunzow, J.R., Grandy, D.K., Langen, H., Monsma Jr., F.J., and Civelli, O. (1995). Orphanin FQ: A neuropeptide that activates an opioid-like G protein-coupled receptor. *Science.* **270,** 792–794.

Relton, J.M., Gee, N.S., Matsas, R., Turner, A.J., and Kenny, A.J. (1983). Purification of endopeptidase 24–11 (enkephalinase) from pig brain by immunoadsorbent chromatography. *Biochem. J.* **215,** 519–523.

Roemer, D., Buscher, H.H., Hill, R.C., Pless, J., Bauer, W., Cardinaux, F., Closse, A., Hauser, D., and Huguenin, R. (1977). A synthetic enkephalin analogue with prolonged parenteral and oral analgesic activity. *Nature (Lond.).* **268,** 547–549.

Roques, B.P. (1991). What are the relevant features of the distribution, selective binding and metabolism of opioid peptides and how can these be applied to drug design? In *Towards a new pharmacotherapy of pain,* ed. A.I. Basbaum and J.M. Besson. New York: John Wiley, pp. 257–278.

Roques, B.P., and Fournié-Zaluski, M.C. (1986). Enkephalin degrading enzyme inhibtors: A physiological way to new analgesics and psychoactive agents. In *Opioid peptides: Molecular, pharmacology, biosynthesis and analysis,* Serie 70, ed. R.S. Rapaka and R.L. Hawks. NIDA Research Monograph, pp. 128–154.

Roques, B.P., Fournié-Zaluski, M.C., Soroca, E., Lecomte, J.M., Malfroy, B., Llorens, C., and Schwartz, J.C. (1980). The enkephalinase inhibitor thiorphan shows antinociceptive activity in mice. *Nature.* **288,** 286–288.

Roques, B.P., Lucas-Soroca, E., Chaillet, P., Costentin, J., and Fournié-Zaluski, M.C. (1983). Complete differentiation between "enkephalinase" and angiotensin converting enzyme inhibition by retro-thiorphan. *Proc. Natl. Acad. Sci. U.S.A.* **80,** 3178–3182.

Roques, B.P., and Noble, F. (1995). Dual inhibitors of enkephalin-degrading enzymes (neutral endopeptidase 24.11 and aminopeptidase N) as potential new medications in the management of pain and opioid addiction. In *Discovery of novel opioid medications,* 147, ed. R.S. Rapaka and H. Sorer. NIDA Research Monograph, pp. 104–145.

Roques, B.P., Noble, F., Daugé, V., Fournié-Zaluski, M.C., and Beaumont, A. (1993). Neutral endopeptidase 24.11: Structure, inhibition, and experimental and clinical pharmacology. *Pharmacol. Rev.* **45,** 87–146.

Ruiz, F., Fournié-Zaluski, M.C., Roques, B.P., and Maldonado, R. (1996). Similar decrease in spontaneous morphine abstinence by methadone and RB 101, an inhibitor of enkephalin catabolism. *Br. J. Pharmcol.* **119,** 174–182.

Ruiz-Gayo, M., Baamonde, A., Turcaud, S., Fournié-Zaluski, M.C., and Roques, B.P. (1992a). In vivo occupation of mouse brain opioid receptors by endogenous enkephalins: Blockade of enkephalin degrading enzymes by RB 101 inhibits [^{3}H]diprenorphine binding. *Brain Res.* **571,** 306–312.

Ruiz-Gayo, M., Durieux, C., Fournié-Zaluski, M.C., and Roques, B.P. (1992b). Stimulation of δ opioid receptors reduces the in vivo binding of the CCK-B selective agonist [^{3}H]pBC264: Evidence for a physiological regulation of CCKergic systems by endogenous enkephalins. *J. Neurochem.* **59,** 1805–1811.

Schmidt, C., Peyroux, J., Noble, F., Fournié-Zaluski, M.C., and Roques, B.P. (1991). Analgesic responses elicited by endogenous enkephalins (protected by mixed peptidase inhibitors) in a variety of morphine-sensitive noxious tests. *Eur. J. Pharmacol.* **192,** 253–262.

Schwartz, J.C. (1983). Metabolism of enkephalins and the inactivating neuropeptidase concept. *Trends Neurosci.* **6,** 45–48.

Seguin, L., Le Marouille-Girardon, S., and Millan, M.J. (1995). Antinociceptive profiles of non-peptidergic neurokinin$_1$ and neurokinin$_2$ receptor antagonists: A comparison to other classes of antinociceptive agent. *Pain.* **61,** 325–343.

Seymour, A.A., Fennell, S.A., and Swerdel, J.N. (1989). Potentiation of renal effects of atrial natriuretic factor-(99–126) by SQ 29072. *Hypertension.* **14,** 87–97.

Smadja, C., Maldonado, R., Turcaud, S., Fournié-Zaluski, M.C., and Roques, B.P. (1995). Opposite role of CCK-A and CCK-B receptors in the modulation of endogenous enkephalin-depressant-like effects. *Psychopharmacology.* **120,** 400–408.

Stanfa, L., Dickenson, A., Xu, X.J., and Wiesenfeld-Hallin, Z. (1994). Cholecystokinin and morphine analgesia. *Trends Pharmacol. Sci.* **15,** 65–66.

Stein, C., Hassan, A.H.S., Lehrberger, K., Giefing, J., and Yassouridis, A. (1993). Local analgesic effect of endogenous opioid peptides. *Lancet.* **342,** 321–324.

Stein, C., Millan, M.J., Shippenberg, T.S., Peter, K., and Herz, A. (1989). Peripheral opioid receptors mediating antinociception in inflammation. Evidence for involvement of mu, delta and kappa receptors. *J. Pharmacol. Exp. Ther.* **248,** 1269–1275.

Stephenson, S.L., and Kenny, A.J. (1987). The hydrolysis of α human atrial natriuretic peptide by pig kidney microvillar membranes is initiated by endopeptidase 24.11. *Biochem. J.* **243,** 183–187.

Sybertz, E.J., Chiu, P.J.S., Vemulapalli, S., Watkins, R., and Haslanger, M.F. (1990). Atrial natriuretic factor-potentiating and hypertensive activity of SCH 34826, an orally active neutral endopeptidase inhibitor. *Hypertension.* **15,** 152–161.

Tölle, T.R., Schadrack, J., Castro-Lopes, J., Evan, G., Roques, B.P., and Zieglgänsberger, W. (1994). Effects of kelatorphan and morphine before and after noxious stimulation on immediate-early gene expression in rat spinal cord neurons. *Pain.* **56,** 103–112.

Valverde, O., Maldonado, R., Fournié-Zaluski, M.C., and Roques, B.P. (1994). Cholecystokinin B antagonists strongly potentiate antinociception mediated by endogenous enkephalins. *J. Pharmacol. Exp. Ther.* **270,** 77–88.

Verge, V.M.K., Wiesenfeld-Hallin, Z., and Hökfelt, T. (1993). Cholecystokinin in mammalian primary sensory neurons and spinal cord: In situ hybridization studies on rat and monkey spinal ganglia. *Eur. J. Neurosci.* **5,** 240–250.

Wagner, J.J., Caudle, R.M., Neumaier, J.F., and Chavkin, C. (1990). Stimulation of endogenous opioid release displaces mu receptor binding in the rat hippocampus. *Neuroscience.* **37,** 45–53.

Waksman, G., Bouboutou, R., Devin, J., Bourgoin, S., Cesselin, F., Hamon, M., Fournié-Zaluski, M.C., and Roques, B.P. (1985). In vitro and in vivo effects of kelatorphan on enkephalin metabolism in rodent brain. *Eur. J. Pharmacol.* **117,** 233–243.

Waksman, G., Hamel, E., Fournié-Zaluski, M.C., and Roques, B.P. (1986). Autoradiographic comparison of the distribution of the neutral endopeptidase "enkephalinase" and of mu and delta opioid receptors in rat brain. *Proc. Natl. Acad. Sci. U.S.A.* **83,** 1523–1527.

Williams, J.T., Christie, M.J., North, R.A., and Roques, B.P. (1987). Potentiation of enkephalin action by peptidase inhibitors in rat locus coeruleus. *J. Pharmacol. Exp. Ther.* **243,** 397–401.

Xie, J., Soleilhac, J.M., Schmidt, C., Peyroux, J., Roques, B.P., and Fournié-Zaluski, M.C. (1989). New kelatorphan related inhibitors of enkephalin metabolism: Improved antinociceptive properties. *J. Med. Chem.* **32,** 1497–1503.

Xu, X.J., Elfvin, A., Hao, J.X., Fournié-Zaluski, M.C., Roques, B.P., and Wiesenfeld-Hallin, Z. (1997). CI-988, an antagonist of the cholecystokinin-B receptor, potentiates endogenous opioid-mediated antinociception at spinal level. *Neuropeptides.* **31,** 287–291.

Xu, X.J., Hao, J.X., Seiger, A., Hughes, J., Hökfelt, T., and Wiesenfeld-Hallin, Z. (1994). Chronic pain-related behaviors in spinally injured rats: Evidence for functional alterations of the endogenous cholecystokinin and opioid systems. *Pain.* **56,** 271–277.

Xu, X.J., Hökfelt, T., Hughes, J., and Wiesenfeld-Hallin, Z. (1994). The CCK-B antagonist CI 988 enhances the reflex-depressive effect of morphine in axotomized rats. *Neuroreport.* **5,** 718–720.

Xu, X.J., Puke, M.J.C., Verge, V.M.K., Wiesenfeld-Hallin, Z., Hughes, J., and Hökfelt, T. (1993). Up-regulation of cholecystokinin in primary sensory neurons is associated with morphine insensitivity in experimental neuropathic pain in the rat. *Neurosci. Lett.* **152,** 129–132.

Yaksh, T.L., and Elde, R.P. (1981). Factors governing release of methionine enkephalin-like immunoreactivity from mesencephalon and spinal cord of the cat in vivo. *J. Neurophysiol.* **46,** 1056–1075.

Zadina, J.E., Hackler, L., Ge, L.J., and Kastin, A.J. (1997). A potent and selective endogenous agonist for the μ-opiate receptor. *Nature (Lond.).* **386,** 499–502.

CHAPTER THREE

Supraspinal Mechanisms of Opioid Analgesia

MARY M. HEINRICHER AND MICHAEL M. MORGAN

The biologic actions of opioids are exerted via interactions with the three major opioid receptor types, μ, δ, and κ, and opioid binding is distributed throughout the central nervous system (Mansour et al., 1988). It is thus not surprising that morphine and other narcotic analgesics produce not only analgesia but changes in respiratory, cardiovascular, gastrointestinal, and neuroendocrine functions when given systemically. For this reason, microinjection mapping studies, in which opioid agonists are applied directly within discrete brain regions, have been used to identify those central nervous system sites at which opioid agonist binding gives rise to analgesia. These studies point to a limited number of brain sites supporting opioid analgesia, the most important and best studied being the midbrain periaqueductal gray (PAG) and rostral ventromedial medulla (RVM) (Mayer and Price, 1976; Yaksh et al., 1988). The PAG and RVM are links in an opioid-sensitive nociceptive modulating network that spans the neuraxis, yet each has within it all of the neuronal machinery necessary to induce analgesia. Understanding that machinery, as well as how the relationships between opioid-sensitive brain regions give rise to the properties of the network as a whole, continues to be a central goal for researchers concerned with nociceptive modulation.

The anatomic organization of this nociceptive modulating network is shown schematically in Figure 3.1. The RVM sends a substantial descending projection through the dorsolateral funiculus to the dorsal horn, with terminations in those layers implicated in nociceptive processing. The PAG does not itself project to the dorsal horn, but sends a large projection to the RVM. Although the details of how the RVM interfaces with dorsal horn systems are not well understood, it is clear that this system influences processing of the nociceptive signal in the dorsal horn, quite likely as early as the first central synapse. Both interoceptive and exteroceptive information can reach the PAG-RVM axis directly and indirectly via higher structures, particularly limbic structures, which have strong reciprocal connections with the PAG.

Christoph Stein, ed., *Opioids in Pain Control: Basic and Clinical Aspects.* Printed in the United States of America.

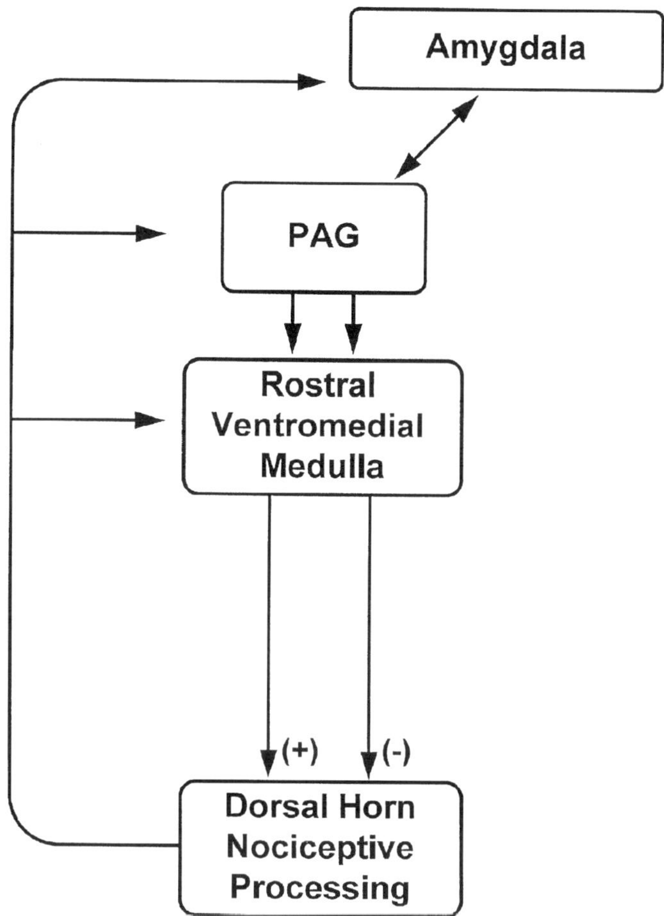

Figure 3.1. Central nociceptive modulatory network with links in the midbrain PAG and RVM. The RVM receives a large input from the PAG and projects to spinal and medullary dorsal horns to modulate processing of nociceptive information. Ascending afferent input can influence activity in this system both directly and indirectly. The PAG-RVM axis receives inputs from spinoreticular and spinomesencephalic systems, and both feedforward and feedback processes can be activated by afferent input. Moreover, processes organized in the limbic forebrain can gain access to nociceptive modulating circuits via projections to the PAG, so that ascending influences converge with inputs from more rostral structures. This system is thus well situated to mediate a complex integration of sensory flow with higher order, particularly limbic, influences.

Activation of Supraspinal Opioid-Sensitive Nociceptive Modulating Network: Basic Principles

There is now overwhelming evidence that the primary mechanism through which opioids act supraspinally to produce antinociception is through activation of brainstem modulatory neurons that exert a net inhibitory effect on spinal nociceptive processing.

Morphine or other μ opioids microinjected within the PAG or RVM suppress nociceptive reflexes organized within the spinal cord (Lewis and Gebhart, 1977; Dickenson, Oliveras, and Besson, 1979; Dickenson, Fardin et al., 1979; Jensen and Yaksh, 1986a, 1986c; Llewelyn et al., 1986; Borszcz, 1995). Similar microinjections can be shown in electrophysiologic experiments to influence the activity of nociceptive dorsal horn neurons (Bennett and Mayer, 1979; Le Bars et al., 1980; Du et al., 1984; Gebhart et al., 1984; Dickenson and Le Bars, 1987; Gebhart and Jones, 1988). In addition, the effects of PAG and RVM opioid microinjections on nociceptive responses are attenuated or blocked by application of monoaminergic antagonists at the level of the spinal cord (Yaksh, 1979; Jensen and Yaksh, 1986b; Aimone et al., 1987; Borszcz et al., 1996). Significantly, the most easily demonstrated effect of direct, nonselective activation of PAG or RVM neurons, using electrical stimulation or microinjection of neuroexcitant agents such as glutamate, is to produce behavioral antinociception and depress activity of nociceptive neurons in the dorsal horn (Mayer and Price, 1976; Zorman et al., 1981; Satoh et al., 1983; Sandkühler and Gebhart, 1984a; Aimone and Gebhart, 1986; Lovick, 1986; Willis, 1988; Jensen and Yaksh, 1989). Conversely, inactivation of the PAG or RVM does not mimic opioid effects in that nociceptive processing is not depressed and may, under some conditions, even be enhanced (Dostrovsky and Deakin, 1977; Yaksh et al., 1977; Proudfit, 1980a, 1980b; Young et al., 1984; Helmstetter and Tershner, 1994). Viewed collectively, these observations indicate that the primary effect of opioids in PAG and RVM is to activate an outflow which exerts a net inhibitory effect on nociceptive processing at the level of the spinal cord.

In addition to recruiting a descending inhibition, opioids acting in PAG and RVM have also been shown to suppress activity in another RVM outflow that likely has a net facilitating effect on spinal nociceptive processing (Fields, 1992; Heinricher et al., 1992, 1994). As will be described, this suppression of nociceptive facilitation parallels, and likely supplements, the better-studied activation discussed above. A third mechanism through which opioids acting in the PAG and RVM are likely to produce analgesia is via controls exerted upon nociceptive processing within the brain itself. Descending controls act only upon the first, spinal, stage of nociceptive processing, whereas ascending mechanisms can alter supraspinally organized responses to noxious stimuli. Although the anatomic and physiologic substrates for such an ascending control mechanism exerted within the brainstem or upon higher structures have not been delineated, behavioral studies indicate that such mechanisms must have some role (Yaksh, 1979; Jensen and Yaksh, 1984; Morgan et al., 1989; Borszcz, 1995; Borszcz et al., 1996).

The Rostral Ventromedial Medulla

As can be seen in Figure 3.1, the descending projections of the opioid-sensitive modulatory system to the dorsal horn originate in the RVM, which is thus the last stage for supraspinal integration of diverse influences related to pain and analgesia. Our understanding of how opioid action within the RVM is translated into a behaviorally measurable analgesia is relatively well advanced. Both μ and δ opioid receptors are found in RVM (Bowker and Dilts, 1988; Mansour et al., 1988, 1994; Delfs et al., 1994). Receptor immunohistochemical studies indicate that μ receptors are localized on RVM neurons, including medullospinal neurons, and that δ receptors are associated with fibers that presumably represent inputs to RVM neurons (Kalyuzhny et al., 1996). Direct local application of the selective μ-receptor agonist DAMGO within the RVM produces behaviorally measurable analgesia, in both awake and lightly anesthetized rats (Dickenson, Fardin et al., 1979; Azami et al., 1982; Fang et al., 1986; Heinricher et al., 1994; Rossi et al., 1994), and μ-receptor mediated effects are apparently paramount in opioid analgesia elicited from this region (Fang et al., 1986). Nevertheless, δ, but not κ, receptors can also support analgesia in RVM (Fang et al., 1986; Jensen and Yaksh, 1986c; Rossi et al., 1994). Recent behavioral studies indicate that the relevant δ receptor is the δ_2, and not the δ_1 (Rossi et al., 1994; Ossipov et al., 1995).

Physiology of RVM: Identification of Facilitating and Inhibiting Outflows

RVM neurons can be divided into three classes in terms of physiology. Together these classes provide a basis for finely tuned modulation of nociception from the RVM (Fields and Heinricher, 1985), and the analgesic actions of opioids within the RVM involve effects on two of these classes, the on-cells and off-cells. On-cells and off-cells were first identified in electrophysiologic studies in lightly anesthetized rats (Fields, Bry et al., 1983). Nociceptive withdrawal reflexes such as the tail-flick reflex, which can be elicited by application of noxious heat to the tail, are preserved in these animals. Off-cells are defined by an abrupt pause in firing that begins just before the tail flick, as well as other nociceptive reflexes (Figure 3.2). On-cells exhibit properties that are in many ways complementary to those of off-cells, and they are characterized by a burst of activity associated with nociceptive reflexes (Figure 3.2). A substantial proportion of cells of each class project to the spinal cord (Vanegas et al., 1984b; Fields et al., 1995).

How do these two cell classes contribute to nociceptive modulation? Given that nonselective activation of RVM neurons is antinociceptive, the characteristic pause of off-cells at the time of nociceptive reflexes suggests that this cell class inhibits nociception under normal conditions. In support of this idea, the tail-flick reflex can be elicited at a lower stimulus temperature at times when off-cells are inactive, either spontaneously or because of a previous noxious stimulus (Heinricher et al., 1989; Ramirez and Vanegas, 1989). More important, blockade of GABA-mediated inhibition within the RVM, by focal infusion of the $GABA_A$ receptor antagonist bicuculline, causes off-cells to become continuously active and produces a profound antinociception (Heinricher and Tortorici, 1994).

In contrast to off-cells, on-cells are likely to have a pronociceptive role. This can be inferred from the fact that these neurons are most active just when the animal is

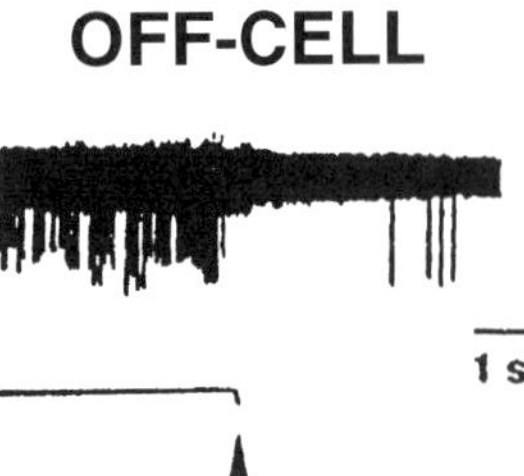

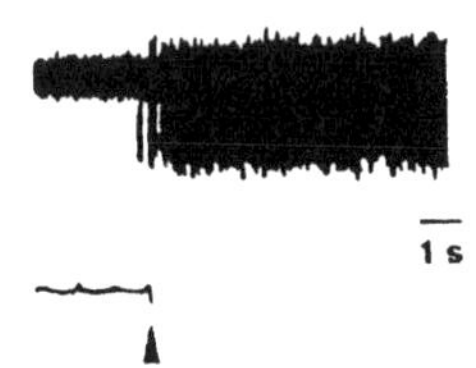

Figure 3.2. On-cells and off-cells. Characteristic tail-flick–related changes in activity of an on-cell and an off-cell. Single 10 s oscilloscope sweeps show cell activity (upper trace) and tail flick (arrowhead in lower trace). Note the abrupt pause (off-cell) and sudden burst (on-cell) associated with the tail flick.

responding to a noxious stimulus – that is, during the tail-flick or other nociceptive reflex. By itself, the reflex-related burst of activity that characterizes these neurons indicates that this cell class must not depress nociceptive processing. Indeed, it suggests that on-cells are more likely to permit, or even facilitate, spinal nociceptive processing.

The idea that the RVM includes a class of neuron that facilitates nociceptive processing may seem inconsistent with evidence presented earlier that nonspecific activation of all RVM neurons gives rise to antinociception. However, disinhibition of off-cells is sufficient to produce analgesia irrespective of whether or not on-cell firing is suppressed (Heinricher and Tortorici, 1994), and it is now clear that the activity of *some* population of RVM neurons does enhance nociceptive processing. Many investigators have noted that at least a small number of spinal neurons are activated by electrical stimulation in the RVM (Fields et al., 1977; Gray and Dostrovsky, 1983; Cervero and Wolstencroft, 1984; Mokha et al., 1985; Light et al., 1986; Tattersall et al., 1986). Using a meticulous microstimulation approach, Zhou and Gebhart (1992) were able to identify sites at which low-stimulation currents produced a descending facilitation of dorsal horn nociceptive neurons. However, as stimulus intensity was increased, inhibition was seen at the same site. A parallel study showed similar descending facilitation of the tail-flick reflex with low-intensity stimulation (Zhuo and Gebhart, 1990). Using c-Fos expression as a marker for dorsal horn activation, Bett and Sandkühler (1995) observed increased expression in superficial dorsal horn following chemical activation of RVM with kainic acid. Finally, hyperalgesia during acute opioid withdrawal is associated with activation of on-cells and is attenuated by inactivation of the RVM (Bederson et al., 1990; Kaplan and Fields, 1991). Taken together, these studies confirm a behaviorally relevant pain-facilitating outflow from the RVM and indicate that the on-cell fills this role.

A third class of RVM neuron, neutral cells, shows no change in activity associated with nociceptive reflexes, and their role, if any, in nociception remains unclear. However, at least some neutral cells have been shown to contain serotonin (Potrebic et al., 1994). Given evidence that spinal serotonin transmission is necessary for opioids acting supraspinally to inhibit spinal nociception (Yaksh, 1979; Besson, 1990; Borszcz et al., 1996), one possibility might be that neutral cell activity enables or "gates" the modulatory actions of on-cell and off-cell firing at the level of the spinal cord.

Opioid Actions within the RVM: Circuit Analysis

The evidence that off-cells exert a net inhibitory effect on nociception whereas on-cells exert a permissive or facilitating effect provides a framework for understanding how opioids act within this region to produce analgesia. When opioid agonists are microinjected within the RVM, off-cells become continuously active, and on-cell firing is suppressed (Heinricher et al., 1994). Because nonselective activation of RVM neurons leads to antinociception whereas inactivation of RVM neurons does not, it can be concluded that the antinociceptive action of opioids within the RVM is best explained as due to activation of off-cells. Suppression of on-cell firing is also likely to contribute, however, reinforcing the effects of off-cell activation.

The opioid inhibition of on-cells is likely direct, since these neurons are also inhibited when morphine is applied to individual on-cells using iontophoretic methods. In contrast, activation of off-cells must be indirect, since off-cells do not respond when morphine is applied by iontophoresis (Heinricher et al., 1992). A circuit that could account for the indirect activation of off-cells by opioids is shown in Figure 3.3. This model is based on the following observations. First, there is strong evidence that the off-cell pause is mediated by GABA (Heinricher et al., 1991), and interfering with GABAergic transmission within the RVM by local application of $GABA_A$ receptor antagonists produces antinociception (Drower and Hammond, 1988; Heinricher and Kaplan, 1991). Moreover, opioids are known to block GABA-mediated inhibitory synaptic potentials in the RVM (Pan et al., 1990). Opioid activation of off-cells would thus be most easily explained as a disinhibition – that is, removing GABA-mediated inhibition (Heinricher and Tortorici, 1994).

The source of the opioid-sensitive GABAergic input to off-cells has not been identified. If inhibitory neurons responsible for the off-cell pause are located within the RVM, they would, by definition, be on-cells in that they would show a burst of activity during the off-cell pause – that is, at the time of the tail flick. Moreover, on-cells are the only RVM neurons known to be directly sensitive to opioids (Heinricher et al., 1992). There is, however, no direct evidence that on-cells are inhibitory interneurons in RVM. A second possibility is that extrinsic GABA-containing termi-

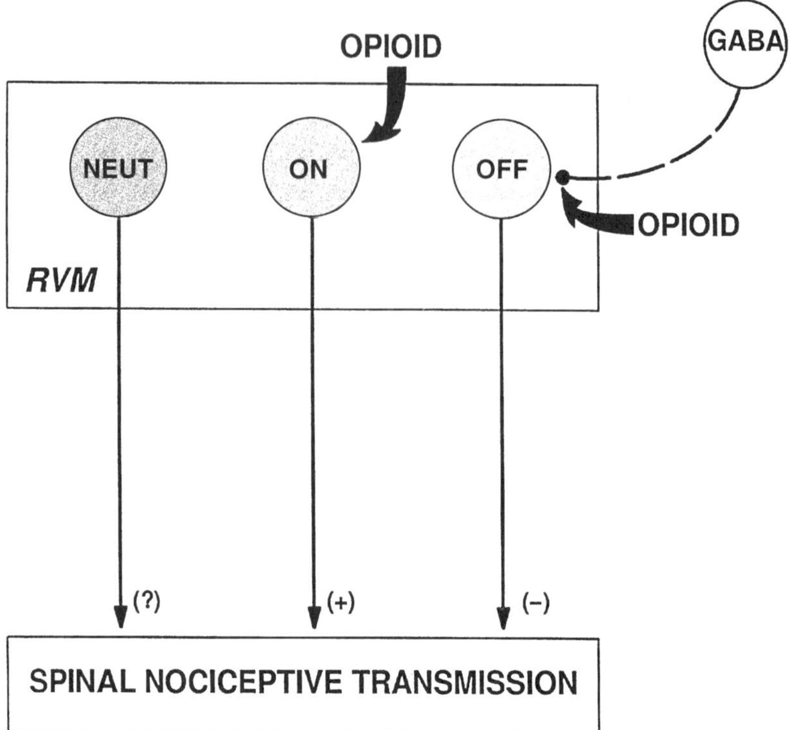

Figure 3.3. Three classes of neurons identified physiologically in RVM have distinct roles in nociceptive modulation. All three project to the dorsal horn. On-cells are likely to exert a net facilitating effect on nociception and are the only RVM neurons directly sensitive to opioids. Some on-cells may serve as inhibitory interneurons, although there is no direct evidence for this. Off-cells, likely to exert a net inhibitory effect on nociception, are activated by opioids. This activation is indirect and is most likely due to presynaptic suppression of GABA-mediated inhibition. Neutral cells are not responsive to opioid analgesics, and their role in nociceptive modulation and relationship to other RVM cell classes is unknown. (Reprinted with permission from Heinricher, M. M., in *Messenger molecules in headache pathogenesis: Monoamines, purines, neuropeptides and nitric oxide* (Frontiers in Headache Research, vol. 7), J. Olesen and P. Tfelt-Hansen, eds. New York: Raven Press, 1997.)

nals synapsing with off-cells are subject to opioid inhibition of transmitter release. If this were the case, opioid actions on the on-cell and off-cell outflows from the RVM would be independent.

When morphine is given systemically, on-cells become silent and off-cells continuously active. Neutral cell firing is unaffected (Fields, Vanegas et al., 1983; Barbaro et al., 1986). Although lesion studies indicate that activity of RVM neurons is not necessary for systemically administered morphine to produce analgesia (Proudfit, 1980a, 1980b), changes in on-cell and off-cell firing likely contribute in some way.

Indeed, if the ability of systemically administered morphine to inhibit on-cell firing is blocked (by local application of the antiopioid peptide cholecystokinin), the antinociceptive effect of the morphine given systemically is also prevented (Heinricher and McGaraughty, 1996). This suggests that on-cell firing interferes with the actions of morphine at the spinal cord or in other brain regions.

The Periaqueductal Gray

Opioid Analgesia from the Periaqueductal Gray

The antinociceptive effects of opioid microinjection into the PAG have been well documented. Administration of opioids into the PAG influences the activity of nociceptive neurons in the dorsal horn (Bennett and Mayer, 1979; Gebhart and Jones, 1988), inhibits nociceptive reflexes (Yaksh et al., 1976; Yaksh, 1979; Depaulis et al., 1987), and suppresses supraspinally organized responses to noxious stimuli (Jensen and Yaksh, 1986a). Although μ, δ, and κ opioid binding sites are found within the PAG (Mansour et al., 1987, 1988, 1994), the antinociceptive effects of opioids acting within the PAG appear to be mediated, as in the RVM, primarily by μ receptors, with an additional contribution of δ_2 receptors (Jensen and Yaksh, 1986c; Smith et al., 1988; Fang et al., 1989; Rossi et al., 1994; Ossipov et al., 1995). Direct administration of κ receptor ligands within the PAG does not produce a behaviorally measurable analgesia (Smith et al., 1988; Fang et al., 1989; Rossi et al., 1994), and the role of these receptors is as yet unknown. The endogenous ligands for μ opioid receptors in the PAG are presumed to be derived from intrinsic enkephalinergic interneurons (Khachaturian et al., 1983; Gioia and Bianchi, 1995) and from a β-endorphin–containing projection arising from the arcuate nucleus (Finley et al., 1981; Sim and Joseph, 1991; Bach and Yaksh, 1995). (It should be noted that β-endorphin has additional pain-modulating actions in PAG mediated via a non-μ receptor [Monroe et al., 1996].)

Neural Circuitry Underlying Opioid Action within the PAG

The neural mechanisms through which opioids in the PAG produce antinociception have not been described in the same detail as in the RVM. Nonetheless, existing evidence suggests a similar disinhibitory mechanism. As with the RVM, direct activation of PAG neurons produces antinociception, whereas lesions do not, indicating that opioids must activate an antinociceptive output from this region (Deakin and Dostrovsky, 1978; Yaksh and Rudy, 1978; Willis, 1988). Opioids hyperpolarize a subset of PAG neurons via a postsynaptic action, but do activate other PAG neurons, albeit indirectly (Behbehani, Jiang, and Chandler, 1990; Chieng and Christie, 1994a). This indirect activation is likely due to a removal of GABAergic inhibition, since opioids are known to block stimulus-evoked GABA-mediated inhibitory potentials in the PAG slice preparation (Chieng and Christie, 1994b). The widespread activation of PAG neurons following local administration of the $GABA_A$ receptor antagonist bicuculline is consistent with this idea of a tonic GABAergic inhibitory control (Behbehani, Jiang et al., 1990; Sandkuhler and Herdegen, 1995). Although the neurons activated by opioids were not functionally identified, the observations that blocking GABAergic transmission in the PAG inhibits the activity of nociceptive neurons in the dorsal horn (Sandkühler et al., 1989) as well as nociceptive reflexes (Moreau and Fields, 1986; Depaulis et al., 1987) demonstrate that this disinhibitory process is relevant to pain modulation. These data, along with anatomic studies indicating that GABAergic interneurons exist in the PAG (Reichling et al., 1988; Reichling and Basbaum, 1990), support a model in which opioids disinhibit PAG output neurons involved in modulating nociception by inhibiting the activity of GABAergic interneurons (see description of RVM circuitry given earlier in this chapter).

Although opioid administration into any region of the PAG produces antinociception, two distinct systems that include a pain-modulating function seem to reside within the PAG. These two systems are organized anatomically as two rostrocaudally oriented columns, one located in the dorsolateral PAG and the other in the ventrolateral PAG. These systems can be distinguished by differences in cytoarchitecture (Beitz, 1985; Beitz and Shepard, 1985; Conti et al., 1988) and connectivity (Rizvi et al., 1991, 1992; Cameron, Khan, Westlund, Cliffer, and Willis, 1995; Cameron, Khan, Westlund, and Willis, 1995) as well as function (Bandler and DePaulis, 1991). Antinociception produced by electrical stimulation in the ventrolateral PAG is attenuated by the opioid antagonist naloxone (Cannon et al., 1982; Thorn et al., 1989), is sensitive to an acute form of tolerance (Morgan and Liebeskind, 1987), and modulates nociception at both spinal and supraspinal sites (Morgan et al., 1989). In contrast, antinociception triggered by stimulating the dorsolateral PAG is relatively insensitive to opioid antagonists, does not show tolerance with continuous stimulation, and modulates nociception only via descending pathways. In addition, cardiovascular and locomotor consequences of ventrolateral and dorsolateral stimulation are distinct. Stimulation of the dorsolateral PAG produces running and jumping, along with an increase in blood pressure, whereas ventrolateral stimulation produces immobility and hypotension (Fardin et al., 1984a, 1984b; Morgan et al., 1987; Carrive, 1991; Depaulis et al., 1994; Davis et al., 1996). These effects are similar to defensive reactions produced by exposure to different threatening situations (Fanselow, 1991). Taken together with the fact that lesions of the PAG attenuate or block some forms of environmentally induced antinociception (Fanselow, 1991; Helmstetter and Tershner, 1994; Bellgowan and Helmstetter, 1996), the co-activation of distinct behavioral reactions in concert with cardiovascular changes and antinociception suggests that a primary function of the PAG is the integration of defensive reactions appropriate to the situation.

Relay of Descending Actions of PAG within the RVM

Descending inhibition of spinal nociceptive processing produced by opioid action within the PAG appears to be mediated in large part through relays in the RVM (Fig. 3.1). Anatomic studies demonstrate that the PAG sends only a sparse projection to the spinal cord, but a large projection to the RVM (Gallager and Pert, 1978; Abols and Basbaum, 1981; Beitz, 1982a, 1982b; Holstege, 1991; Van Bockstaele et al., 1991; Cameron, Khan, Westlund, and Willis, 1995). Among the neurotransmitters that have been identified in PAG-RVM projection neurons are excitatory amino acids, neurotensin, serotonin, and somatostatin (Beitz, 1982b; Beitz et al., 1983; Clements et al., 1987; Wiklund et al., 1988). Electrical stimulation in the PAG excites the great majority of RVM neurons, including identified on-cells and off-cells (Pomeroy and Behbehani, 1979; Vanegas et al., 1984a; Willis et al., 1984; Lovick, 1992), and the threshold current for activating RVM neurons with PAG stimulation was shown to be indistinguishable from that required to produce behaviorally measurable antinociception (Vanegas et al., 1984a). An important role for the RVM in mediating antinociception from the PAG is further supported by lesion studies. Inactivation of the RVM, using either electrolytic lesions or a local anesthetic infusion, attenuates descending inhibition from the PAG (Behbehani and Fields, 1979; Gebhart et al., 1983; Prieto et al., 1983; Sandkühler and Gebhart, 1984b; Young et al., 1984; Lovick, 1985; Aimone and Gebhart, 1986). The entire RVM must apparently be inactivated (Gebhart et al., 1983; Sandkühler and Gebhart, 1984b; Aimone and Gebhart, 1986), a finding consistent with anatomic studies demonstrating an overlapping projection from both dorsal and lateral/ventrolateral PAG across the entire medio-lateral extent of the RVM (Van Bockstaele et al., 1991).

When opioids are applied by microinjection within the PAG, off-cells become continuously active and on-cells silent (Cheng et al., 1986; Morgan et al., 1992). Thus, opioids acting in the PAG give rise to a behaviorally measurable analgesia by inducing changes in RVM cell activity that are indistinguishable from those seen following either RVM or systemic opioid administration.

As already mentioned, the neural basis for opioid action within the PAG is not well understood. However, electrical stimulation in the PAG gives rise to a short-latency excitation of both on-cells and off-cells in the RVM, suggesting that both cell classes receive an excitatory input from the PAG (Vanegas et al., 1984a). In contrast, opioid microinjection activates off-cells, but inhibits on-cells (Morgan et al., 1992). This disparity between the effects of electrical and opioid actions within the PAG indicates that the population of PAG neurons projecting to the RVM is not homogeneous, a conclusion consistent with the fact that only a subset of PAG-RVM projection neurons are subject to direct opioid influence (Osborne et al., 1990; Williams and Beitz, 1990). One possibility is that the population of PAG-RVM projection neurons receiving opioid input have an excitatory influence on on-cell firing in RVM.

This cell population would thus be activated by PAG electrical stimulation, but inhibited by local opioid administration. Presumably, PAG output neurons projecting to off-cells are also activated by electrical stimulation and disinhibited by opioid administration. In both cases the net effect is activation of off-cells and, consequently, measurable antinociception.

Relationships among Opioid-Sensitive Sites: Synergy

The evidence from focal application experiments reviewed earlier demonstrates that the PAG and RVM each contains all of the neuronal machinery required to produce a behaviorally measurable opioid antinociception. However, when given systemically, morphine has parallel actions at more than one site within the brain, as well as at the spinal cord and in the periphery. The relative contributions of these different sites, especially the relative roles of supraspinal and spinal actions, has been the subject of some debate. In early experiments, Tsou (1963) and later Yeung and Rudy (1980b) showed that supraspinal administration of an opiate antagonist could attenuate systemic morphine analgesia. Azami et al. (1982) reported that application of naloxone within the RVM reversed the analgesic effect of systemically administered morphine. These observations seemingly led to the conclusion that a supraspinal site of action is primary in the analgesic effects of systemically administered morphine. This notion was further supported by reports that the analgesic actions of systemically administered morphine on spinal reflexes were attenuated by spinalization or by cutting the dorsolateral funiculus, which includes the descending projection from the RVM to the spinal cord (Basbaum et al., 1977; Barton et al., 1980; Advokat and Burton, 1987; Herrero and Headley, 1991).

Controversy arose when it became clear that blocking opioid actions at the level of the spinal cord, using intrathecal administration of naloxone, also completely antagonized the effects of systemically administered morphine (Yaksh and Rudy, 1977). This observation seemed to indicate that the primary site of opiate action was in fact not supraspinal but spinal. This apparent disparity was resolved by subsequent demonstrations that spinal and supraspinal sites interact in a supra-additive fashion, so that removal of either the spinal or the supraspinal component produced a substantial attenuation of the opiate effect (Yeung and Rudy, 1980a; Roerig and Fujimoto, 1989; Roerig et al., 1991). This spinal/supraspinal synergy was subsequently shown to be mediated by the μ_2 opioid receptor (Pick et al., 1992). Further study demonstrated similar synergy among brainstem opioid-sensitive sites, with supra-additive effects of co-administration of morphine within the PAG and RVM (Rossi et al., 1993, 1994).

Thus, when given systemically, morphine induces mutually reinforcing effects at multiple central nervous system sites in parallel. The question of the relative contribution of different opioid-sensitive central sites to the analgesia produced by systemically administered morphine seems therefore to have little meaning. Analysis of the relationships among the various opioid-sensitive sites may prove more useful. In behavioral studies, the effects of supraspinal agonist administration are attenuated by opiate antagonists given intrathecally (Levine et al., 1982). Conversely, the analgesic effect of intrathecal morphine are attenuated by ICV administration of an opiate antagonist (Miaskowski and Levine, 1992). These behavioral studies are consistent with a single-cell recording study in which it was shown that morphine administration either intrathecally or within the PAG activated off-cells and depressed activity of on-cells in RVM (Cheng et al., 1986; Drasner and Fields, 1988), suggesting that opioid administration at one site recruits other opioid-sensitive sites. Significantly, the depressive effects produced by intrathecal and PAG morphine involve different mechanisms (Morgan et al., 1992), and PAG, but not spinal, morphine appears to involve release of an endogenous opioid within the RVM (Gear and Levine, 1995; Pan and Fields, 1996; Roychowdhury and Fields, 1996).

Ascending Modulation

To this point, our analysis of the means through which the PAG-RVM axis modulates nociception has emphasized descending control mechanisms. However, behavioral studies provide some indication that, in addition to its well-studied effects at spinal levels, this system can modulate subsequent, supraspinal, stages of nociceptive processing. In these studies, investigators have generally compared the effects of PAG or RVM manipulations on spinally and supraspinally organized responses to noxious stimulation. The ability of supraspinal opioids to suppress supraspinally organized responses was, at least in some experiments, spared when descending influences were removed. For example, in early studies, intrathecal administration of monoamine antagonists attenuated the ability of morphine or PAG or RVM stimulation to inhibit spinally organized withdrawal reflexes, but did not block inhibition of supraspinally organized responses (Yaksh, 1979; Jensen and Yaksh, 1984). Unfortunately, different noxious stimuli and stimulation sites were used to elicit the spinal and supraspinal responses in those studies, a factor that confounds interpretation of the results (Borszcz, 1995; Fang and Proudfit, 1996). However, in a more recent study using electric tail shock to evoke distinct responses organized at spinal cord, brainstem, and forebrain levels, Borszcz et al. (1996) showed that intrathecal administration of monoamine antagonists had differential effects on the ability of supraspinal morphine to inhibit responses organized within the cord or supraspinally. Moreover, Morgan et al. (1989) demonstrated that a lesion which transected the descending outflow from the PAG did not block stimulation-produced inhibition of the hot-plate response, a supraspinally organized response, whereas antinociceptive effects on the tail-flick response (a spinal reflex) were abolished.

Behavioral studies thus point to a significant contribution of ascending, as well as descending, modulation in supraspinal opioid effects. The neural circuits mediating ascending modulation have not been determined, however. The PAG in particular has extensive ascending projections, with targets in both diencephalic and telencephalic regions known to be involved in nociceptive processing (Mantyh, 1983; Eberhart et al., 1985; Carstens et al., 1990; Rizvi et al., 1991; Coffield et al., 1992; Cameron, Khan, Westlund, Cliffer, and Willis, 1995). The specific role of any of these connections in ascending modulation is as yet unknown.

Other Supraspinal Sites Supporting Opioid Analgesia

In addition to the PAG and RVM, a number of other supraspinal sites support opioid analgesia, among them the ventral tegmental area, globus pallidus, hypothalamus, and a circumscribed region within insular cortex (Anagnostakis et al., 1992; Manning et al., 1994; Fuchs and Melzack, 1995; Burkey et al., 1996). However, the physiology of opioid-sensitive neurons and whether opioids produce their effects in these regions via activation of the PAG-RVM axis or through independent pathways have not yet been investigated.

The amygdala is one forebrain region in which an analgesic action of opioids has received significant attention. The amygdala has reciprocal connections with the PAG, and some nuclei display very high levels of μ, δ, and κ binding. The greatest density of μ binding is in lateral, basolateral, medial, and cortical nuclei, and these same nuclei display moderate to dense δ and κ binding. The central nucleus shows little or no μ or δ binding, but moderate κ binding (Mansour et al., 1987). Direct local administration of morphine or opioid peptides into some nuclei impairs measures of conditioned fear and produces measurable antinociception in both awake and lightly anesthetized animals (Rodgers, 1978; Yaksh et al., 1988; Helmstetter et al., 1993; Good and Westbrook, 1995; Helmstetter et al., 1995; Pavlovic et al., 1995). As might be predicted from the binding studies, this effect is most robust in the basolateral nucleus, although cortical and/or medial nuclei have also been reported to support opioid hypoalgesia (Rodgers, 1978; Helmstetter et al., 1993). In the basolateral nucleus, the analgesic effect is mediated by an action at the μ receptor and not the δ or κ receptors (Helmstetter et al., 1995). In vitro, opioids hyperpolarize a substantial proportion of neurons in the lateral amygdala and attenuate GABA-mediated synaptic potentials (Sugita and North, 1993; Sugita et al., 1993), suggesting that, as in the RVM (Pan et al., 1990; Heinricher et al., 1992, 1994), increased activity exhibited by some amygdala neurons following systemic morphine administration (Chou and Wang, 1977) is indirect.

In addition to any effects of opioids within the amygdala itself, the amygdala may be important in the analgesia produced by systemically administered morphine. Thus, lesions or inactivation of the central nucleus, but not basolateral or medial nuclei, were recently reported to attenuate the analgesic effects of systemically administered morphine on both tail-flick and formalin tests (Manning and Mayer, 1995a, 1995b), although in previous work such lesions had no effect on systemic morphine analgesia (Calvino et al., 1982). Nevertheless, it is possible that the integrity of the central nucleus is important for full expression of systemic morphine analgesia. Finally, the amygdala is implicated in the aversive motivational state associated with opiate withdrawal (Stinus et al., 1990; Koob et al., 1992).

Summary

When given systemically, opioid analgesics act at multiple sites in the brain as well as in the spinal cord. In the spinal cord, although the receptor may be located on primary afferent terminals or on interneurons or spinofugal projection neurons, the net effect is to decrease the ascending traffic. In the brain, the situation is more complex, but the primary supraspinal mechanism underlying opioid analgesia is to activate a nociceptive modulatory network with links in the PAG and RVM and a descending projection to the spinal cord. This network is also likely to influence nociceptive processing at supraspinal levels. Although physiologic mechanisms linking opioid-sensitive sites are as yet poorly understood, behavioral studies indicate that synergistic interactions among supraspinal and spinal opioid-sensitive sites are likely to be crucial in the analgesic effects of systemically administered opioids.

REFERENCES

Abols, I.A., and Basbaum, A.I. (1981). Afferent connections of the rostral medulla of the cat: A neural substrate for midbrain-medullary interactions in the modulation of pain. *J. Comp. Neurol.* **201,** 285–297.

Advokat, C., and Burton, P. (1987). Antinociceptive effect of systemic and intrathecal morphine in spinally transected rats. *Eur. J. Pharmacol.* **139,** 335–343.

Aimone, L.D., and Gebhart, G.F. (1986). Stimulation-produced spinal inhibition from the midbrain in the rat is mediated by an excitatory amino acid neurotransmitter in the medial medulla. *J. Neurosci.* **6,** 1803–1813.

Aimone, L.D., Jones, S.L., and Gebhart, G.F. (1987). Stimulation-produced descending inhibition from the periaqueductal gray and nucleus raphe magnus in the rat: Mediation by spinal monoamines but not opioids. *Pain.* **31,** 123–136.

Anagnostakis, Y., Zis, V., and Spyraki, C. (1992). Analgesia induced by morphine injected into the pallidum. *Behav. Brain Res.* **48,** 135–143.

Azami, J., Llewelyn, M.B., and Roberts, M.H. (1982). The contribution of nucleus reticularis paragigantocellularis and nucleus raphe magnus to the analgesia produced by systemically administered morphine, investigated with the microinjection technique. *Pain.* **12,** 229–246.

Bach, F.W., and Yaksh, T.L. (1995). Release into ventriculo-cisternal perfusate of beta-endorphin- and Met-enkephalin-immunoreactivity: Effects of electrical stimulation in the arcuate nucleus and periaqueductal gray of the rat. *Brain Res.* **690,** 167–176.

Bandler, R., and DePaulis, A. (1991). Midbrain periaqueductal gray control of defensive behavior in cat and rat. In DePaulis, A., and Bandler, R. (eds.), *The midbrain periaqueductal gray matter.* New York: Plenum, pp. 175–198.

Barbaro, N.M., Heinricher, M.M., and Fields, H.L. (1986). Putative pain modulating neurons in the rostral ventral medulla: Reflex-related activity predicts effects of morphine. *Brain Res.* **366,** 203–210.

Barton, C., Basbaum, A.I., and Fields, H.L. (1980). Dissociation of supraspinal and spinal actions of morphine: A quantitative evaluation. *Brain Res.* **188,** 487–498.

Basbaum, A.I., Marley, N.J., O'Keefe, J., and Clanton, C.H. (1977). Reversal of morphine and stimulus-produced analgesia by subtotal spinal cord lesions. *Pain.* **3,** 43–56.

Bederson, J.B., Fields, H.L., and Barbaro, N.M. (1990). Hyperalgesia during naloxone-precipitated withdrawal from morphine is associated with increased on-cell activity in the rostral ventromedial medulla. *Somatosen. Mot. Res.* **7,** 185–203.

Behbehani, M.M., and Fields, H.L. (1979). Evidence that an excitatory connection between the periaqueductal gray and nucleus raphe magnus mediates stimulation produced analgesia. *Brain Res.* **170,** 85–93.

Behbehani, M.M., Jiang, M., and Chandler, S.D. (1990). The effect of [Met]enkephalin on the periaqueductal gray neurons of the rat: An in vitro study. *Neuroscience.* **38,** 373–380.

Behbehani, M.M., Jiang, M.R., Chandler, S.D., and Ennis, M. (1990). The effect of GABA and its antagonists on midbrain periaqueductal gray neurons in the rat. *Pain.* **40,** 195–204.

Beitz, A.J. (1982a). The nuclei of origin of brain stem enkephalin and substance P projections to the rodent nucleus raphe magnus. *Neuroscience.* **7,** 2753–2768.

Beitz, A.J. (1982b). The sites of origin of brain stem neurotensin and serotonin projections to the rodent nucleus raphe magnus. *J. Neurosci.* **2,** 829–842.

Beitz, A.J. (1985). The midbrain periaqueductal gray in the rat. I. Nuclear volume, cell number, density, orientation, and regional subdivisions. *J. Comp. Neurol.* **237,** 445–459.

Beitz, A.J., and Shepard, R.D. (1985). The midbrain periaqueductal gray in the rat. II. A Golgi analysis. *J. Comp. Neurol.* **237,** 460–475.

Beitz, A.J., Shepard, R.D., and Wells, W.E. (1983). The periaqueductal gray-raphe magnus projection contains somatostatin, neurotensin and serotonin but not cholecystokinin. *Brain Res.* **261,** 132–137.

Bellgowan, P.S., and Helmstetter, F.J. (1996). Neural systems for the expression of hypoalgesia during nonassociative fear. *Behav. Neurosci.* **110,** 727–736.

Bennett, G.J., and Mayer, D.J. (1979). Inhibition of spinal cord interneurons by narcotic microinjection and focal electrical stimulation in the periaqueductal central gray matter. *Brain Res.* **172,** 243–257.

Besson, J.M. (1990). *Serotonin and pain.* New York: Excerpta Medica.

Bett, K., and Sandkühler, J. (1995). Map of spinal neurons activated by chemical stimulation in the nucleus raphe magnus of the unanesthetized rat. *Neuroscience.* **67,** 497–504.

Borszcz, G.S. (1995). Increases in vocalization and motor reflex thresholds are influenced by the site of morphine microinjection: Comparisons following administration into the periaqueductal gray, ventral medulla, and spinal subarachnoid space. *Behav. Neurosci.* **109,** 502–522.

Borszcz, G.S., Johnson, C.P., and Thorp, M.V. (1996). The differential contribution of spinopetal projections to increases in vocalization and motor reflex thresholds generated by the microinjection of morphine into the periaqueductal gray. *Behav. Neurosci.* **110,** 368–388.

Bowker, R.M., and Dilts, R.P. (1988). Distribution of μ-opioid receptors in the nucleus raphe magnus and nucleus gigantocellularis: A quantitative autoradiographic study. *Neurosci. Lett.* **88,** 247–252.

Burkey, A.R., Carstens, E., Wenniger, J.J., Tang, J., and Jasmin, L. (1996). An opioidergic cortical antinociception triggering site in the agranular insular cortex of the rat that contributes to morphine antinociception. *J. Neurosci.* **16,** 6612–6623.

Calvino, B., Levesque, G., and Besson, J.M. (1982). Possible involvement of the amygdaloid complex in morphine analgesia as studied by electrolytic lesions in rats. *Brain Res.* **233,** 221–226.

Cameron, A.A., Khan, I.A., Westlund, K.N., Cliffer, K.D., and Willis, W.D. (1995). The efferent projections of the periaqueductal gray in the rat: A Phaseolus vulgaris-leucoagglutinin study. I. Ascending projections. *J. Comp. Neurol.* **351,** 568–584.

Cameron, A.A., Khan, I.A., Westlund, K.N., and Willis, W.D. (1995). The efferent projections of the periaqueductal gray in the rat: A Phaseolus vulgaris-leucoagglutinin study. II. Descending projections. *J. Comp. Neurol.* **351,** 585–601.

Cannon, J.T., Prieto, G.J., Lee, A., and Liebeskind, J.C. (1982). Evidence for opioid and non-opioid forms of stimulation-produced analgesia in the rat. *Brain Res.* **243,** 315–321.

Carrive, P. (1991). Functional organization of PAG neurons controlling regional vascular beds. In DePaulis, A., and Bandler, R. (eds.), *The midbrain periaqueductal gray matter.* New York: Plenum Press, pp. 67–100.

Carstens, E., Leah, J., Lechner, J., and Zimmermann, M. (1990). Demonstration of extensive brainstem projections to medial and lateral thalamus and hypothalamus in the rat. *Neuroscience.* **35,** 609–626.

Cervero, F., and Wolstencroft, J.H. (1984). A positive feedback loop between spinal cord nociceptive pathways and antinociceptive areas of the cat's brain stem. *Pain.* **20,** 125–138.

Cheng, Z.F., Fields, H.L., and Heinricher, M.M. (1986). Morphine microinjected into the periaqueductal gray has differential effects on 3 classes of medullary neurons. *Brain Res.* **375,** 57–65.

Chieng, B., and Christie, M.J. (1994a). Hyperpolarization by opioids acting on mu-receptors of a sub-population of rat periaqueductal gray neurones in vitro. *Br. J. Pharmacol.* **113,** 121–128.

Chieng, B., and Christie, M.J. (1994b). Inhibition by opioids acting on mu-receptors of GABAergic and glutamatergic postsynaptic potentials in single rat periaqueductal gray neurones in vitro. *Br. J. Pharmacol.* **113,** 303–309.

Chou, D.T., and Wang, S.C. (1977). Unit activity of amygdala and hippocampal neurons: Effects of morphine and benzodiazepines. *Brain Res.* **126,** 427–440.

Clements, J.R., Madl, J.E., Johnson, R.L., Larson, A.A., and Beitz, A.J. (1987). Localization of glutamate, glutaminase, aspartate and aspartate aminotransferase in the rat midbrain periaqueductal gray. *Exp. Brain Res.* **67,** 594–602.

Coffield, J.A., Bowen, K.K., and Miletic, V. (1992). Retrograde tracing of projections between the nucleus submedius, the ventrolateral orbital cortex, and the midbrain in the rat. *J. Comp. Neurol.* **321,** 488–499.

Conti, F., Barbaresi, P., and Fabri, M. (1988). Cytochrome oxidase histochemistry reveals regional subdivisions in the rat periaqueductal gray matter. *Neuroscience.* **24,** 629–633.

Davis, P.J., Zhang, S.P., and Bandler, R. (1996). Midbrain and medullary regulation of respiration and vocalization. *Prog. Brain Res.* **107,** 315–325.

Deakin, J.F., and Dostrovsky, J.O. (1978). Involvement of the periaqueductal grey matter and spinal 5-hydroxytryptaminergic pathways in morphine analgesia: Effects of lesions and 5-hydroxytryptamine depletion. *Br. J. Pharmacol.* **63,** 159–165.

Delfs, J.M., Kong, H., Mestek, A., Chen, Y., Yu, L., Reisine, T., and Chesselet, M.F. (1994). Expression of mu opioid receptor mRNA in rat brain: An in situ hybridization study at the single cell level. *J. Comp. Neurol.* **345,** 46–68.

Depaulis, A., Keay, K.A., and Bandler, R. (1994). Quiescence and hyporeactivity evoked by activation of cell bodies in the ventrolateral midbrain periaqueductal gray of the rat. *Exp. Brain Res.* **99,** 75–83.

Depaulis, A., Morgan, M.M., and Liebeskind, J.C. (1987). GABAergic modulation of the analgesic effects of morphine microinjected in the ventral periaqueductal gray matter of the rat. *Brain Res.* **436,** 223–228.

Dickenson, A.H., Fardin, V., Le Bars, D., and Besson, J.M. (1979). Antinociceptive action following microinjection of methionine-enkephalin in the nucleus raphe magnus of the rat. *Neurosci. Lett.* **15,** 265–270.

Dickenson, A.H., and Le Bars, D. (1987). Supraspinal morphine and descending inhibitions acting on the dorsal horn of the rat. *J. Physiol.* **384,** 81–107.

Dickenson, A.H., Oliveras, J.L., and Besson, J.M. (1979). Role of the nucleus raphe magnus in opiate analgesia as studied by the microinjection technique in the rat. *Brain Res.* **170,** 95–111.

Dostrovsky, J.O., and Deakin, J.F.W. (1977). Periaqueductal gray lesions reduce morphine analgesia in the rat. *Neurosci. Lett.* **4,** 99–103.

Drasner, K., and Fields, H.L. (1988). Synergy between the antinociceptive effects of intrathecal clonidine and systemic morphine in the rat. *Pain.* **32,** 309–312.

Drower, E.J., and Hammond, D.L. (1988). GABAergic modulation of nociceptive threshold: Effects of THIP and bicuculline microinjected in the ventral medulla of the rat. *Brain Res.* **450,** 316–324.

Du, H.J., Kitahata, L.M., Thalhammer, J.G., and Zimmermann, M. (1984). Inhibition of nociceptive neuronal responses in the cat's spinal dorsal horn by electrical stimulation and morphine microinjection in nucleus raphe magnus. *Pain.* **19,** 249–257.

Eberhart, J.A., Morrell, J.I., Krieger, M.S., and Pfaff, D.W. (1985). An autoradiographic study of projections ascending from the midbrain central gray, and from the region lateral to it, in the rat. *J. Comp. Neurol.* **241,** 285–310.

Fang, F.G., Fields, H.L., and Lee, N.M. (1986). Action at the *mu* receptor is sufficient to explain the supraspinal analgesic effect of opiates. *J. Pharmacol. Exp. Ther.* **238,** 1039–1044.

Fang, F.G., Haws, C.M., Drasner, K., Williamson, A., and Fields, H.L. (1989). Opioid peptides (DAGO-enkephalin, dynorphin A(1–13), BAM 22P) microinjected into the rat brainstem: Comparison of their antinociceptive effect and their effect on neuronal firing in the rostral ventromedial medulla. *Brain Res.* **501,** 116–128.

Fang, F., and Proudfit, H.K. (1996). Spinal cholinergic and monoamine receptors mediate the antinociceptive effect of morphine microinjected in the periaqueductal gray on the rat tail, but not the feet. *Brain Res.* **722,** 95–108.

Fanselow, M.S. (1991). The midbrain periaqueductal gray as a coordinator of action in response to fear and anxiety. In DePaulis, A., and Bandler, R. (eds.), *The midbrain periaqueductal gray matter.* New York: Plenum, pp. 151–173.

Fardin, V., Oliveras, J.L., and Besson, J.M. (1984a). A reinvestigation of the analgesic effects induced by stimulation of the periaqueductal gray matter in the rat. I. The production of behavioral side effects together with analgesia. *Brain Res.* **306,** 105–123.

Fardin, V., Oliveras, J.L., and Besson, J.M. (1984b). A reinvestigation of the analgesic effects induced by stimulation of the periaqueductal gray matter in the rat. II. Differential characteristics of the analgesia induced by ventral and dorsal PAG stimulation. *Brain Res.* **306,** 125–139.

Fields, H.L. (1992). Is there a facilitating component to central pain modulation? *APS Journal.* **1,** 71–78.

Fields, H.L., Basbaum, A.I., Clanton, C.H., and Anderson, S.D. (1977). Nucleus raphe magnus inhibition of spinal cord dorsal horn neurons. *Brain Res.* **126,** 441–453.

Fields, H.L., Bry, J., Hentall, I., and Zorman, G. (1983a). The activity of neurons in the rostral medulla of the rat during withdrawal from noxious heat. *J. Neurosci.* **3,** 2545–2552.

Fields, H.L., and Heinricher, M.M. (1985). Anatomy and physiology of a nociceptive modulatory system. *Philos. Trans. Roy. Soc. Lond. B.* **308,** 361–374.

Fields, H.L., Malick, A., and Burstein, R. (1995). Dorsal horn projection targets of on and off cells in the rostral ventromedial medulla. *J. Neurophysiol.* **74,** 1742–1759.

Fields, H.L., Vanegas, H., Hentall, I.D., and Zorman, G. (1983b). Evidence that disinhibition of brain stem neurones contributes to morphine analgesia. *Nature.* **306,** 684–686.

Finley, J.C., Maderdrut, J.L., and Petrusz, P. (1981). The immunocytochemical localization of enkephalin in the central nervous system of the rat. *J. Comp. Neurol.* **198,** 541–565.

Fuchs, P.N., and Melzack, R. (1995). Analgesia induced by morphine microinjection into the lateral hypothalamus of the rat. *Exp. Neurol.* **134,** 277–280.

Gallager, D.W., and Pert, A. (1978). Afferents to brain stem nuclei (brain stem raphe, nucleus reticularis, pontis caudalis and nucleus gigantocellularis) in the rat as demonstrated by microiontophoretically applied horseradish peroxidase. *Brain Res.* **144,** 257–275.

Gear, R.W., and Levine, J.D. (1995). Antinociception produced by an ascending spino-supraspinal pathway. *J. Neurosci.* **15,** 3154–3161.

Gebhart, G.F., and Jones, S.L. (1988). Effects of morphine given in the brain stem on the activity of dorsal horn nociceptive neurons. *Prog. Brain Res.* **77,** 229–243.

Gebhart, G.F., Sandkühler, J., Thalhammer, J.G., and Zimmermann, M. (1983). Inhibition of spinal nociceptive information by stimulation in midbrain of the cat is blocked by lidocaine microinjected in nucleus raphe magnus and medullary reticular formation. *J. Neurophysiol.* **50,** 1446–1459.

Gebhart, G.F., Sandkühler, J., Thalhammer, J.G., and Zimmermann, M. (1984). Inhibition in spinal cord of nociceptive information by electrical stimulation and morphine microinjection at identical sites in midbrain of the cat. *J. Neurophysiol.* **51,** 75–89.

Gioia, M., and Bianchi, R. (1995). Enkephalin in thc caudal PAG of rat: An immunocytochemical electron microscopic study. *J. Hirnforsch.* **36,** 421–431.

Good, A.J., and Westbrook, R.F. (1995). Effects of a microinjection of morphine into the amygdala on the acquisition and expression of conditioned fear and hypoalgesia in rats. *Behav. Neurosci.* **109,** 631–641.

Gray, B.G., and Dostrovsky, J.O. (1983). Descending inhibitory influences from periaqueductal gray, nucleus raphe magnus, and adjacent reticular formation. I. Effects on lumbar spinal cord nociceptive and nonnociceptive neurons. *J. Neurophysiol.* **49,** 932–947.

Heinricher, M.M., Barbaro, N.M., and Fields, H.L. (1989). Putative nociceptive modulating neurons in the rostral ventromedial medulla of the rat: Firing of on- and off-cells is related to nociceptive responsiveness. *Somatosen. Mot. Res.* **6,** 427–439.

Heinricher, M.M., Haws, C.M., and Fields, H.L. (1991). Evidence for GABA-mediated control of putative nociceptive modulating neurons in the rostral ventromedial medulla: Iontophoresis of bicuculline eliminates the off-cell pause. *Somatosen. Mot. Res.* **8,** 215–225.

Heinricher, M.M., and Kaplan, H.J. (1991). GABA-mediated inhibition in rostral ventromedial medulla: Role in nociceptive modulation in the lightly anesthetized rat. *Pain.* **47,** 105–113.

Heinricher, M.M., and McGaraughty, S. (1996). CCK modulates the antinociceptive actions of opioids by an action within the rostral ventromedial medulla: A combined electrophysiological and behavioral study. International Association for the Study of Pain, 8th World Congress, Vancouver, B.C., Canada.

Heinricher, M.M., Morgan, M.M., and Fields, H.L. (1992). Direct and indirect actions of morphine on medullary neurons that modulate nociception. *Neuroscience.* **48,** 533–543.

Heinricher, M.M., Morgan, M.M., Tortorici, V., and Fields, H.L. (1994). Disinhibition of off-cells and antinociception produced by an opioid action within the rostral ventromedial medulla. *Neuroscience.* **63,** 279–288.

Heinricher, M.M., and Tortorici, V. (1994). Interference with GABA transmission in the rostral ventromedial medulla: Disinhibition of off-cells as a central mechanism in nociceptive modulation. *Neuroscience.* **63,** 533–546.

Helmstetter, F.J., Bellgowan, P.S., and Poore, L.H. (1995). Microinfusion of mu but not delta or kappa opioid agonists into the basolateral amygdala results in inhibition of the tail flick reflex in pentobarbital-anesthetized rats. *J. Pharmacol. Exp. Ther.* **275,** 381–388.

Helmstetter, F.J., Bellgowan, P.S., and Tershner, S.A. (1993). Inhibition of the tail flick reflex following microinjection of morphine into the amygdala. *Neuroreport.* **4,** 471–474.

Helmstetter, F.J., and Tershner, S.A. (1994). Lesions of the periaqueductal gray and rostral ventromedial medulla disrupt antinociceptive but not cardiovascular aversive conditional responses. *J. Neurosci.* **14,** 7099–7108.

Herrero, J.F., and Headley, P.M. (1991). The effects of sham and full spinalization on the systemic potency of mu- and kappa-opioids on spinal nociceptive reflexes in rats. *Br. J. Pharmacol.* **104,** 166–170.

Holstege, G. (1991). Descending pathways from the periaqueductal gray and adjacent areas. In DePaulis, A., and Bandler, R. (eds.), *The midbrain periaqueductal gray matter.* New York: Plenum, pp. 239–265.

Jensen, T.S., and Yaksh, T.L. (1984). Spinal monoamine and opiate systems partly mediate the antinociceptive effects produced by glutamate at brainstem sites. *Brain Res.* **321,** 287–297.

Jensen, T.S., and Yaksh, T.L. (1986a). Comparison of antinociceptive action of morphine in the periaqueductal gray, medial and paramedial medulla in rat. *Brain Res.* **363,** 99–113.

Jensen, T.S., and Yaksh, T.L. (1986b). Examination of spinal monoamine receptors through which brainstem opiate-sensitive systems act in the rat. *Brain Res.* **363,** 114–127.

Jensen, T.S., and Yaksh, T.L. (1986c). III. Comparison of the antinociceptive action of mu and delta opioid receptor ligands in the periaqueductal gray matter, medial and paramedial ventral medulla in the rat as studied by the microinjection technique. *Brain Res.* **372,** 301–312.

Jensen, T.S., and Yaksh, T.L. (1989). Comparison of the antinociceptive effect of morphine and glutamate at coincidental sites in the periaqueductal gray and medial medulla in rats. *Brain Res.* **476,** 1–9.

Kalyuzhny, A.E., Arvidsson, U., Wu, W., and Wessendorf, M.W. (1996). μ-Opioid and δ-opioid receptors are expressed in brainstem antinociceptive circuits: Studies using immunocytochemistry and retrograde tract-tracing. *J. Neurosci.* **16,** 6490–6503.

Kaplan, H., and Fields, H.L. (1991). Hyperalgesia during acute opioid abstinence: Evidence for a nociceptive facilitating function of the rostral ventromedial medulla. *J. Neurosci.* **11,** 1433–1439.

Khachaturian, H., Lewis, M.E., and Watson, S.J. (1983). Enkephalin systems in diencephalon and brainstem of the rat. *J. Comp. Neurol.* **220,** 310–320.

Koob, G.F., Maldonado, R., and Stinus, L. (1992). Neural substrates of opiate withdrawal. *Tr. Neurosci.* **15,** 186–191.

Le Bars, D., Dickenson, A.H., and Besson, J.M. (1980). Microinjection of morphine within nucleus raphe magnus and dorsal horn neurone activities related to nociception in the rat. *Brain Res.* **189,** 467–481.

Levine, J.D., Lane, S.R., Gordon, N.C., and Fields, H.L. (1982). A spinal opioid synapse mediates the interaction of spinal and brain stem sites in morphine analgesia. *Brain Res.* **236,** 85–91.

Lewis, V.A., and Gebhart, G.F. (1977). Evaluation of the periaqueductal central gray (PAG) as a morphine-specific locus of action and examination of morphine-induced and stimulation-produced analgesia at coincident PAG loci. *Brain Res.* **124,** 283–303.

Light, A.R., Casale, E.J., and Menetrey, D.M. (1986). The effects of focal stimulation in nucleus raphe magnus and periaqueductal gray on intracellularly recorded neurons in spinal laminae I and II. *J. Neurophysiol.* **56,** 555–571.

Llewelyn, M.B., Azami, J., and Roberts, M.H. (1986). Brainstem mechanisms of antinociception. Effects of electrical stimulation and injection of morphine into the nucleus raphe magnus. *Neuropharmacology.* **25,** 727–735.

Lovick, T.A. (1985). Ventrolateral medullary lesions block the antinociceptive and cardiovascular responses elicited by stimulating the dorsal periaqueductal grey matter in rats. *Pain.* **21,** 241–252.

Lovick, T.A. (1986). Analgesia and the cardiovascular changes evoked by stimulating neurones in the ventrolateral medulla in rats. *Pain.* **25,** 259–268.

Lovick, T.A. (1992). Midbrain influences on ventrolateral medullo-spinal neurones in the rat. *Exp. Brain Res.* **90,** 147–152.

Manning, B.H., and Mayer, D.J. (1995a). The central nucleus of the amygdala contributes to the production of morphine antinociception in the tail flick test. *J. Neurosci.* **15,** 8199–8213.

Manning, B.H., and Mayer, D.J. (1995b). The central nucleus of the amygdala contributes to the production of morphine antinociception in the tail flick test. *Pain.* **63,** 141–152.

Manning, B.H., Morgan, M.J., and Franklin, K.B. (1994). Morphine analgesia in the formalin test: Evidence for forebrain and midbrain sites of action. *Neuroscience.* **63,** 289–294.

Mansour, A., Fox, C.A., Burke, S., Meng, F., Thompson, R.C., Akil, H., and Watson, S.J. (1994). Mu, delta, and kappa opioid receptor mRNA expression in the rat CNS: An in situ hybridization study. *J. Comp. Neurol.* **350,** 412–438.

Mansour, A., Khachaturian, H., Lewis, M.E., Akil, H., and Watson, S.J. (1987). Autoradiographic differentiation of mu, delta, and kappa opioid receptors in the rat forebrain and midbrain. *J. Neurosci.* **7,** 2445–2464.

Mansour, A., Khachaturian, H., Lewis, M.E., Akil, H., and Watson, S.J. (1988). Anatomy of CNS opioid receptors. *Tr. Neurosci.* **11,** 308–314.

Mantyh, P.W. (1983). Connections of midbrain periaqueductal gray in the monkey. I. Ascending efferent projections. *J. Neurophysiol.* **49,** 567–581.

Mayer, D.J., and Price, D.D. (1976). Central nervous system mechanisms of analgesia. *Pain.* **2,** 379–404.

Miaskowski, C., and Levine, J.D. (1992). Inhibition of spinal opioid analgesia by supraspinal administration of selective opioid antagonists. *Brain Res.* **596,** 41–45.

Mokha, S.S., McMillan, J.A., and Iggo, A. (1985). Descending control of spinal nociceptive transmission. Actions produced on spinal multireceptive neurones from the nuclei locus coeruleus (LC) and raphe magnus (NRM). *Exp. Brain Res.* **58,** 213–226.

Monroe, P.J., Hawranko, A.A., Smith, D.L., and Smith, D.J. (1996). Biochemical and pharmacological characterization of multiple β-endorphinergic antinociceptive systems in the rat periaqueductal gray. *J. Pharmacol. Exp. Ther.* **276,** 65–73.

Moreau, J.L., and Fields, H.L. (1986). Evidence for GABA involvement in midbrain control of medullary neurons that modulate nociceptive transmission. *Brain Res.* **397,** 37–46.

Morgan, M.M., Depaulis, A., and Liebeskind, J.C. (1987). Diazepam dissociates the analgesic and aversive effects of periaqueductal gray stimulation in the rat. *Brain Res.* **423,** 395–398.

Morgan, M.M., Heinricher, M.M., and Fields, H.L. (1992). Circuitry linking opioid-sensitive nociceptive modulatory systems in periaqueductal gray and spinal cord with rostral ventromedial medulla. *Neuroscience.* **47,** 863–871.

Morgan, M.M., and Liebeskind, J.C. (1987). Site specificity in the development of tolerance to stimulation-produced analgesia from the periaqueductal gray matter of the rat. *Brain Res.* **425,** 356–359.

Morgan, M.M., Sohn, J.H., and Liebeskind, J.C. (1989). Stimulation of the periaqueductal gray matter inhibits nociception at the supraspinal as well as spinal level. *Brain Res.* **502,** 61–66.

Osborne, P.B., Vaughan, C.W., Wilson, H.I., and Christie, M. (1990). Opioid inhibition of rat periaqueductal gray neurons with identified projections to rostral ventromedial medulla *in vitro. J. Physiol.* **490,** 383–389.

Ossipov, M.H., Kovelowski, C.J., Nichols, M.L., Hruby, V.J., and Porreca, F. (1995). Characterization of supraspinal antinociceptive actions of opioid delta agonists in the rat. *Pain.* **62,** 287–293.

Pan, Z.Z., and Fields, H.L. (1996). Endogenous opioid-mediated inhibition of putative pain-modulating neurons in rat rostral ventromedial medulla. *Neuroscience.* **74,** 855–862.

Pan, Z.Z., Williams, J.T., and Osborne, P.B. (1990). Opioid actions on single nucleus raphe magnus neurons from rat and guinea-pig *in vitro. J. Physiol.* **427,** 519–532.

Pavlovic, Z.W., Cooper, M.L., and Bodnar, R.J. (1995). Opioid antagonists in the periaqueductal gray inhibit morphine analgesia elicited from the amygdala. *Soc. Neurosci. Abstr.* **21,** 362.

Pick, C.G., Roques, B., Gacel, G., and Pasternak, G.W. (1992). Supraspinal mu 2-opioid receptors mediate spinal/supraspinal morphine synergy. *Eur. J. Pharmacol.* **220,** 275–277.

Pomeroy, S.L., and Behbehani, M.M. (1979). Physiologic evidence for a projection from periaqueductal gray to nucleus raphe magnus in the rat. *Brain Res.* **176,** 143–147.

Potrebic, S.B., Fields, H.L., and Mason, P. (1994). Serotonin immunoreactivity is contained in one physiological cell class in the rat rostral ventromedial medulla. *J. Neurosci.* **14,** 1655–1665.

Prieto, G.J., Cannon, J.T., and Liebeskind, J.C. (1983). N. raphe magnus lesions disrupt stimulation-produced analgesia from ventral but not dorsal midbrain areas in the rat. *Brain Res.* **261,** 53–57.

Proudfit, H.K. (1980a). Effects of raphe magnus and raphe pallidus lesions on morphine-induced analgesia and spinal cord monoamines. *Pharmacol. Biochem. Behav.* **13,** 705–714.

Proudfit, H.K. (1980b). Reversible inactivation of raphe magnus neurons: Effects on nociceptive threshold and morphine-induced analgesia. *Brain Res.* **201,** 459–464.

Ramirez, F., and Vanegas, H. (1989). Tooth pulp stimulation advances both medullary off-cell pause and tail flick. *Neurosci. Lett.* **100,** 153–156.

Reichling, D.B., and Basbaum, A.I. (1990). Contribution of brainstem GABAergic circuitry to descending antinociceptive controls: I. GABA-immunoreactive projection neurons in the periaqueductal gray and nucleus raphe magnus. *J. Comp. Neurol.* **302,** 370–377.

Reichling, D.B., Kwiat, G.C., and Basbaum, A.I. (1988). Anatomy, physiology and pharmacology of the periaqueductal gray contribution to antinociceptive controls. *Prog. Brain Res.* **77,** 31–46.

Rizvi, T.A., Ennis, M., Behbehani, M.M., and Shipley, M.T. (1991). Connections between the central nucleus of the amygdala and the midbrain periaqueductal gray: Topography and reciprocity. *J. Comp. Neurol.* **303,** 121–131.

Rizvi, T.A., Ennis, M., and Shipley, M.T. (1992). Reciprocal connections between the medial preoptic area and the midbrain periaqueductal gray in rat: A WGA-HRP and PHA-L study. *J. Comp. Neurol.* **315,** 1–15.

Rodgers, R.J. (1978). Influence of intra-amygdaloid opiate injections on shock thresholds, tail-flick latencies and open field behaviour in rats. *Brain Res.* **153,** 211–216.

Roerig, S.C., and Fujimoto, J.M. (1989). Multiplicative interaction between intrathecally and intracerebroventricularly administered mu opioid agonists but limited interactions between delta and kappa agonists for antinociception in mice. *J. Pharmacol. Exp. Ther.* **249,** 762–768.

Roerig, S.C., Hoffman, R.G., Takemori, A.E., Wilcox, G.L., and Fujimoto, J.M. (1991). Isobolographic analysis of analgesic interactions between intrathecally and intracerebroventricularly administered fentanyl, morphine and D-Ala2-D-Leu5-enkephalin in morphine-tolerant and nontolerant mice. *J. Pharmacol. Exp. Ther.* **257,** 1091–1099.

Rossi, G.C., Pasternak, G.W., and Bodnar, R.J. (1993). Synergistic brainstem interactions for morphine analgesia. *Brain Res.* **624,** 171–180.

Rossi, G.C., Pasternak, G.W., and Bodnar, R.J. (1994). Mu and delta opioid synergy between the periaqueductal gray and the rostro-ventral medulla. *Brain Res.* **665,** 85–93.

Roychowdhury, S.M., and Fields, H.L. (1996). Endogenous opioids acting at a medullary mu-opioid receptor contribute to the behavioral antinociception produced by GABA antagonism in the midbrain periaqueductal gray. *Neuroscience.* **74,** 863–872.

Sandkühler, J., and Gebhart, G.F. (1984a). Characterization of inhibition of a spinal nociceptive reflex by stimulation medially and laterally in the midbrain and medulla in the pentobarbital-anesthetized rat. *Brain Res.* **305,** 67–76.

Sandkühler, J., and Gebhart, G.F. (1984b). Relative contributions of the nucleus raphe magnus and adjacent medullary reticular formation to the inhibition by stimulation in the periaqueductal gray of a spinal nociceptive reflex in the pentobarbital-anesthetized rat. *Brain Res.* **305,** 77–87.

Sandkühler, J., and Herdegen, T. (1995). Distinct patterns of activated neurons throughout the rat midbrain periaqueductal gray induced by chemical stimulation within its subdivisions. *J. Comp. Neurol.* **357,** 546–553.

Sandkühler, J., Willmann, E., and Fu, Q.G. (1989). Blockade of $GABA_A$ receptors in the midbrain periaqueductal gray abolishes nociceptive spinal dorsal horn neuronal activity. *Eur. J. Pharmacol.* **160,** 163–166.

Satoh, M., Oku, R., and Akaike, A. (1983). Analgesia produced by microinjection of L-glutamate into the rostral ventromedial bulbar nuclei of the rat and its inhibition by intrathecal alpha-adrenergic blocking agents. *Brain Res.* **261,** 361–364.

Sim, L.J., and Joseph, S.A. (1991). Arcuate nucleus projections to brainstem regions which modulate nociception. *J. Chem. Neuroanatom.* **4,** 97–109.

Smith, D.J., Perrotti, J.M., Crisp, T., Cabral, M.E., Long, J.T., and Scalzitti, J.M. (1988). The mu opiate receptor is responsible for descending pain inhibition originating in the periaqueductal gray region of the rat brain. *Eur. J. Pharmacol.* **156,** 47–54.

Stinus, L., Le Moal, M., and Koob, G.F. (1990). Nucleus accumbens and amygdala are possible substrates for the aversive stimulus effects of opiate withdrawal. *Neuroscience.* **37,** 767–773.

Sugita, S., and North, R.A. (1993). Opioid actions on neurons of rat lateral amygdala in vitro. *Brain Res.* **612,** 151–155.

Sugita, S., Tanaka, E., and North, R.A. (1993). Membrane properties and synaptic potentials of three types of neurone in rat lateral amygdala. *J. Physiol.* **460,** 705–718.

Tattersall, J.E., Cervero, F., and Lumb, B.M. (1986). Viscerosomatic neurons in the lower thoracic spinal cord of the cat: Excitations and inhibitions evoked by splanchnic and somatic nerve volleys and by stimulation of brain stem nuclei. *J. Neurophysiol.* **56,** 1411–1423.

Thorn, B.E., Applegate, L., and Johnson, S.W. (1989). Ability of periaqueductal gray subdivisions and adjacent loci to elicit analgesia and ability of naloxone to reverse analgesia. *Behav. Neurosci.* **103,** 1335–1339.

Tsou, K. (1963). Antagonism of morphine analgesia by the intracerebral micorinjection of nalorphine. *Acta Physiol. Sinica* **26,** 332–337.

Van Bockstaele, E.J., Aston-Jones, G., Pieribone, V.A., Ennis, M., and Shipley, M.T. (1991). Subregions of the periaqueductal gray topographically innervate the rostral ventral medulla in the rat. *J. Comp. Neurol.* **309,** 305–327.

Vanegas, H., Barbaro, N.M., and Fields, H.L. (1984a). Midbrain stimulation inhibits tail-flick only at currents sufficient to excite rostral medullary neurons. *Brain Res.* **321,** 127–133.

Vanegas, H., Barbaro, N.M., and Fields, H.L. (1984b). Tail-flick related activity in medullospinal neurons. *Brain Res.* **321,** 135–141.

Wiklund, L., Behzadi, G., Kalen, P., Headley, P.M., Nicolopoulos, L.S., Parsons, C.G., and West, D.C. (1988). Autoradiographic and electrophysiological evidence for excitatory amino acid transmission in the periaqueductal gray projection to nucleus raphe magnus in the rat. *Neurosci. Lett.* **93,** 158–163.

Williams, F.G., and Beitz, A.J. (1990). Ultrastructural morphometric analysis of enkephalin-immunoreactive terminals in the ventrocaudal periaqueductal gray: Analysis of their relationship to periaqueductal gray-raphe magnus projection neurons. *Neuroscience.* **38,** 381–394.

Willis, W.D., Jr. (1988). Anatomy and physiology of descending control of nociceptive responses of dorsal horn neurons: Comprehensive review. *Prog. Brain Res.* **77,** 1–29.

Willis, W.D., Gerhart, K.D., Willcockson, W.S., Yezierski, R.P., Wilcox, T.K., and Cargill, C.L. (1984). Primate raphe- and reticulospinal neurons: Effects of stimulation in periaqueductal gray or VPLc thalamic nucleus. *J. Neurophysiol.* **51,** 467–480.

Yaksh, T.L. (1979). Direct evidence that spinal serotonin and noradrenaline terminals mediate the spinal antinociceptive effects of morphine in the periaqueductal gray. *Brain Res.* **160,** 180–185.

Yaksh, T.L., al-Rodhan, N.R., and Jensen, T.S. (1988). Sites of action of opiates in production of analgesia. *Prog. Brain Res.* **77,** 371–394.

Yaksh, T.L., Plant, R.L., and Rudy, T.A. (1977). Studies on the antagonism by raphe lesions of the antinociceptive action of systemic morphine. *Eur. J. Pharmacol.* **41,** 399–408.

Yaksh, T.L., and Rudy, T.A. (1977). Studies on the direct spinal action of narcotics in the production of analgesia in the rat. *J. Pharmacol. Exp. Ther.* **202,** 411–428.

Yaksh, T.L., and Rudy, T.A. (1978). Narcotic analgestics: CNS sites and mechanisms of action as revealed by intracerebral injection techniques. *Pain.* **4,** 299–359.

Yaksh, T.L., Yeung, J.C., and Rudy, T.A. (1976). Systematic examination in the rat of brain sites sensitive to the direct application of morphine: Observation of differential effects within the periaqueductal gray. *Brain Res.* **114,** 83–103.

Yeung, J.C., and Rudy, T.A. (1980a). Multiplicative interaction between narcotic agonisms expressed at spinal and supraspinal sites of antinociceptive action as revealed by concurrent intrathecal and intracerebroventricular injections of morphine. *J. Pharmacol. Exp. Ther.* **215,** 633–642.

Yeung, J.C., and Rudy, T.A. (1980b). Sites of antinociceptive action of systemically injected morphine: Involvement of supraspinal loci as revealed by intracerebroventricular injection of naloxone. *J. Pharmacol. Exp. Ther.* **215,** 626–632.

Young, E.G., Watkins, L.R., and Mayer, D.J. (1984). Comparison of the effects of ventral medullary lesions on systemic and microinjection morphine analgesia. *Brain Res.* **290,** 119–129.

Zhuo, M., and Gebhart, G.F. (1990). Characterization of descending inhibition and facilitation from the nuclei reticularis gigantocellularis and gigantocellularis pars alpha in the rat. *Pain.* **42,** 337–350.

Zhuo, M., and Gebhart, G.F. (1992). Characterization of descending facilitation and inhibition of spinal nociceptive transmission from the nuclei reticularis gigantocellularis and gigantocellularis pars alpha in the rat. *J. Neurophysiol.* **67,** 1599–1614.

Zorman, G., Hentall, I.D., Adams, J.E., and Fields, H.L. (1981). Naloxone-reversible analgesia produced by microstimulation in the rat medulla. *Brain Res.* **219,** 137–148.

CHAPTER FOUR

Spinal Mechanisms of Opioid Analgesia

FRANÇOIS CESSELIN, JEAN-JACQUES BENOLIEL, SILVIE BOURGOIN, ELISABETH COLLIN, MICHEL POHL, AND MICHEL HAMON

Introduction

Besides supraspinal (see Heinricher and Morgan, Chap. 3 this vol.) and peripheral sites (see Stein, Cabot, and Schäfer, Chap. 5 this vol.), the dorsal horn (DH) of the spinal cord is a major area in which opioids exert their analgesic action. Thus, opioids administered at the spinal level produce a powerful analgesia in animals and humans (see Yaksh, 1997). Furthermore, whatever its route of administration, the most often used analgesic agent, morphine, exerts part of its antinociceptive effects by acting at spinal opioid receptors (Le Bars et al., 1976).

Opioid receptors of the μ, δ, and κ types have been cloned (see Gavériaux-Ruff and Kieffer, Chap. 1, this vol.). The existence of subclasses of these receptors: μ_1 and μ_2, δ_1 and δ_2, κ_1, κ_2, and κ_3, has been postulated on the basis of pharmacologic data, but molecular biology investigations have not yet provided support for this hypothesis (see Dhawan et al., 1996). Possible variations in the post-translational processing of the receptor proteins might account for this pharmacologic heterogeneity, which has led to the distinction of receptor subtypes, notably in the spinal cord. Endogenous ligands for opioid receptors (see Roques, Noble, and Fournié-Zaluski Chap. 2 this vol.) are also present at the spinal level. In particular, endogenous opioid systems are strategically located in the DH, where primary afferent fibers (PAF), whose cell bodies are located in dorsal root ganglia (DRG), convey nociceptive messages from the periphery. These fibers contain excitatory amino acids and several neuropeptides such as substance P (SP) and calcitonin gene-related peptide (CGRP) (see Weihe, 1992).

Important conclusions regarding the functions of endogenous opioid peptides have been drawn from experiments that consisted of blocking their degradation by peptidase inhibitors (see Roques et al., Chap. 2 this vol.). However, only a few studies have specifically examined the functions of spinal opioidergic systems under actual physiologic conditions – that is, in the absence of drugs. Further investigations are clearly needed in this respect since disruption of the gene that encodes one of the families of opioid peptides, for example, the preproenkephalin A (PA) gene,

Christoph Stein, ed., *Opioids in Pain Control: Basic and Clinical Aspects*. Printed in the United States of America.

has been shown to affect supraspinal, but not spinal, responses to painful stimuli in mice (König et al., 1996). However, the latter findings must be interpreted with caution because possible adaptive changes of the other endogenous opioidergic systems, able to compensate for the disruption of the PA gene, were not investigated.

This review first summarizes anatomic and biochemical data concerning the spinal opioidergic systems. Thereafter, the control by opioids of the activity of some neurones involved in the spinal processing of nociception are described. To date, the most appropriate method to estimate the activity of a given population of neurones consists of measuring the release of their neurotransmitter(s). We thus examine the main findings reported in the literature about the spinal release of SP, CGRP, cholecystokinin (CCK), and Met-enkephalin (ME), which (except CGRP) can arise from various categories of neurones within the DH. Investigations on the modulations by opioids of the release of these peptides have provided new insights into both the involvement of endogenous opioid peptides in the physiologic control of nociception and the mechanisms of action of exogenous opioid analgesics at the spinal level.

Anatomic and Biochemical Data

Opioid Peptides

The spinal gray matter is divided into 10 laminae, the first five of which are located in the DH. Laminae I, II, and V are rich in enkephalinergic neurones (Hunt et al., 1980; Sumal et al., 1982; Conrath-Verrier et al., 1983; Glazer and Basbaum, 1983; La Motte and de Lanerolle, 1983; Basbaum and Fields, 1984; Gruz and Basbaum, 1985; Harlan et al., 1987). The distribution of dynorphinergic neurones is more restricted because most of these cells are found in lamina I (Cruz and Basbaum, 1985; Basbaum et al., 1986; Ruda et al., 1988). Some dynorphin-immunoreactive (IR) cell bodies, dendrites, and terminals are postsynaptic to PAF terminals (Basbaum et al., 1986; Carlton and Hayes, 1989; Cho and Basbaum, 1989). Conversely, enkephalin and dynorphin terminals do not provide a significant presynaptic input to PAF (Hunt et al., 1980; Sumal et al., 1982; Glazer and Basbaum, 1983; La Motte and de Lanerolle, 1983; Cho and Basbaum, 1989). In contrast, opioid-IR axonal boutons contact spinal projection neurones (Ruda, 1982; Ruda et al., 1984; Nahin et al., 1992). Some terminals of bulbospinal neurones contain both enkephalin- and dynorphin-IR (Blomqvist et al., 1994; see Weihe, 1992). In addition, PAF issued from PA- and prodynorphin-containing cells in the DRG also contribute to a portion of opioid-IR terminals in the DH (Botticelli et al., 1981; Sweetnam et al., 1986; Weihe et al., 1988; Pohl et al., 1994, 1997; Carlton and Coggeshall, 1997).

Although most enkephalin-IR cells in the DH are local interneurones, certain opioidergic neurones are at the origin of ascending projections to the brain (Cruz and Basbaum, 1985; Basbaum et al., 1986; Coffield and Miletic, 1987; Leah et al., 1988). At least in the cat, most of the nociceptive neurones (either specifically nociceptive cells or wide dynamic-range neurones) contain enkephalin-IR (Ribeiro-Da-Silva et al., 1992; Ma et al., 1997). It is thus not surprising that acute noxious stimuli trigger the release of opioid peptides at the spinal level in various species (see Hamon et al., 1988). Also, the characteristics of spinal endogenous opioid systems have been shown to exhibit marked changes in animal models of chronic pain. Thus, increases in the levels of PA- and prodynorphin-derived peptides (Cesselin et al., 1980, 1988; Millan et al., 1985, 1986, 1988; Nahin et al., 1989; Weihe et al., 1989; Kar et al., 1991, 1994; Pohl et al., 1997) and of their encoding mRNAs (Höllt et al., 1987; Iadarola et al., 1988; Ruda et al., 1988; Draisei et al., 1991; Noguchi et al., 1992; Przewlocka et al., 1992; Pohl et al., 1997) have been found in the DH of rats subjected to chronic peripheral inflammation. These observations support the idea that spinal opioidergic systems are activated during chronic inflammatory pain. Indeed, an increased spinal release of dynorphin has been reported in polyarthritic rats (Pohl et al., 1997). However, other observations do not support this hypothesis because, in contrast, a decreased release of PA-derived peptides has been shown to occur at the spinal level in rats suffering from chronic inflammatory pain (Bourgoin et al., 1988; Cesselin et al., 1988; Przewlocka et al., 1992; Pohl et al., 1997). This paradoxical change is probably explained by the fact that PA-mRNA levels are dramatically reduced in the DRG of polyarthritic rats (Pohl et al., 1997). The close parallel between the reduction in the spinal release of PA-derived peptides and the decrease in the levels of PA-mRNA in the DRG of polyarthritic rats suggests that the activity of enkephalin-containing PAF decreases markedly during chronic inflammatory pain. In addition, these observations support the case that ME originating from PAF terminals represents an important part of the peptide that is released at the spinal level, even if the contribution of PAF to the ME content of the DH is low (Pohl et al., 1990, 1997).

Opioid Receptors

The three major types of opioid receptors are present in the DH (Besse et al., 1990). Autoradiographic investigations showed that the binding of μ and κ ligands is limited for the most part to the upper laminae, particularly the substantia gelatinosa (lamina II) (Gouardères et al., 1985; Morris and Herz, 1987; Stevens et al., 1991; Gouardères et al., 1993), where small afferent fibers conveying nociceptive messages are mainly projecting. In contrast, δ receptors are distributed not only in the upper laminae but also in the deeper laminae of the dorsal horn and in the ventral horn (Gouardères et al., 1993). The absolute densities of the μ, δ, and κ binding sites in laminae I and II vary from one study to another, but, at least in rodents, μ receptors are always found to be the most abundant. Recently, the key role of this receptor type in mediating morphine-induced analgesia, at both supraspinal and spinal sites, has been elegantly confirmed. Indeed, the antinociceptive effects of the alkaloid are abolished in mice lacking the μ receptor gene (Matthes et al., 1996; Sora et al., 1997).

Recent in situ hybridization studies with molecular probes, and immunocytochemical investigations with specific antibodies raised against the receptor proteins, provided new data about the expression and location of opioid receptors in the spinal cord. Thus, in the rat, cells expressing μ receptor mRNA are localized in laminae IV, V, VII, VIII, and X. Contradictory results have been published concerning the intensity of its expression in laminae I and II (Maekawa et al., 1994; Mansour et al., 1994). Cells expressing δ receptor mRNA are scattered in the dorsal and ventral horn, but they are more specifically localized in laminae IV, V, and VII–X (Mansour et al., 1994). Kappa-receptor mRNA is distributed over neurones throughout the DH; as for μ receptor mRNA, there are discrepancies about its presence in laminae I and II (Maekawa et al., 1994; Mansour et al., 1994; Schäfer et al., 1994).

Immunohistochemical studies confirmed that the superficial DH of the rat contains a dense network of μ receptor-IR, which is present on the plasma membrane of somata and dendrites as well as on unmyelinated axons and axon terminals (Arvidsson, Riedl et al., 1995; Cheng et al., 1996; Moriwaki et al., 1996). Coexistence of μ receptor-IR and opioid-IR in somata and dendrites has been occasionally reported (Cheng et al., 1996). Commonly, mismatches between enkephalin-IR varicosities and μ receptor-IR labeling are found (Arvidsson, Riedl et al., 1995; Cheng et al., 1996). Mu receptor-IR labeling is essentially extrasynaptic (Arvidsson, Riedl et al., 1995; Cheng et al., 1996; Moriwaki et al., 1996), indicating that opioids acting at μ receptors could be involved in a diffuse mode of neurotransmission on surrounding elements (see Fuxe and Agnati, 1991). Delta receptor-IR has been found in fibers and axon terminals that are distributed throughout the spinal cord gray matter, with highest densities in the superficial DH (Arvidsson, Dado et al., 1995; Cheng et al., 1995). Some varicosities co-express μ receptor-IR and δ receptor-IR (Arvidsson, Riedl et al., 1995). A subset of terminals showing δ receptor-IR also contains ME-IR, and, conversely, most terminals showing ME-IR also show δ receptor-IR. Few postsynaptic densities on dendrites are immunolabeled by anti-δ receptor antibodies. Thus, δ receptors may serve autoreceptor functions on ME terminals as well as presynaptic modulation of the release of other neurotransmitters (Zerari et al., 1994; Cheng et al., 1995). Kappa receptor-IR, which is especially dense in the substantia gelatinosa, extends to laminae III–VII and X, where it is localized predominantly on fibers. In addition, κ receptor-IR perikarya are also detected in laminae I, II, V, and VII (Mansour et al., 1996).

In the primate *Macaca fascicularis,* μ and δ receptor-IR form a dense plexus of small profiles within the superficial DH, which differs from that observed in the rat. Indeed, in the monkey, δ receptor-IR is found in laminae I and II, whereas μ receptor-IR is confined mostly to lamina II (Honda and Arvidsson, 1995).

In the rat, some of the μ receptor-IR axon terminals derive from DRG cells since a dorsal rhizotomy decreases the staining in laminae I and outer II (Arvidsson, Riedl et al., 1995). This confirms autoradiographic data which indicated that dorsal rhizotomy in various species results in a significant reduction (variable from one study to another, but in a 50–75% range) of the specific binding of opioid radioligands in the DH, suggesting that a significant proportion of μ, δ, and κ binding sites are associated with the degenerating PAF (La Motte et al., 1976; Jessell et al., 1979; Fields et al., 1980; Daval et al., 1987; Zajac et al., 1989; Besse et al., 1990; Stevens and Seybold, 1995). In line with these observations, in situ hybridization studies showed that opioid receptors are expressed in DRG cells (Young et al., 1980; Ninkovic et al., 1982; Maekawa et al., 1994; Mansour et al., 1994; Schäfer et al., 1994) at the origin of PAF. Indeed, in the rat DRG, these studies indicated that μ receptor mRNA is localized in medium-sized and large cells, κ receptor mRNA in small and medium neurones, and δ receptor mRNA in predominantly large-diameter cells (Mansour et al., 1994; Schäfer et al., 1994). Some neurones in rat DRG were also found to be positively stained with an antiserum raised against the cloned μ receptor. Interestingly, the latter neurones were essentially negative for RT97, a marker of large, myelinated PAF. Thus, in discordance with the in situ hybridization data, this finding suggests that μ receptor-IR is mainly localized to small-diameter PAF. Delta receptor-IR cells are found in DRG, some of which also exhibit a positive staining with an antiserum to the μ receptor (Arvidsson et al., 1995). Kappa receptor-IR is localized in two populations of DRG cells: a small-diameter, densely stained population that corresponds to those cells expressing κ receptor mRNA and a second, larger-diameter, faintly stained population that does not (Mansour et al., 1996).

Thus, in spite of some discrepancies concerning their presence in particular cell types, autoradiographic, immunohistochemical, and in situ hybridization data all indicate that opioid receptors are located both on neuronal elements intrinsic to the spinal cord and on terminals of PAF. Consequently, the analgesic effects of intrathecal administration of opioids, which have been observed in a great variety of animal models of acute or chronic pain (see Yaksh, 1997), could be due to a presynaptic modulation of the activity of PAF (see Cesselin et al., 1993) and/or postsynaptic influences on other spinal neurones.

For reasons of space, electrophysiologic data will not be summarized. However, they lead to the same conclusions by providing support for both pre- (notably for agonists at δ receptors) (Murase et al., 1982; Hori et al., 1992; Glaum et al., 1994) and postsynaptic (particularly for μ agonists) (Belcher and Ryall, 1978; Zieglgänsberger and Tulloch, 1979; Murase et al., 1982; Yoshimura and North, 1983; Willcokson et al., 1984; Besson and Chaouch, 1987; Jeftinija, 1988; Glaum et al., 1994; Grudt and Williams, 1994) sites of action for opioid receptor ligands at the spinal level. Various transduction mechanisms, triggered by agonist occupancy of opioid receptors (see Dhawan, 1996; Gavériaux-Ruff and Kieffer, Chap. 1 this vol.), finally lead to modulations of the release of various neurotransmitters within the DH.

Effects of Opioids on the Spinal Release of Neuropeptides

Substance P

Numerous convergent studies have shown that stimulation of δ receptors inhibits the spinal release of substance P (SP) (Go and Yaksh, 1987; Mauborgne et al., 1987; Aimone and Yaksh, 1989; Pohl, Mauborgne et al., 1989; Collin et al., 1991; Suarez-

Roca and Maixner, 1992b; Zachariou and Goldstein, 1996b), whereas their blockade increases it (Collin et al., 1991; Zachariou and Goldstein, 1996b). Thus, endogenous opioids acting at these receptors exert a tonic inhibitory control on SP-containing fibers. In the DH, SP, together with most neurotransmitters, with the notable exception of CGRP, can arise not only from PAF terminals but also from other neuronal elements – that is, intrinsic spinal interneurones and descending fibers (Hökfeet et al., 1977; Chung et al., 1988; Kruger et al., 1988; Pohl et al., 1990; Weihe, 1992; Ahmed et al., 1995). However, the control of SP release by δ receptors very likely concerns only the peptide in PAF, which supports the concept of a presynaptic action of opioids. Thus, δ agonists are especially efficient in depressing SP release that is evoked selectively from those fibers by capsaicin (Aimone and Yaksh, 1989; Pohl, Mauborgne et al., 1989). Conversely, no opioid control is observed on the spinal release of SP in rats whose unmyelinated PAF had been destroyed by a neonatal administration of capsaicin (Pohl, Mauborgne et al., 1989).

In contrast to the clear situation for δ receptors, the involvement of the other opioid receptor types in the control of SP release is controversial. Both excitatory (Mauborgne et al., 1987; Pohl, Mauborgne et al., 1989; Collin, Mauborgne et al., 1992) and inhibitory (Aimone and Yaksh, 1989) influences of μ receptor stimulation on the peptide release have been reported. Similarly, although most investigations have shown that the activation of κ receptors exerts no significant action on the spinal release of SP (Go and Yaksh, 1987; Mauborgne et al., 1987; Aimone and Yaksh, 1989; Pohl, Mauborgne et al., 1989; Collin, Mauborgne et al., 1992), some inhibitory (Chang et al., 1989) or rather complex effects have also been reported (Suarez-Roca and Maixner, 1993; Zachariou and Goldstein, 1996a). Interestingly, κ-receptor stimulation influences the effect of μ-receptor stimulation on the peptide release. Thus, in halothane-anesthetized rats, Collin, Mauborgne et al. (1992) showed the κ agonist U-50488-H (see Dhawan et al., 1996) not only suppresses the stimulatory effect of the μ agonist DAGO (Dhawan et al., 1996) on SP release, but reverses it, leading to a significant decrease in SP release upon the concomitant perfusion of the subarachnoid space with both compounds.

These data emphasize the complexity of the control of spinal SP-containing neurones by opioids. Since morphine is able to stimulate μ, δ, and κ receptors (see Dhawan et al., 1996), interactions between them could account for the reported differences in the magnitude and direction of the effects of this alkaloid on the release of SP. Indeed, data in the literature vary from a complete inhibition (Jessell and Iversen, 1977; Yaksh et al., 1980), a partial reduction (Hirota et al., 1985; Lembeck and Donnerer, 1985; Pang and Vasko, 1986; Go and Yaksh, 1987; Aimone and Yaksh, 1989; Chang et al., 1989), no effect (Mauborgne et al., 1987; Morton et al., 1990), or even a facilitation (Pohl, Mauborgne et al., 1989) of SP release by morphine. In fact, the alkaloid seems to exert variable effects depending on its concentration (Suarez-Roca et al., 1992; Suarez-Roca and Maixner, 1992a, 1995). In any case, in contrast to the concept originally proposed by Jessell and Iversen (1977), it is no longer relevant to consider that morphine exerts a simple, monophasic, inhibitory influence on the spinal release of SP.

Calcitonin Gene-Related Peptide

As already noted, because of the exclusive location of calcitonin gene-related peptide (CGRP) in PAF terminals within the DH, the release of this peptide is probably a better index of PAF activity and of the transmission of pain messages than would be the release of any other neurotransmitter. Consequently, a presynaptic site of action should presumably be responsible for the modulation by opioids of the spinal release of CGRP.

Surprisingly, however, whereas in vitro investigations showed that the spinal release of CGRP can be modulated by opioids (Pohl, Lombard et al., 1989), in vivo studies concluded that neither morphine (by intravenous or intrathecal route) nor selective agonists at μ, δ, and κ receptors (administered intrathecally) decrease the spinal release of the peptide (Morton and Hutchison, 1990; Morton et al., 1991; Collin, Frechilla et al., 1993) (Fig. 4.1). In sharp contrast, stimulation of δ receptors unexpectedly has been found to increase the spinal release of CGRP (Fig. 4.1). However, the *simultaneous* stimulation of μ and κ receptors markedly inhibits the spinal release of CGRP. In fact, the activation of δ receptors by morphine prevents this drug from inhibiting CGRP release through the stimulation of *both* μ and κ receptors. Thus, morphine exerts a clear-cut inhibitory influence on the spinal release of CGRP when δ receptors are blocked by naltrindole (see Dhawan et al., 1996), which is inactive by itself (Collin et al., 1993). By contrast, the blockade of μ or κ receptors increases the release of CGRP (Collin, Frechilla et al., 1993; Yu et al., 1995; Malcangio and Bowery, 1996) (Fig. 4.2), indicating that endogenous opioids acting at these receptors exert a tonic inhibitory influence on the spinal release of the peptide.

Interestingly, CGRP-containing PAF are under a stronger tonic opioid inhibitory control in polyarthritic rats than in controls. Although the blockade of κ receptors

---

Opposite

Figure 4.1. Effects of opioid receptor agonists on the spinal release of CGRP in control and polyarthritic rats. The intrathecal space of control and polyarthritic (subjected to an intradermal injection of complete Freund's adjuvant near the base of the tail 4 weeks prior to the experiment) halothane-anasthetized rats was perfused with an artificial CSF at a flow rate of 0.1 ml/minute, and 1.5 mL fractions were collected on dry ice 30–45 minutes after starting the perfusion. CGRP content of each fraction was estimated using a specific radioimmunoassay. The mean release of the peptide was approximately 15-fold higher in polyarthritic animals (61 ± 5 pg/minute) than in controls (4.0 ± 0.5 pg/minute). Each compound was added (at 10 μM) to the perfusing CSF during the collection of fractions 4 to 6. Each bar is the mean ± S.E.M. ($n \geq 9$ independent determinations) of the CGRP content of each fraction expressed as a percentage of the mean levels in the first three fractions. ★ $P < 0.05$, ★★ $P < 0.01$, ★★★ $P < 0.001$ as compared to CGRP levels in fractions 1–3. The effects of all agonists except U 50488H were significantly different ($P < 0.05$) in polyarthritic rats and in controls.

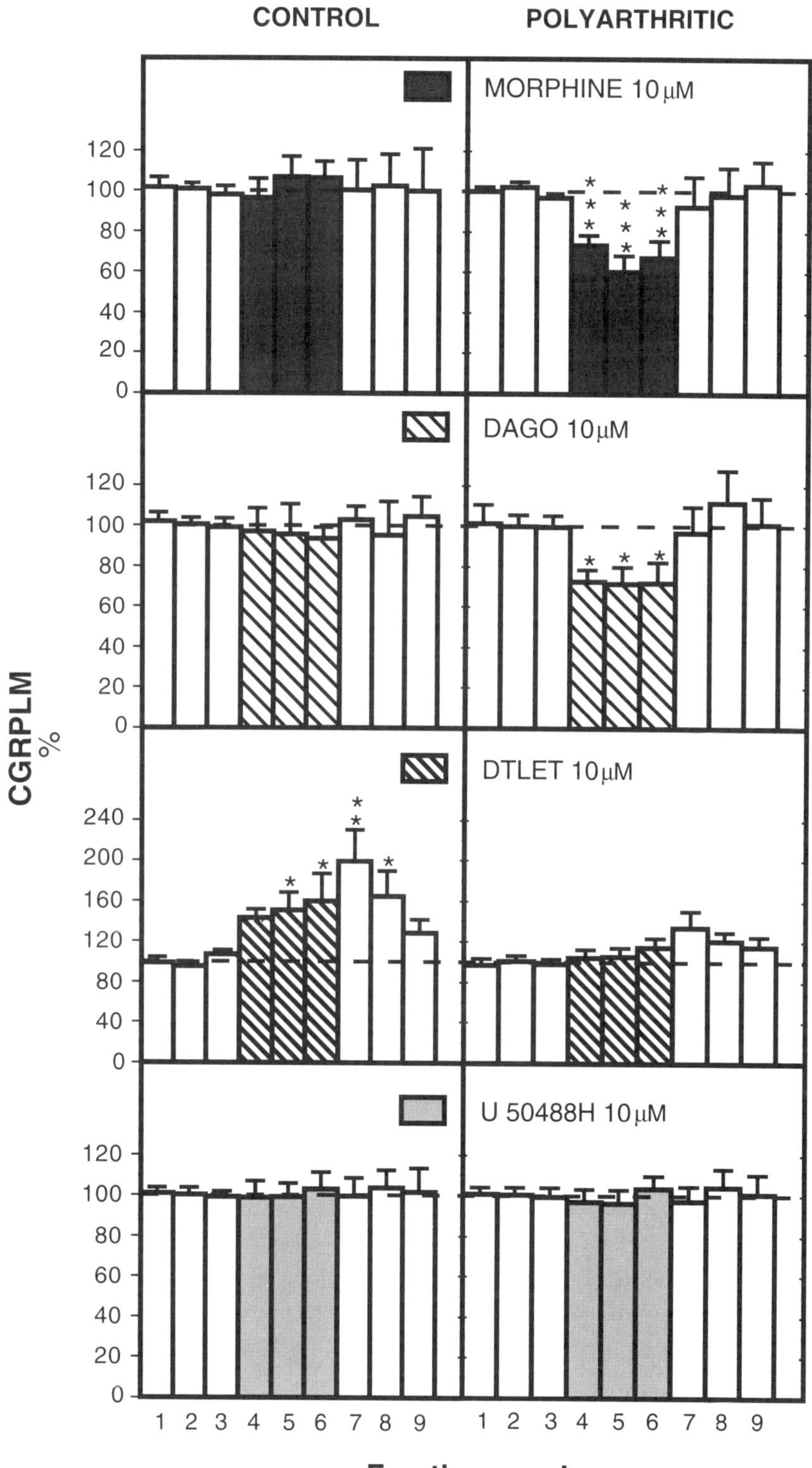

CONTROL
POLYARTHRITIC
MORPHINE 10µM
DAGO 10µM
DTLET 10µM
U 50488H 10µM
CGRPLM %
Fraction number

increases the spinal release of CGRP to the same extent in both groups of animals, the blockade of μ receptors produces a larger increase in the CGRP outflow in polyarthritic rats than in controls (Collin, Mantelet et al., 1993). In addition, intrathecal perfusion with naltrindole increases CGRP release in polyarthritic rats (Fig. 4.2). Nevertheless, the efficiency of this control remains limited because the absolute rate of CGRP release from the spinal cord in polyarthritic animals is markedly higher than in controls (Nanayama et al., 1989; Garry and Hargreaves, 1992; Collin, Mantelet et al., 1993; Schaible et al., 1994; Galeazza et al., 1995). Differences between polyarthritic and control rats are also observed in experiments with opioid receptor agonists. Indeed, DAGO and morphine significantly reduce the peptide outflow, whereas δ receptor stimulation is inactive in polyarthritic rats (Ballet et al., unpublished observations) (Fig. 4.1).

Cholecystokinin

Cholecystokinin (CCK) appears to play a role in nociception by modulating the action of opioids (see Baber et al., 1989; Cesselin, 1995). Interactions between opioids and CCK take place notably at the level of the spinal cord where CCK is contained in interneurones (Vanderhaegen et al., 1982; Conrath-Verrier et al., 1984), and, for a lower part, in descending (Skirboll et al., 1983; Maciewicz et al., 1984) and ascending (Leah et al., 1988; Zouaoui et al., 1991) pathways. However, in contrast to SP and CGRP, CCK is absent in terminals of capsaicin-sensitive PAF in the rat (Pohl et al., 1990; Zouaoui et al., 1990).

Numerous behavioral data have shown that CCK reduces, whereas CCK receptor antagonists enhance, the antinociceptive effects of both exogenous and endogenous opioids. Accordingly, opioids may activate CCKergic systems, leading to increased extracellular levels of CCK, which counteract the antinociceptive actions of opioids. Other behavioral data support the idea that, reciprocally, CCK can activate opioid systems and thus exert naloxone-reversible antinociceptive effects (see Cesselin, 1995).

The ability of opioids and CCK to mutually modulate their spinal release has been investigated in few studies. Relevant data showed that μ agonists exert an inhibitory

Opposite

Figure 4.2. Effects of opioid receptor antagonists on the spinal release of CGRP in control and polyarthritic rats. The same protocol as that described for Figure 4.1 was used. Each bar is the mean ± S.E.M. ($n \geq 9$ independent determinations) of the CGRP content of each fraction expressed as a percentage of the mean levels in the first three fractions. ★ $P < 0.05$, ★★ $P < 0.01$, ★★★ $P < 0.001$, ★★★★ $P < 0.0001$ as compared to CGRP levels in fractions 1–3. The effects of naloxone and naltrindole, but not those of nor-binaltorphimine, were significantly different (P < 0.05) in polyarthritic rats and in controls.

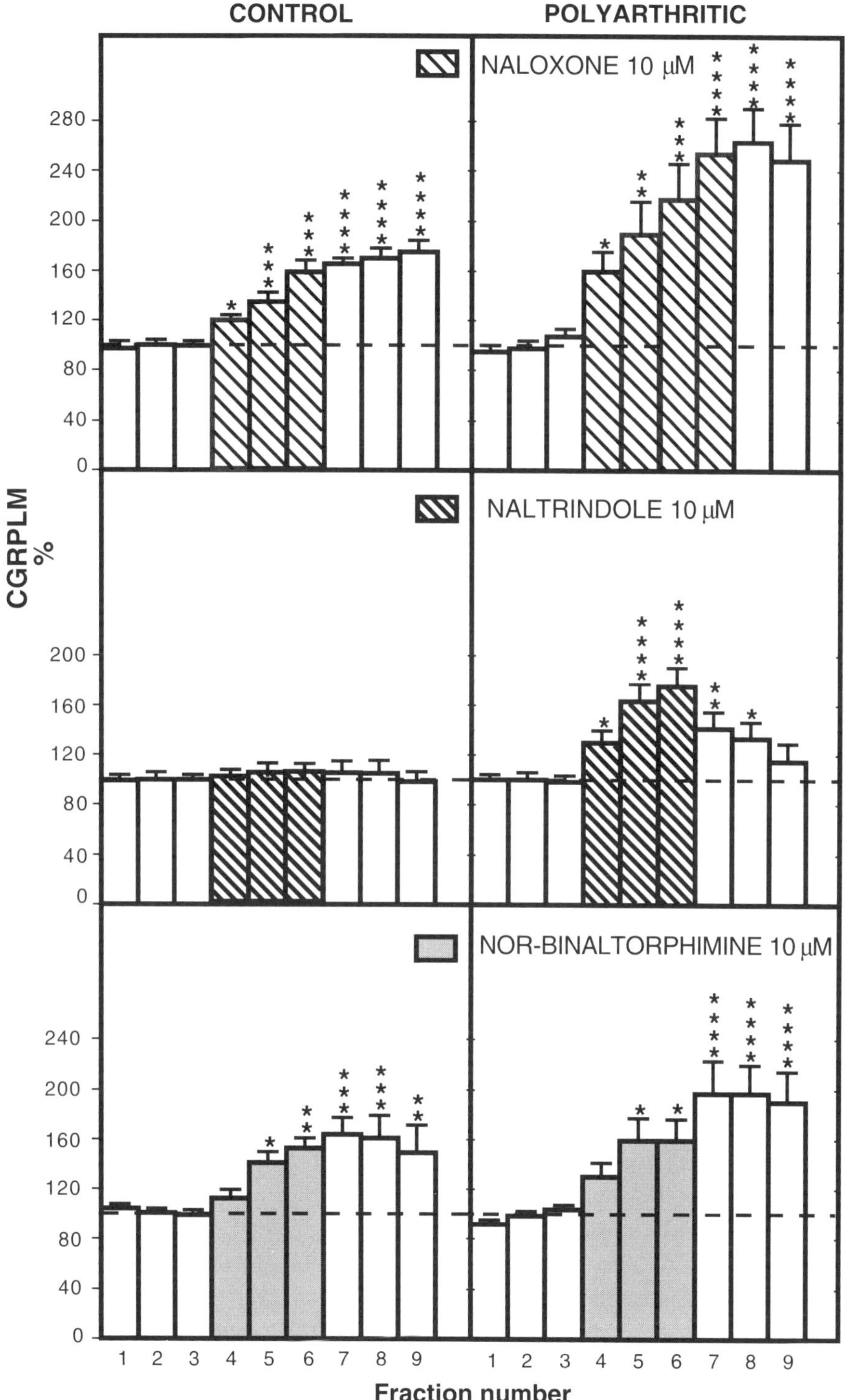

CONTROL
POLYARTHRITIC
NALOXONE 10 μM
NALTRINDOLE 10 μM
NOR-BINALTORPHIMINE 10 μM
CGRPLM %
Fraction number

influence on the spinal release of CCK, whereas, in contrast, morphine and δ agonists can increase the peptide outflow (Rodriguez and Sacristan, 1989; Benoliel et al., 1991, 1994; Zhou et al., 1993; Tang et al., 1984). Indeed, complex, biphasic effects were noted with the latter two compounds: when applied at low concentrations (0.1 nM–1 μM), both morphine and the δ agonist DTLET induce a decrease in spinal CCK release, whereas, at higher concentrations (≥ 10 μM), the reverse is found: CCK release is enhanced (Benoliel et al., 1994). Recent investigations have shown that the opioid receptors whose stimulation triggers a reduction in the spinal release of CCK are the μ and the δ_1 subtypes, whereas δ_2 receptor stimulation is responsible for the increase in the peptide release due to high concentrations of morphine and DTLET. Similarly, endogenous opioids also appear to exert both inhibitory and excitatory tonic influences on CCK release through the stimulation of δ_1 and δ_2 receptors, respectively (Benoliel et al., unpublished observations) (Fig. 4.3). Further emphasizing the complexity of the opioid control of spinal CCK release, interactions between κ (whose stimulation is inactive on its own) and μ receptors can also play a role in this control (Benoliel et al., 1991), similar to that previously noted about the opioid control of SP and CGRP release.

Reciprocally, recent data from our laboratory have confirmed and extended earlier findings indicating that CCK actually modulates the spinal release of ME (Cesselin et al., 1984). Indeed, an increase of the spinal release of ME is noted upon stimulation of CCK-A receptors, whereas their blockade markedly decreases the release of the opioid peptide. These data suggest that endogenous CCK exerts a tonic stimulatory influence on spinal ME-containing neurones through the activation of CCK-A receptors (Fig. 4.3).

Met-enkephalin

As mentioned earlier, the potential sources of Met-enkephalin (ME) in the DH are multiple and include not only intrinsic spinal neurones but also terminals of ME-containing PAF. In addition, we also noted that μ and δ receptors may serve autoreceptor functions in spinal opioidergic neurones.

Indeed, whereas the stimulation of κ receptors has no effect, μ and δ agonists inhibit the spinal release of ME (Bourgoin et al., 1991; Collin, Bourgoin et al., 1992). Interestingly, under in vitro conditions, the inhibition due to the stimulation of μ or δ receptors persists in the presence of the Na^+ channel blocker tetrodotoxin, as expected of the location of the receptors on the terminals of enkephalinergic neurones themselves. Intrathecal morphine also reduces the spinal release of ME (Yaksh and Elde, 1981; Jhamandas et al., 1984; Collin, Mauborgne et al., 1994). Further supporting the idea that presynaptic autoreceptors on ME-containing neurones are of the δ type, the inhibitory effect of morphine on the release of ME can be totally abolished by the δ antagonist naltrindole, but remains unaffected by μ receptor blockade. However, when both δ and κ receptors are blocked, morphine still reduces the spinal

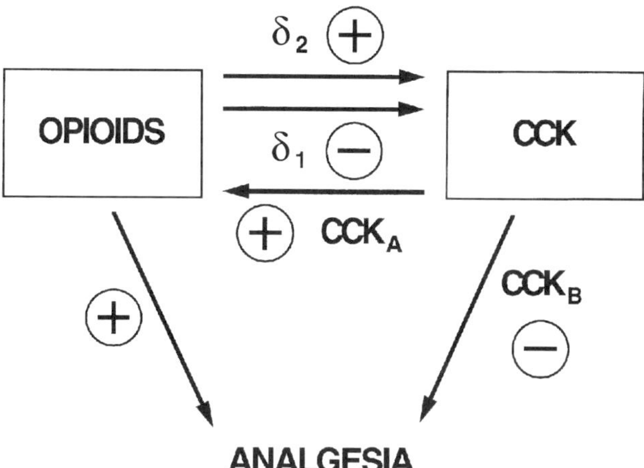

Figure 4.3. Schematic representation of the interactions between endogenous opioids and CCK in the spinal cord. Endogenous opioids exert both excitatory and inhibitory tonic influence on CCKergic systems, through the stimulation of δ_2 and δ_1 receptors, respectively, and CCK, through CCK-B receptors, can reduce the analgesic effects of opioids. In turn, endogenous CCK, through an action at CCK-A receptors, tonically increases the release of endogenous opioids (namely, Met-enkephalin) and thus can facilitate opioid-mediated analgesia.

release of ME, showing that its action at μ receptors might also be relevant to its inhibitory influence on enkephalinergic neurones (Collin et al., 1994). In line with the observations reported earlier in this chapter concerning the opioid control of the spinal release of SP, CGRP, and CCK, interactions between the receptor types are also involved in the opioid control of ME release. Thus, with morphine alone, the stimulation of κ receptors prevents the μ-dependent inhibitory effect of the drug, allowing only the expression of its δ-mediated inhibitory influence on the spinal release of ME (Collin et al., 1994). Once more, this emphasizes the importance of the interactions among the μ, κ, and/or δ receptors in the central effects of exogenous and endogenous opioids.

When applied alone, antagonists of the three types of opioid receptors exert no influence on the spinal release of ME, demonstrating the lack of a tonic control by opioids on this process (Burgoin et al., 1991; Collin, Burgoin et al., 1992). However, a feedback control of ME release can occur under certain circumstances. Thus, the enhancement of spinal ME extracellular levels that results from the blockade of its degrading peptidases (Bourgoin et al., 1986) can be further increased by the addition of naltrindole to the artificial cerebrospinal fluid perfusing the intrathecal space in anesthetized rats (Collin, Bourgoin et al., 1992). Similarly, intrathecal perfusion with porcine calcitonin produces (via an indirect mechanism that involves bulbospinal serotoninergic neurones) (see Bourgoin et al., 1988) a marked increase in the spinal outflow of ME, which is further enhanced by naltrindole (Collin et al., 1989; Collin, Bourgoin et al., 1992). These data suggest that the spinal release of ME can be under an inhibitory control exerted by endogenous opioids acting at δ receptors only when the extracellular concentrations of the latter peptides are increased up to a critical threshold level.

Summary

The presence within the DH of endogenous opioid peptides in various neuronal elements, including PAF, interneurones, and (nociceptive) spinothalamic neurones, and the location of μ, δ, and κ receptors at both pre- and postsynaptic sites very likely accounts for the complexity of spinal opioid actions, notably the opioid modulation of the release of SP, CGRP, CCK, and ME. However, several (provisional) conclusions can be drawn from the data summarized above.

The first conclusion concerns the functional correlate of the opioid control of peptides' release with regard to nociception. Thus, in control animals, endogenous opioids can modulate the transfer of (acute) nociceptive messages by PAF, via a δ receptor-mediated inhibitory control of SP release and a μ/κ receptor-mediated tonic inhibitory influence on the release of CGRP. Probably, and more interestingly from a clinical point of view, at least for CGRP-containing PAF, this tonic inhibitory control is increased in chronic suffering (polyarthritic) rats where it involves μ and δ receptors. This observation is in line with the fact that naloxone induces an enhancement of hyperalgesia and of activity of DH nociceptive neurones in polyarthritic rats (Oliveras et al., 1979; Kaiser and Guilbaud, 1981; Lombard and Besson, 1989; Millan and Colpaert, 1991). However, such a stronger tonic opioid inhibitory control of PAF in polyarthritic rats, which does not prevent the spinal release of CGRP from being higher in these animals than in controls, is not easily attributable to known changes in the activity of spinal endogenous opioid systems in chronic inflammatory pain. Indeed, the spinal extracellular levels of enkephalins (which bind preferentially to μ and δ receptors) (see Dhawan et al., 1996) is markedly diminished in polyarthritic rats. However, it should be noted that some endogenous ligands for μ and δ receptors may still be unrevealed. This is illustrated by the very recent discovery of potent and selective endogenous agonists for the μ receptors, called endomorphins 1 and 2 (Zadina et al., 1997), the presence of which in the spinal cord, and possible changes in chronic inflammatory pain, remain to be studied.

It could appear surprising that the control of spinal CGRP release due to endogenous opioids acting at κ receptors is not modified in polyarthritic rats. Indeed, (1) an increased activity of spinal dynorphinergic neurones is clearly demonstrated in these animals; (2) dynorphin is one of the endogenous ligands of κ receptors (see Dhawan et al., 1996); and (3) several reports suggest that an enhanced κ opioidergic control of nociception, behavior, and pathology occurs in response to inflammatory pain (see, e.g., Millan et al., 1985, 1987, 1988; Millan and Colpaert, 1991; Stiller et al.,

1993). In fact, the blockade of κ receptors in polyarthritic rats significantly decreases the response threshold for pressure, but does not affect the heat threshold (Millan et al., 1985, 1987, 1988). Interestingly, spinal CGRP release in the rat is increased by noxious heat, but not by noxious mechanical stimuli (Pohl et al., 1992). Thus, blockade of κ receptors has consequences on behavioral responses to noxious mechanical stimuli that do not involve CGRP, but does not modify in polyarthritic animals the response to acute noxious heat, a stimulus that does imply CGRP. These observations further support the idea that κ receptor-mediated analgesic effects of opioids are independent of the presynaptic control by these compounds of CGRP-containing PAF at the spinal level.

In addition to the increased inhibitory control of spinal CGRP release by endogenous opioids (through the activation of μ and δ receptors) in polyarthritic rats as compared to controls, differences between the two groups of rats also exist with regard to the effects of exogenous opioid receptor agonists. Indeed, the μ agonist DAGO, and the nonselective agonist morphine, decrease the spinal outflow of CGRP in polyarthritic rats but not in control animals. Furthermore, the δ-preferring agonist DTLET loses in polyarthritic rats its capability to enhance the spinal release of the peptide, which is observed in control animals. Such functional alterations of μ and δ receptors in polyarthritic animals can be neither simply related to established changes in the extracellular levels of identified endogenous opioids (see earlier) nor assigned to modifications of opioid binding sites since, except those of Millan et al. (1986), all investigations failed to reveal any modification in the density and/or affinity of opioid receptors in the spinal cord of such chronic suffering animals (Cesselin et al., 1980, 1988; Delay-Goyet et al., 1989; Besse et al., 1992). However, functional alterations of opioid receptors are in line with behavioral data showing that chronic inflammatory pain is associated with supersensitivity to opioids (Pircio et al., 1975; Oliveras et al., 1979; Kayser and Guilbaud, 1983; Przewlocki et al., 1984; Millan et al., 1986, 1987; Neil et al., 1986; Kayser et al., 1991; Millan and Colpaert, 1991; Stiller et al., 1993), notably when these compounds are administered directly at the spinal level (Hylden et al., 1991). Whatever the explanation(s) of the apparent changes in the sensitivity of μ and δ receptors in polyarthritic rats, the opioid-induced decrease of the spinal release of CGRP might contribute to the high analgesic efficiency of morphine and other opioids in these chronic suffering animals. Indeed, the marked activation of CGRP-containing fibers observed in polyarthritic rats is recognized to play an important role in the generation and expression of the inflammation-evoked increase in responsiveness of the spinal nociceptive neurones (see Neugebauer et al., 1996). Since CGRP in synovial fluid from knee joints is found in higher concentrations in patients suffering from rheumatoid arthritis than in subjects with osteoarthritis (Hernanz et al., 1993), it can be hypothesized that an activation of CGRP-containing PAF also occurs in humans with inflammatory pain and that its reduction by opioids contributes to the marked analgesic action of these compounds.

The second conclusion is that interactions between μ and κ receptors are involved in the opioidergic modulation of the spinal release of neuropeptides. In particular, in control rats, the aforementioned tonic inhibitory control of spinal CGRP release by opioids requires the concomitant stimulation of these two types of receptors. Moreover, the changes in neuropeptide release in response to μ receptor stimulation, whatever their direction (reduction or enhancement), can be altered by the concomitant stimulation of κ receptors. Such interactions could be of particular benefit regarding opioid-induced analgesia. Thus, μ receptor stimulation alone produces both a decrease in ME release and an increase in SP release, two changes opposite to those expected for an antinociceptive action. In contrast, the concomitant stimulation of μ and κ receptors not only abolishes the μ-mediated reduction in ME release and converts the enhancement to a diminution of SP release, but also induces a decrease in CGRP release, all these changes converging to reduce pain transmission at the spinal level.

Interactions between μ and κ receptors also account for the net effect of morphine (which can activate μ, δ, and κ receptors) on the spinal release of the four peptides examined in the present review. As discussed above, such interactions very likely explain the failure of morphine to reduce the spinal release of CGRP in control animals as well as its ability to do so in polyarthritic rats. Depending on these interactions and on the proper effects of the stimulation of a given receptor, the opioid receptor(s) that seem(s) to be involved in the action of the alkaloid vary(ies) from one neuropeptide to another. For instance, morphine acts as a δ agonist to reduce the spinal release of ME, and as a μ and/or a δ agonist (depending on its concentration) to affect the release of CCK. Such a complexity explains why the mechanisms of action of this drug are still a matter of debate. Yet, the multiple actions of morphine at the three classes of opioid receptors very probably account for its remarkable efficiency in relieving pain. Thus, for instance, the alkaloid can reduce the release of SP to a very large extent through the inhibitory effects of both δ and μ + κ receptor stimulation. In addition, as a result of the κ/μ interactions, morphine may lead to a decrease in the activity of spinal ME neurones that is less pronounced than that due to the selective stimulation of μ and/or δ opioid (auto)receptors, therefore favoring the antinociceptive action of endogenous ME. Finally, at the doses used for relieving pain, morphine can also inhibit (via the stimulation of μ receptors) the activity of spinal CCK-containing neurones, thereby reducing the "antagonism" that CCK exerts toward opioid-induced analgesia. However, when morphine is administered chronically at a high dose, it can trigger the activity of spinal CCKergic neurones (via the stimulation of δ_2 receptors), which would contribute, through the activation of CCK-B receptors (see Cesselin, 1995), to reducing the efficiency of the alkaloid.

The last conclusion is that these pharmacologic CCK-opioid interactions mimic those that occur between endogenous CCK and opioids (Fig. 4.3). This supports the hypothesis that under certain circumstances, such as neuropathic pain, increased activity of CCKergic neurones could antagonize the actions of opioid analgesics either released endogenously or applied exogenously, resulting in their limited efficiency (see Stanfa et al., 1994). This suggests that CCK-B receptor antagonists should be appropriate drugs to restore the sensitivity of neurogenic pain to opioids (see Zhang et al., 1993).

REFERENCES

Ahmed, M., Bjuholm, A., Srinivasan, G.R., Lundeberg, T., Theodorsson, E., Schultzberg, M., and Kreicbergs, A. (1995). Capsaicin effects on substance P and CGRP in rat adjuvant arthritis. *Regul. Pept.* **55,** 85–102.

Aimone, L.D., and Yaksh, T.L. (1989). Opioid modulation of capsaicin-evoked release of substance P from rat spinal cord in vivo. *Peptides.* **10,** 1127–1131.

Arvidsson, U., Dado, R.J., Riedl, M., Lee, J.H., Law, P.Y., Loh, H.H., Elde, R., and Wessendorf, M.W. (1995). Delta-opioid receptor immunoreactivity: Distribution in brainstem and spinal cord, and relationship to biogenic amines and enkephalin. *J. Neurosci.* **15,** 1215–1235.

Arvidsson, U., Riedl, M., Chakrabarti, S., Lee, J.H., Nakano, A.H., Dado, R.J., Loh, H.H., Law, P.Y., Wessendorf, M.W., and Elde, R. (1995). Distribution and targeting of a μ-opioid receptor (MOR1) in brain and spinal cord. *J. Neurosci.* **15,** 3328–3341.

Baber, N.S., Dourish, C.T., and Hill, D.R. (1989). The role of CCK, caerulein, and CCK antagonists in nociception. *Pain.* **39,** 307–328.

Basbaum, A.I., Cruz, L., and Weber, E. (1986). Immunoreactive dynorphin B in sacral primary afferent fibres of the cat. *J. Neurosci.* **6,** 127–133.

Basbaum, A.I., and Fields, H.C. (1984). Endogenous pain control systems: Brainstem spinal pathways and endorphin circuitry. *Ann. Rev. Neurosci.* **7,** 309–338.

Belcher, G., and Ryall, R.W. (1978). Differential excitatory and inhibitory effects of opiates on non-nociceptive and nociceptive neurones in the spinal cord of the cat. *Brain Res.* **145,** 303–314.

Benoliel, J.J., Bourgoin, S., Mauborgne, A., Legrand, J.C., Hamon, M., and Cesselin, F. (1991). Differential inhibitory/stimulatory modulation of spinal CCK release by μ and δ opioid agonists, and selective blockade of μ-dependent inhibition by κ receptor stimulation. *Neurosci. Lett.* **124,** 204–207.

Benoliel, J.J., Collin, E., Mauborgne, A., Bourgoin, S., Legrand, J.C., Hamon, M., and Cesselin, F. (1994). Mu and delta opioid receptors mediate opposite modulations by morphine of the spinal release of cholecystokinin-like material. *Brain Res.* **653,** 916–922.

Besse, D., Lombard, M.C., Zajac, J.M., Roques, B.P., and Besson, J.M. (1990). Pre- and postsynaptic distribution of μ, δ and κ opioid receptors in the superficial layers of the cervical dorsal horn of the rat spinal cord. *Brain Res.* **521,** 15–22.

Besse, D., Weil-Fugazza, J., Lombard, M.C., Butler, S.H., and Besson, J.M. (1992). Monoarthritis induces complex changes in μ-, δ- and κ-opioid binding sites in the superficial dorsal horn of the rat spinal cord. *Eur. J. Pharmacol.* **223,** 123–131.

Besson, J.M., and Chaouch, A. (1987). Peripheral and spinal mechanisms of nociception. *Physiol. Rev.* **67,** 67–186.

Blomqvist, A., Hermanson, O., Ericson, H., and Larhammar, D. (1994). Activation of a bulbospinal opioidergic projection by pain stimuli in the awake rat. *Neuroreport.* **5,** 461–464.

Botticelli, L.J., Cox, B.M., and Goldstein, A. (1981). Immunoreactive dynorphin in mammalian spinal cord and dorsal root ganglia. *Proc. Natl. Acad. Sci. U.S.A.* **78,** 7783–7786.

Bourgoin, S., Collin, E., Benoliel, J.J., Chantrel, D., Mauborgne, A., Pohl, M., Hamon, M., and Cesselin, F. (1991). Opioid control of the release of Met-enkephalin-like material from the rat spinal cord. *Brain Res.* **551,** 178–184.

Bourgoin, S., Le Bars, D., Artaud, F., Clot, A.M., Bouboutou, R., Fournié-Zaluski, M.C., Roques, B.P., Hamon, M., and Cesselin, F. (1986). Effects of kelatorphan and other peptidase inhibitors on the in vivo and in vitro release of methionine-enkephalin-like material from the rat spinal cord. *J. Pharmacol. Exp. Ther.* **238,** 360–366.

Bourgoin, S., Le Bars, D., Clot, A.M., Hamon, M., and Cesselin, F. (1988). Spontaneous and evoked release of met-enkephalin-like material from the spinal cord of arthriric rats *in vivo. Pain.* **32,** 107–114.

Bourgoin, S., Pohl, M., Hirsch, M., Mauborgne, A., Cesselin, F., and Hamon, M. (1988). Direct stimulatory effect of calcitonin on [^{3}H]5-hydroxytryptamine release from the rat spinal cord. *Eur. J. Pharmacol.* **156,** 13–23.

Carlton, S.M., and Coggeshall, R.E. (1997). Immunohistochemical localization of enkephalin in peripheral sensory axons in the rat. *Neurosci. Lett.* **221,** 121–124.

Carlton, S.M., and Hayes, E.S. (1989). Dynorphin A(1–8) immunoreactive cell bodies, dendrites and terminals are postsynaptic to calcitonin gene-related peptide primary afferent terminals in the monkey dorsal horn. *Brain Res.* **504,** 124–128.

Cesselin, F. (1995). Opioid and anti-opioid peptides. *Fundam. Clin. Pharmacol.* **9,** 409–433.

Cesselin, F., Bourgoin, S., Artaud, F., and Hamon, M. (1984). Basic and regulatory mechanisms of in vitro release of met-enkephalin from the dorsal zone of the rat spinal cord. *J. Neurochem.* **43,** 763–773.

Cesselin, F., Bourgoin, S., Le Bars, D., and Hamon, M. (1988). Central met-enkephalinergic systems in arthritic rats. In *The arthritic rat as a model of clinical pain?,* ed. J.M. Besson and G. Guilbaud. Amsterdam, New York, and Oxford: Excerpta Medica-Elsevier, pp. 185–202.

Cesselin, F., Collin, E., Bourgoin, S., Pohl, M., Mauborgne, A., Benoliel, J.J., and Hamon, M. (1993). Pharmacological and physiological modulations of the release of peptides from nociceptors. In *Peripheral neurons in nociception: Physio-pharmacological aspects,* ed. J.M. Besson, G. Guilbaud, and H. Ollat. Paris: John Libbey Eurotext, pp. 255–271.

Cesselin, F., Montastruc, J.L., Gros, C., Bourgoin, S., and Hamon, M. (1980). Met-enkephalin levels and opiate receptors in the spinal cord of chronic suffering rats. *Brain Res.* **191,** 25–31.

Chang, H.M., Berde, C.B., Holz, G.G., Stewart, G.F., and Kream, R.M. (1989). Sufentanyl, morphine, met-enkephalin, and κ-agonist (U 50,488H) inhibit substance P release from primary sensory neurons: A model for presynaptic spinal opioid actions. *Anesthesiology* **70,** 672–677.

Cheng, P.Y., Moriwaki, A., Wang, J.B., Uhl, G.R., and Pickel, V.M. (1996). Ultrastructural localization of μ-opioid receptors in the superficial layers of the rat cervical spinal cord: Extrasynaptic localization and proximity to Leu^5-enkephalin. *Brain Res.* **731,** 141–154.

Cheng, P.Y., Svingos, A.L., Wang, H., Clarke, C.L., Jenab, S., Beczkowska, I.W., Inturrisi, C.E., and Pickel, V.M. (1995). Ultrastructural immunolabeling shows prominent presynaptic vesicular localization of delta-opioid receptor within both enkephalin- and nonenkephalin-containing axon terminals in the superficial layers of the rat cervical spinal cord. *J. Neurosci.* **15,** 5976–5988.

Cho, H.J., and Basbaum, A.I. (1989). Ultrastructural analysis of dynorphin B-immunoreactive cells and terminals in the superficial dorsal horn of the deafferented spinal cord of the rat. *J. Comp. Neurol.* **281,** 193–205.

Chung, K., Lee, W.T., and Carlton, S.M. (1988). The effects of dorsal rhizotomy and spinal cord isolation on calcitonin gene-related peptide-labeled terminals in the lumbar dorsal horn. *Neurosci. Lett.* **90,** 27–32.

Coffield, J.A., and Miletic, V. (1987). Immunoreactive enkephalin is contained within some trigeminal and spinal neurons projecting to the rat medial thalamus. *Brain Res.* **425,** 380–383.

Collin, E., Bourgoin, S., Gorce, P., Hamon, M., and Cesselin, F. (1989). Intrathecal porcine calcitonin enhances the release of [Met^5]-enkephalin-like material from the rat spinal cord. *Eur. J. Pharmacol.* **168,** 201–208.

Collin, E., Bourgoin, S., Mantelet, S., Hamon, M., and Cesselin, F. (1992). Feedback inhibition of Met-enkephalin release from the rat spinal cord in vivo. *Synapse.* **11,** 76–84.

Collin, E., Frechilla, D., Pohl, M., Bourgoin, S., Le Bars, D., Hamon, M., and Cesselin, F. (1993). Opioid control of the release of calcitonin gene-related peptide-like material from the rat spinal cord in vivo. *Brain Res.* **609,** 211–222.

Collin, E., Mantelet, S., Frechilla, D., Pohl, M., Bourgoin, S., Hamon, M., and Cesselin, F. (1993). Increased in vivo release of calcitonin gene-related peptide-like material from the spinal cord in arthritic rats. *Pain.* **54,** 203–211.

Collin, E., Mauborgne, A., Bourgoin, S., Benoliel, J.J., Hamon, M., and Cesselin, F. (1994). Morphine reduces the release of Met-enkephalin-like material from the rat spinal cord in vivo by acting at δ opioid receptors. *Neuropeptides.* **27,** 75–83.

Collin, E., Mauborgne, A., Bourgoin, S., Chantrel, D., Hamon, M., and Cesselin, F. (1991). In vivo tonic inhibition of substance P (like material) release by endogenous opioid(s) acting at δ receptors. *Neuroscience.* **44,** 725–731.

Collin, E., Mauborgne, A., Bourgoin, S., Mantelet, S., Ferhat, L., Hamon, M., and Cesselin, F. (1992). Kappa/mu-receptor interactions in the opioid control of the in vivo release of substance P-like material from the rat spinal cord. *Neuroscience.* **332,** 347–355.

Conrath-Verrier, M., Dietl, M., Arluison, M., Cesselin, F., Bourgoin, S., and Hamon, M. (1983). Localization of met-enkephalin-like immunoreactivity within pain-related nuclei of cervical spinal cord, brainstem and midbrain in the cat. *Brain Res. Bull.* **11,** 587–604.

Conrath-Verrier, M., Dietl, M., and Tramu, G. (1984). Cholecystokinin-like immunoreactivity in the dorsal horn of the spinal cord of the rat: A light and electron microscopic study. *Neuroscience.* **13,** 871–885.

Cruz, L., and Basbaum, A. (1985). Multiple opioid peptides and the modulation of pain: Immunohistochemical analysis of dynorphin and enkephalin in the trigeminal nucleus caudalis and spinal cord of the rat. *J. Comp. Neurol.* **240,** 331–348.

Daval, G., Vergé, D., Basbaum, A.L., Bourgoin, S., and Hamon, M. (1987). Autoradiographic evidence of serotonin binding sites on primary afferent fibres in the dorsal horn of the rat spinal cord. *Neurosci. Lett.* **83,** 71–76.

Delay-Goyet, P., Kayser, V., Zajac, J.M., Guilbaud, G., Besson, J.M., and Roques, B.P. (1989). Lack of significant changes in mu, delta opioid binding sites and neutral endopeptidase EC 3.4.24.11 in the brain and spinal cord of arthritic rats. *Neuropharmacology.* **28,** 1341–1348.

Dhawan, B.N., Cesselin, F., Raghubir, R., Reisine, T., Bradley, P.B., Portoghese, P.S., and Hamon, M. (1996). International Union of Pharmacology. XII. Classification of opioid receptors. *Pharmacol. Rev.* **48,** 567–592.

Draisci, G., Kajander, K.C., Dubner, R., Bennett, G.J., and Iadarola, M.J. (1991). Up-regulation of opioid gene expression in spinal cord evoked by experimental nerve injuries and inflammation. *Brain Res.* **560,** 86–192.

Fields, H.L., Emson, P.C., Leigh, B.K., Gilbert, R.T.F., and Iversen, L.L. (1980). Multiple opiate receptors on primary afferent fibres. *Nature.* **284,** 351–353.

Fuxe, K., and Agnati, L.F. (1991). Advances in neuroscience, Volume transmission in the brain: Novel mechanisms for neuronal transmission. New York: Raven Press.

Galeazza, M.T., Garry, M.G., Yost, H.J., Strait, K.A., Hargreaves, K.M., and Seybold, V.S. (1995). Plasticity in the synthesis and storage of substance P and calcitonin gene-related peptide in primary afferent neurons during peripheral inflammation. *Neuroscience.* **66,** 443–458.

Garry, M.G., and Hargreaves, K.M. (1992). Enhanced release of immunoreactive CGRP and substance P from spinal dorsal horn slices occurs during carrageenan inflammation. *Brain Res.* **582,** 139–142.

Gavériaux-Ruff, C., and Kieffer, B.L. Opioid receptors: Gene structure and function. Chapter 1 this volume.

Glaum, S.R., Miller, R.J., and Hammond, D.L. (1994). Inhibitory actions of δ_1-, δ_2-, and μ-opioid receptor agonists on excitatory transmission in lamina II neurons of adult rat spinal cord. *J. Neurosci.* **14,** 4965–4971.

Glazer, E.J., and Basbaum, A.I. (1983). Opioid neurons and pain modulation: An ultrastructural analysis of enkephalin in cat superficial dorsal horn. *Neuroscience.* **10,** 357–376.

Go, V.L.W., and Yaksh, T.L. (1987). Release of substance P from the cat spinal cord. *J. Physiol. (Lond.).* **391,** 141–167.

Gouardères, C., Cros, J., and Quirion, R. (1985). Autoradiographic localization of μ, δ and κ receptor binding sites in rat and guinea pig spinal cord. *Neuropeptides.* **5,** 331–342.

Gouardères, C., Tellez, S., Tafani, J.A.M., and Zajac, J.M. (1993). Quantitative autoradiographic mapping of delta-opioid receptors in the rat central nervous system using $[^{125}I][D.Ala^2]$deltorphin-I. *Synapse.* **13,** 231–240.

Grudt, T.J., and Williams, J.T. (1994). μ-Opioid agonists inhibit spinal trigeminal substantia gelatinosa neurons in guinea pig and rat. *J. Neurosci.* **14,** 1646–1654.

Hamon, M., Bourgoin, S., Le Bars, D., and Cesselin, F. (1988). In vivo and in vitro release of central neurotransmitters in relation to pain and analgesia. *Progr. Brain Res.* **77,** 433–446.

Harlan, R.E., Shivers, B.D., Romano, G.J., Howells, R.D., and Pfaff, D.W. (1987). Localization of proenkephalin mRNA in the rat brain and spinal cord by in situ hybridization. *J. Comp. Neurol.* **258,** 159–184.

Heinricher, M.M., and Morgan, M.M. Supraspinal mechanisms of opioid analgesia. Chapter 3 this volume.

Hernanz, A., De Miguel, E., Romera, N., Perez-Ayala, C., Gijon, J., and Arnalich, F. (1993). Calcitonin gene-related peptide II, substance P and vasoactive intestinal peptide in plasma and synovial fluid from patients with inflammatory joint disease. *Br. J. Rheumatol.* **32,** 31–35.

Hirota, N., Kuraishi, Y., Hino, Y., Sato, M., and Takagi, H. (1985). Met-enkephalin and morphine but not dynorphin inhibit noxious stimuli-induced release of substance P from rabbit dorsal horn in situ. *Neuropharmacology.* **24,** 567–570.

Hökfelt, T., Ljungdahl, A., Terenius, L., Elde, R., and Nilsson, G. (1977). Immunohistochemical analysis of peptide pathways possibly related to pain and analgesia: Enkephalin and substance P. *Proc. Natl. Acad. Sci. U.S.A.* **74,** 3081–3085.

Höllt, V., Haarmann, I., Millan, M.J., and Herz, A. (1987). Prodynorphin gene expression is enhanced in the spinal cord of chronic arthritic rats. *Neurosci. Lett.* **73,** 90–94.

Honda, C.N., and Arvidsson, U. (1995). Immunohistochemical localization of delta- and mu-opioid receptors in primate spinal cord. *Neuroreport.* **6,** 1025–1028.

Hori, Y., Endo, K., and Takahashi, T. (1992). Presynaptic inhibitory action of enkephalin on excitatory transmission in superficial dorsal horn of rat spinal cord. *J. Physiol (Lond.).* **450,** 673–685.

Hunt, S.P., Kelly, J.S., and Emson, P.C. (1980). The electron-microscopic localization of methionine enkephalin within the superficial layers (I and II) of the spinal cord. *Neuroscience.* **5,** 1871–1890.

Hylden, J.L.K., Thomas, D.A., Iadarola, M.J., Nahin, R.L., and Dubner, R. (1991). Spinal opioid analgesic effects are enhanced in a model of unilateral inflammation/hyperalgesia: Possible involvement of noradrenergic mechanisms. *Eur. J. Pharmacol.* **194,** 135–143.

Iadarola, M.J., Brady, L.S., Draisci, G., and Dubner, R. (1988). Enhancement of dynorphin gene expression in spinal cord following experimental inflammation: Stimulus specificity, behavioral parameters and opioid receptor binding. *Pain.* **35,** 313–326.

Jeftinija, S. (1988). Enkephalins modulate excitatory synaptic transmission in the superficial dorsal horn by acting at μ-opioid receptor sites. *Brain Res.* **460,** 260–268.

Jessell, T.M., and Iversen, L.L. (1977). Opiate analgesics inhibit substance P release from rat trigeminal nucleus. *Nature.* **268,** 549–551.

Jessell, T., Tsunoo, A., Kanazawa, I., and Otsuka, M. (1979). Substance P: Depletion in the dorsal horn of rat spinal cord after section of the peripheral processes of primary sensory neurons. *Brain Res.* **168,** 247–259.

Jhamandas, K., Yaksh, T.L., and Go, V.L.W. (1984). Acute and chronic morphine modifies the in vivo release of methionine enkephalin-like immunoreactivity from the cat spinal cord and brain. *Brain Res.* **297,** 91–103.

Kar, S., Gibson, S.J., Rees, R.G., Jura, W.G.Z.O., Brewerton, D.A. and Polak, J.M. (1991). Increased calcitonin gene-related peptide (CGRP), substance P, and enkephalin immunoreactivities in dorsal spinal cord and loss of CGRP-immunoreactive motoneurons in arthritic rats depend on intact peripheral nerve supply. *J. Mol. Neurosci.* **3,** 7–18.

Kar, S., Rees, R.G., and Quirion, R. (1994). Altered calcitonin gene-related peptide, substance P and enkephalin immunoreactivities and receptor binding sites in the dorsal spinal cord of the polyarthritic rat. *Eur. J. Pharmacol.* **6,** 345–354.

Kayser, V., Besson, J.M., and Guilbaud, G. (1991). Effects of the analgesic agent tramadol in normal and arthritic rats: Comparison with the effects of different opioids, including tolerance and cross-tolerance to morphine. *Eur. J. Pharmacol.* **195,** 37–45.

Kayser, V., and Guilbaud, G. (1981). Dose-dependent analgesic and hyperalgesic effects of systemic naloxone in arthritic rats. *Brain Res.* **226,** 344–348.

Kayser, V., and Guilbaud, G. (1983). The analgesic effects of morphine, but not those of the enkephalinase inhibitor thiorphan, are enhanced in arthritic rats. *Brain Res.* **267,** 131–138.

König, M., Zimmer, A.M., Steiner, H., Holmes, P.V., Crawley, J.N., Brownstein, M.J., and Zimmer, A. (1996). Pain responses, anxiety and aggression in mice deficient in preproenkephalin. *Nature.* **383,** 535–538.

Kruger, L., Stermini, C., Becha, N.C., and Mantyh, P. (1988). Distribution of calcitonin gene-related peptide immunoreactivity in relation to the rat central somatosensory projection. *J. Comp. Neurol.* **273,** 149–162.

La Motte, C.C., and de Lanerolle, N.C. (1983). Ultrastructure of chemically defined systems in the dorsal horn of the monkey. II. Methionine-enkephalin immunoreactivity. *Brain Res.* **274,** 51–63.

La Motte, C., Pert, C.B., and Snyder, S.H. (1976). Opiate receptor binding in primate spinal cord. Distribution and changes after dorsal root section. *Brain Res.* **112,** 407–412.

Le Bars, D., Guilbaud, G., Jurna, I., and Besson, J.M. (1976). Differential effects of morphine on responses of dorsal horn lamina V type cells elicited by A and C fibre stimulation in the spinal cat. *Brain Res.* **115,** 518–524.

Leah, J., Ménétrey, D., and de Pommery, J. (1988). Neuropeptides in long ascending spinal tract cells in the rat: Evidence for parallel processing of ascending information. *Neuroscience.* **24,** 195–207.

Lembeck, F., and Donnerer, J. (1985). Opioid control of the primary afferent substance P fibres. *Eur. J. Pharmacol.* **114,** 190–195.

Lombard, M.C., and Besson, J.M. (1989). Electrophysiological evidence for a tonic activity of the spinal cord intrinsic opioid systems in a chronic pain model. *Brain Res.* **447,** 48–56.

Ma, W., Ribeiro-Da-Silva, A., De Koninck, Y., Radhakrishnan, V., Cuello, A.C., and Henry, J.P. (1997). Substance P and enkephalin immunoreactivities in axonal boutons presynaptic to physiologically identified dorsal horn neurons. An ultrastructural multiple-labelling study in the cat. *Neuroscience.* **77,** 793–811.

Maciewicz, M., Phillips, B.S., Grenier, Y., and Poletti, C.E. (1984). Edinger-Westphal nucleus: Cholecystokinin immunochemistry and projections to spinal cord and trigeminal nucleus of the cat. *Brain Res.* **299,** 139–145.

Maekawa, K., Minami, M., Yabuuchi, K., Katao, Y., Hosoi, Y., Onogi, T., and Satoh, M. (1994). In situ hybridization study of mu- and kappa-opioid receptor mRNAs in the rat spinal cord and dorsal root ganglia. *Neurosci. Lett.* **168,** 97–100.

Malcangio, M., and Bowery, N.G. (1996). Calcitonin gene-related peptide content, basal outflow and electrically-evoked release from monoarthritic rat spinal cord in vitro. *Pain.* **66,** 351–358.

Mansour, A., Burke, S., Pavlic, R.J., Akil, H., and Watson, S.J. (1996). Immunohistochemical localization of the cloned κ_1 receptor in the rat CNS and pituitary. *Neuroscience.* **71,** 671–690.

Mansour, A., Fox, C.A., Burke, S., Meng, F., Thompson, R.C., Akil, H., and Watson, S.J. (1994). Mu, delta, and kappa opioid receptor mRNA expression in the rat CNS: An in situ hybridization study. *J. Comp. Neurol.* **350,** 412–438.

Matthes, H.W.D., Maldonado, R., Simonin, F., Valverde, O., Slowe, S., Kitchen, I., Befort, K., Dierich, A., Le Meur, M., Dollé, P., Tzavara, E., Hanoune, J., Roques, B.P., and Kieffer, B.L. (1996). Loss of morphine-induced analgesia, reward effect and withdrawal symptoms in mice lacking the μ-opioid receptor gene. *Nature.* **383,** 819–823.

Mauborgne, A., Lutz, O., Legrand, J.C., Hamon, M., and Cesselin, F. (1987). Opposite effects of δ and μ opioid receptor agonists on the in vitro release of substance P-like material from the rat spinal cord. *J. Neurochem.* **48,** 529–537.

Millan, M.J., and Colpaert, F.C. (1991). Opioid systems in the response to inflammatory pain: Sustained blockade suggests role of κ- but not μ-opioid receptors in the modulation of nociception, behaviour and pathology. *Neuroscience.* **42,** 541–553.

Millan, M.J., Czlonkowski, A., Morris, B., Stein, C., Arendt, R., Huber, A., Höllt, V., and Herz, A. (1988). Inflammation of the hindlimb as a model of unilateral, localized pain: Influence on multiple opioid systems in the spinal cord of the rat. *Pain.* **35,** 299–312.

Millan, M.J., Czlonkowski, A., Pilcher, C.W.T., Almeida, O.F.X., Millan, M.H., Colpaert, F.C., and Herz, A. (1987). A model of chronic pain in the rat: Functional correlates of alterations in the activity of opioid systems. *J. Neurosci.* **7,** 77–87.

Millan, M.J., Millan, M.H., Czlonkowski, A., Höllt, V., Pilcher, C.W., Herz, A., and Colpaert, F.C. (1986). A model of chronic pain in the rat: Response of multiple opioid systems to adjuvant-induced arthritis. *J. Neurosci.* **6,** 899–906.

Millan, M.J., Millan, M.H., Pilcher, C.W.T., Czlonkowski, A., Herz, A., and Colpaert, F.C.

(1985). Spinal cord dynorphin may modulate nociception via a κ-opioid receptor in chronic arthritic rats. *Brain Res.* **340,** 156–159.

Moriwaki, A., Wang, J.B., Svingos, A., Vanbockstaele, E., Cheng, P., Pickel, V., and Uhl, G.R. (1996). Mu opiate receptor immunoreactivity in rat central nervous system. *Neurochem. Res.* **21,** 1315–1331.

Morris, B.J., and Herz, A. (1987). Distinct distribution of opioid receptor types in rat lumbar spinal cord. *Naunyn-Schmiedeberg's Arch. Pharmacol.* **336,** 240–243.

Morton, C.R., and Hutchison, W.D. (1990). Morphine does not reduce the intraspinal release of calcitonin gene-related peptide in the cat. *Neurosci. Lett.* **117,** 319–324.

Morton, C.R., Hutchison, W.D., Duggan, A.W., and Hendry, I.A. (1990). Morphine and substance P release in the spinal cord. *Exp. Brain Res.* **82,** 89–96.

Morton, C.R., Hutchison, W.D., and Hendry, I.A. (1991). Intraspinal release of substance P and calcitonin gene-related peptide during opiate dependence and withdrawal. *Neuroscience.* **43,** 593–600.

Murase, K., Ndeljkov, V., and Randic, M. (1982). The actions of neuropeptides on dorsal horn neurons in the rat spinal cord slice preparation: An intracellular study. *Brain Res.* **234,** 170–176.

Nahin, R.L., Hylden, J.L.K., and Humphrey, E. (1992). Demonstration of dynorphin A 1–8 immunoreactive axons contacting spinal cord projection neurons in a rat model of peripheral inflammation and hyperalgesia. *Pain.* **51,** 135–143.

Nahin, R.L., Hylden, J.L.K., Iadarola, M.J., and Dubner, R. (1989). Peripheral inflammation is associated with increased dynorphin immunoreactivity in both projection and local circuit neurons in the superficial dorsal horn of the rat lumbar spinal cord. *Neurosci. Lett.* **96,** 247–252.

Nanayama, T., Kuraishi, Y., Ohno, H., and Satoh, M. (1989). Capsaicin-induced release of calcitonin gene-related peptide from dorsal horn slices is enhanced in adjuvant arthritic rats. *Neurosci. Res.* **6,** 569–572.

Neil, A., Kayser, V., Gacel, G., Besson, J.M., and Guilbaud, G. (1986). Opioid receptor types and antinociceptive activity in chronic inflammation: Both κ- and μ-opiate agonistic effects are enhanced in arthritic rats. *Eur. J. Pharmacol.* **130,** 203–208.

Neugebauer, V., Rümenapp, P., and Schaible, H.G. (1996). Calcitonin gene-related peptide is involved in the spinal processing of mechanosensory input from the rat's knee joint and in the generation and maintenance of hyperexcitability of dorsal horn neurons during development of acute inflammation. *Neuroscience.* **71,** 1095–1109.

Ninkovic, M., Hunt, S.P., and Gleaves, J.R.W. (1982). Localization of opiate and histamine H^1 receptors in the primate sensory ganglia and spinal cord. *Brain Res.* **241,** 197–206.

Noguchi, K., Kowalski, K., Traub, R., Solodkin, A., Iadarola, M.J., and Ruda, M.A. (1992). Dynorphin expression and fos-like immunoreactivity following inflammation induced hyperalgesia are colocalized in spinal cord neurons. *Mol. Brain Res.* **10,** 227–233.

Oliveras, J.L., Bruxelle, J., Clot, A.M., and Besson, J.M. (1979). Effects of morphine and naloxone on painful reaction in normal and chronic suffering rats. *Neurosci. Lett.* **3,** S263.

Pang, I.H., and Vasko, M.R. (1986). Morphine and norepinephrine but not 5-hydroxytryptamine and γ-aminobutyric acid inhibit the potassium-stimulated release of substance P from rat spinal cord slices. *Brain Res.* **376,** 268–279.

Pircio, A.W., Fedele, C.T., and Bierwagen, M.E. (1975). A new method for the evaluation of analgesic activity using adjuvant-induced arthritis in the rat. *Eur. J. Pharmacol.* **31,** 207–215.

Pohl, M., Ballet, S., Collin, E., Mauborgne, A., Bourgoin, S., Benoliel, J.J., Hamon, M., and

Cesselin, F. (1997). Enkephalinergic and dynorphinergic neurons in the spinal cord and dorsal root ganglia of the polyarthritic rat – in vivo release and cDNA hybridization studies. *Brain Res.* **749,** 18–28.

Pohl, M., Benoliel, J.J., Bourgoin, S., Lombard, M.C., Mauborgne, A., Taquet, H., Carayon, A., Besson, J.M., Cesselin, F., and Hamon, M. (1990). Regional distribution of calcitonin gene-related peptide-, substance P-, cholecystokinin-, Met^5-enkephalin-, and dynorphin A(1–8)-like materials in the spinal cord and dorsal root ganglia of adult rats: Effects of dorsal rhizotomy and neonatal capsaicin. *J. Neurochem.* **55,** 1122–1130.

Pohl, M., Collin, E., Bourgoin, S., Clot, A.M., Hamon, M., Cesselin, F., and Le Bars, D. (1992). *In vivo* release of calcitonin gene-related peptide-like material from the cervicotrigeminal area in the rat. Effects of electrical and noxious stimulation of the muzzle. *Neuroscience.* **50,** 697–706.

Pohl, M., Collin, E., Bourgoin, S., Conrath, M., Benoliel, J.J., Nevo, I., Hamon, M., Giraud, P., and Cesselin, F. (1994). Expression of preproenkephalin A gene and presence of met-enkephalin in dorsal root ganglia of the adult rat. *J. Neurochem.* **63,** 1226–1234.

Pohl, M., Lombard, M.C., Bourgoin, S., Carayon, A., Benoliel, J.J., Mauborgne, A., Besson, J.M., Hamon, M., and Cesselin, F. (1989). Opioid control of the in vitro release of calcitonin gene-related peptide from primary afferent fibres projecting in the rat cervical cord. *Neuropeptides.* **14,** 151–159.

Pohl, M., Mauborgne, A., Bourgoin, S., Benoliel, J.J., Hamon, M., and Cesselin, F. (1989). Neonatal capsaicin treatment abolishes the modulations by opioids of substance P release from rat spinal cord slices. *Neurosci. Lett.* **96,** 102–107.

Przewlocka, B., Lason, W., and Przewlocki, R. (1992). Time-dependent changes in the activity of opioid systems in the spinal cord of monoarthritic rats – A release and in situ hybridization study. *Neuroscience.* **46,** 209–216.

Przewlocki, R., Przewlocka, B., Lason, W., Garzon, J., Stala, L., and Herz, A. (1984). Opioid peptides, particularly dynorphin, and chronic pain. In *Spinal opioids and the relief of pain,* ed. J.M. Besson and Y. Lazorthes. Paris: INSERM, 159–170.

Ribeiro-Da-Silva, A., De Koninck, Y., Cuello, A.C., and Henry, J.L. (1992). Enkephalin-immunoreactive nociceptive neurons in the cat spinal cord. *Neuroreport.* **3,** 25–28.

Rodriguez, R.E., and Sacristan, M.P. (1989). In vivo release of CCK-8 from the dorsal horn of the rat: Inhibition by DAGOL. *FEBS Lett.* **250,** 215–217.

Roques, B.P., Noble, F., and Fournié-Zaluski, M.-C. Endogenous opioid peptides and analgesia. Chapter 2 this volume.

Ruda, M.A. (1982). Opiates and pain pathways: Demonstration of enkephalin synapses on dorsal horn projection neurons. *Science.* **215,** 1523–1525.

Ruda, M.A., Coffield, J., and Dubner, R. (1984). Demonstration of postsynaptic opioid modulation of thalamic projection neurons by the combined techniques of retrograde horseradish peroxidase and enkephalin immunocytochemistry. *J. Neurosci.* **4,** 2117–2132.

Ruda, M.A., Iadarola, M.J., Cohen, L.V., and Young, W.S. (1988). In situ hybridization histochemistry and immunocytochemistry reveal an increase in spinal dynorphin bioynthesis in a rat model of peripheral inflammation and hyperalgesia. *Proc. Natl. Acad. Sci. U.S.A.* **85,** 622–626.

Schäfer, M.K.H., Bette, M., Romeo, H., Schwaeble, W., and Weihe, E. (1994). Localization of κ-opioid receptor mRNA in neuronal subpopulations of rat sensory ganglia and spinal cord. *Neurosci. Lett.* **167,** 137–140.

Schaible, H.G., Freudenberger, U., Neugebauer, V., and Stiller, R.U. (1994). Intraspinal release of immunoreactive calcitonin gene-related peptide during development of inflammation in the joint *in vivo* – A study with antibody microprobes in cat and rat. *Neuroscience.* **62,** 1293–1305.

Skirboll, L., Hökfelt, T., Dockray, G., Rehfeld, J.F., Brownstein, M., and Cuello, A.C. (1983). Evidence of periaqueductal cholecystokinin-substance P neurons projecting to the spinal cord. *Neuroscience.* **3,** 1151–1158.

Sora, I., Takahashi, N., Funada, M., Ujike, H., Revay, R.S., Donovan, D.M., Miner, L.L., and Uhl, G.R. (1997). Opiate receptor knockout mice define μ receptor roles in endogenous nociceptive responses and morphine-induced analgesia. *Proc. Natl. Acad. Sci. U.S.A.* **94,** 1544–1549.

Stanfa, L., Dickenson, A., Xu, X.J., and Wiesenfeld-Hallin, Z. (1994). Cholecystokinin and morphine analgesia: Variations on a theme. *Trends Neurosci.* **15,** 65–66.

Stein, C., Cabot, P.J., and Schäfer, M. Peripheral opioid analgesia – Mechanisms and clinical applications. Chapter 5 this volume.

Stevens, C.W., Lacey, C.B., Miller, K.E., Elde, R.P., and Seybold, V.S. (1991). Biochemical characterization and regional quantification of mu, delta and kappa opioid binding sites in rat spinal cord. *Brain Res.* **550,** 77–85.

Stevens, C.W., and Seybold, V.S. (1995). Changes in opioid binding density in the rat spinal cord following unilateral dorsal rhizotomy. *Brain Res.* **687,** 53–62.

Stiller, R.U., Grubb, B.D., and Schaible, H.G. (1993). Neurophysiological evidence for increased kappa opioidergic control of spinal cord neurons in rats with unilateral inflammation of the ankle. *Eur. J. Neurosci.* **5,** 1520–1527.

Suarez-Roca, H., Abdullah, L., Zuniga, J., Madison, S., and Maixner, W. (1992). Multiphasic effect of morphine on the release of substance P from trigeminal nucleus slices. *Brain Res.* **579,** 187–194.

Suarez-Roca, H., and Maixner, W. (1992a). Morphine produces a multiphasic effect on the release of substance P from rat trigeminal nucleus slices by activating different opioid receptor subtypes. *Brain Res.* **576,** 195–203.

Suarez-Roca, H., and Maixner, W. (1992b). δ-Opioid-receptor activation by [D-Pen^2, D-Pen^5] enkephalin and morphine inhibits substance P release from trigeminal nucleus slices. *Eur. J. Pharmacol.* **229,** 1–7.

Suarez-Roca, H., and Maixner, W. (1993). Activation of kappa opioid receptors by U50488H and morphine enhances the release of substance P from rat trigeminal nucleus slices. *J. Pharmacol. Exp. Ther.* **264,** 648–653.

Suarez-Roca, H., and Maixner, W. (1995). Morphine produces a biphasic modulation of substance P release from cultured dorsal root ganglion neurons. *Neurosci. Lett.* **194,** 41–44.

Sumal, K.K., Pickel, V.M., Miller, R.J., and Reis, D.J. (1982). Enkephalin-containing neurons in substantia gelatinosa of trigeminal complex: Ultrastructure and synaptic interaction with primary sensory afferents. *Brain Res.* **248,** 223–236.

Sweetnam, P.M., Wrathall, J.R., and Neale, J.H. (1986). Localization of dynorphin gene product-immunoreactivity in neurons from spinal cord and dorsal root ganglia. *Neuroscience.* **18,** 947–955.

Tang, J., Chou, J., Iadarola, M., Yang, H.Y.T., and Costa, E. (1984). Proglumide prevents and curtails acute tolerance to morphine in rats. *Neuropharmacology.* **23,** 715–718.

Vanderhaegen, J.J., Deschepper, C., Lostra, F., and Schonen, J. (1982). Immunocytochemical evidence for cholecystokinin-like peptides in neuronal cell bodies of the rat spinal cord. *Cell Tissue Res.* **223,** 463–467.

Weihe, E. (1992). Neurochemical anatomy of the mammalian spinal cord: Functional implications. *Ann. Anat.* **174,** 89–118.

Weihe, E., Millan, M.J., Höllt, V., Nohr, D., and Herz, A. (1989). Induction of the gene encoding pro-dynorphin by experimentally induced arthritis enhances staining for dynorphin in the spinal cord of rats. *Neuroscience.* **31,** 77–95.

Weihe, E., Nohr, D., and Hartschuh, W. (1988). Immunohistochemical evidence for a co-transmitter role of opioid peptides in primary sensory neurons. *Prog. Brain Res.* **74,** 189–199.

Willcokson, W.S., Chung, J.M., Hori, Y., Lee, K.H., and Willis, W.D. (1984). Effects of iontophoretically released peptides on primate spinothalamic tract cells. *J. Neurosci.* **4,** 741–750.

Yaksh, T.L. (1997). Pharmacology and mechanisms of opioid analgesic activity. *Acta Anaesthesiol. Scand.* **41,** 94–111.

Yaksh, T.L., and Elde, R.P. (1981). Factors governing release of methionine enkephalin-like immunoreactivity from mesencephalon and spinal cord of the cat in vivo. *J. Neurophysiol.* **46,** 1056–1075.

Yaksh, T.L., Jessell, T.M., Gamse, R., Mudge, A.W., and Leeman, S.E. (1980). Intrathecal morphine inhibits substance P release from mammalian spinal cord in vivo. *Nature.* **286,** 155–157.

Yoshimura, M., and North, R.A. (1983). Substantia gelatinosa neurons hyperpolarized in vitro by enkephalin. *Nature.* **305,** 529–530.

Young, W.S., Wamsley, J.K., Zarbin, M.A., and Kuhar, M.J. (1980). Opioid receptors undergo axonal flow. *Science.* **210,** 76–78.

Yu, L.C., Hansson, P., and Lundeberg, T. (1995). Opioid antagonists naloxone, beta-funaltrexamine and naltrindole, but not nor-binaltorphimine, reverse the increased hindpaw withdrawal latency in rats induced by intrathecal administration of the calcitonin gene-related peptide antagonist CGRP8–37. *Brain Res.* **698,** 23–29.

Zachariou, V., and Goldstein, B.D. (1996a). Kappa-opioid receptor modulation of the release of substance P in the dorsal horn. *Brain Res.* **706,** 80–88.

Zachariou, V., and Goldstein, B.D. (1996b). δ-Opioid receptor modulation of the release of substance P-like immunoreactivity in the dorsal horn of the rat following mechanical or thermal noxious stimulation. *Brain Res.* **736,** 305–314.

Zadina, J.E., Hackler, L., Ge, L.J., and Kastin, A.J. (1997). A potent and selective endogenous agonist for the μ-opiate receptor. *Nature.* **386,** 499–502.

Zajac, J.M., Lombard, M.C., Peschanski, M., Besson, J.M., and Roques, B.P. (1989). Autoradiographic study of μ and δ opioid binding sites and neutral endopeptidase-24–11 in rat after dorsal root rhizotomy. *Brain Res.* **477,** 400–403.

Zerari, F., Zouaoui, D., Gastard, M., Apartis, E., Fischer, J., Herbrecht, F., Cupo, A., Cucumel, K., and Conrath, M. (1994). Ultrastructural study of δ-opioid receptors in the dorsal horn of the rat spinal cord using monoclonal anti-idiotypic antibodies. *J. Chem. Neuroanat.* **7,** 159–170.

Zhang, X., Dagerlind, A., Elde, R.P., Catel, M.N., Broberger, C., Wiesenfeld-Hallin, Z., and Hökfelt, T. (1993). Marked increase in cholecystokinin B receptor messenger RNA levels in rat dorsal root ganglia after peripheral axotomy. *Neuroscience,* **57,** 227–233.

Zhou, Y., Sun, Y.H., Zhang, Z.W., and Han, J.S. (1993). Increased release of immunoreactive cholecystokinin octapeptide by morphine and potentiation of μ-opioid analgesia by CCKB receptor antagonist L-365,260 in rat spinal cord. *Eur. J. Pharmacol.* **234,** 147–154.

Zieglgänsberger, W., and Tulloch, I.F. (1979). The effects of methionine- and leucine-enkephalin on spinal neurones of the cat. *Brain Res.* **167,** 53–64.

Zouaoui, D., Benoliel, J.J., Cesselin, F., and Conrath, M. (1991). Cholecystokinin-like immunoreactivity in the rat spinal cord: Effects of thoracic transection. *Brain Res. Bull.* **26,** 543–547.

Zouaoui, D., Benoliel, J.J., Conrath, M., and Cesselin, F. (1990). Cholecystokinin-like immunoreactivity in the dorsal horn of the rat spinal cord: An attempt to analyse contradictory results between immunocytochemistry and radioimmunoassay. *Neuropeptides.* **17,** 177–185.

CHAPTER FIVE

Peripheral Opioid Analgesia: Mechanisms and Clinical Implications

CHRISTOPH STEIN, PETER J. CABOT, AND MICHAEL SCHAFER

Introduction

In contrast to the traditional view that opioid antinociception is mediated exclusively within the central nervous system, peripheral opioid receptors have been discovered and shown to mediate analgesic effects when activated by locally applied exogenous opioid agonists. Such effects are particularly prominent in painful inflammatory conditions and have been demonstrated in both animals and humans (Barber and Gottschlich, 1992; Stein, 1995). Opioid receptors are present on peripheral sensory nerves and are up-regulated during the development of inflammation. Their endogenous ligands, opioid peptides, are expressed in resident immune cells within peripheral inflamed tissue. Environmental stimuli (stress) and releasing agents (corticotropin-releasing factor, cytokines) can liberate these opioid peptides to elicit local analgesia, and suppression of the immune system abolishes these effects. These findings have led to the concept that endogenous opioid peptides can be secreted from immunocytes, occupy opioid receptors on sensory nerves, and produce analgesia by inhibiting either the excitability of these nerves or the release of excitatory, proinflammatory neuropeptides. This chapter summarizes the discoveries that led to the formulation of this concept and discusses therapeutic implications resulting therefrom.

Peripheral Analgesic Effects of Exogenous Opioids

The basis for the concept just described has emerged from animal experiments investigating local analgesic actions of opioids in peripheral tissues. Interestingly, almost all of these studies have used models of inflammation. In those models exogenous opioid agonists produce potent local antinociception. Different strategies have been used to exclude central effects – for example, compounds that do not cross the blood-brain barrier (Chang et al., 1996) or the local versus systemic application of equivalent doses of agents (Stein, 1993; Stein et al., 1997). Rigorous criteria such as reversibility by standard opioid antagonists (e.g., naloxone), dose dependency, and stereospecificity have been applied to demonstrate the opioid receptor-specificity of these peripheral effects.

Christoph Stein, ed., *Opioids in Pain Control: Basic and Clinical Aspects*. Printed in the United States of America.

The comparison of agonists with differing affinities for the three types of opioid receptors (μ, δ, κ) has shown that ligands with a preference for μ receptors are generally the most potent, but δ and κ ligands are active as well. Considering the different characteristics of the various inflammatory models, it is conceivable that, depending on the nature and stage of the inflammatory reaction, different types of local opioid receptors become active. Thus, depending on the particular circumstances, all three receptor types can be present and functionally active in peripheral tissues (for details, see Stein, 1993).

Peripheral Opioid Receptors

Early studies have produced evidence for opioid binding in the dorsal root ganglion and on central terminals of primary afferent neurons (LaMotte et al., 1976). More recently, opioid receptors were demonstrated on peripheral sensory nerve terminals in rats (Stein et al., 1990; Hassan et al., 1993) and humans (Stein et al., 1996) (Fig. 5.1). Pharmacologic experiments indicate that the characteristics of these receptors are very similar to those in the brain (Hassan et al., 1993). The advent of opioid receptor cloning (Gavériaux-Ruff and Kieffer, Chap. 1 this volume) has made it possible to generate specific antisera to identify μ, δ, and κ opioid receptors in the dorsal root ganglia and on small-diameter primary afferent nerve fibers (Ji et al., 1995; Zhang et

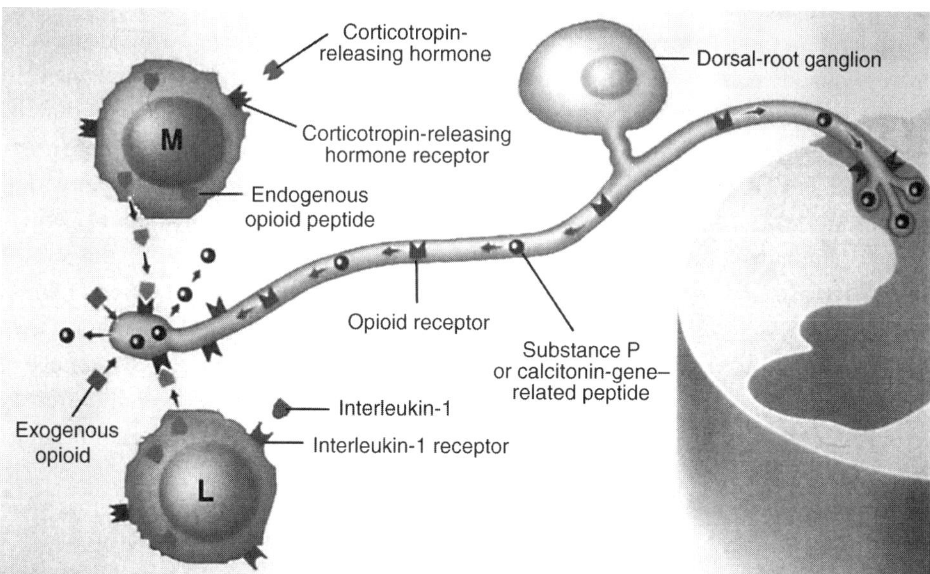

Figure 5.1. A primary afferent sensory neuron with its cell body situated in the dorsal root ganglion. Opioid receptors are transported toward its central (right) and peripheral (left) terminals. After stimulation with IL-1 or corticotropin-releasing-hormone, opioid peptides are released from monocytic cells (M) or lymphocytes (L). Occupation of the neuronal opioid receptors by these endogenous or exogenous ligands decreases the release of excitatory (proinflammatory) neuropeptides (e.g., substance P or calcitonin–gene-related peptide) and reduces the excitability of the primary afferent neuron.

al., 1996). In line with these findings are in vivo studies indicating that capsaicin-sensitive primary afferents indeed mediate the peripheral antinociceptive effects of morphine (Bartho et al., 1990) and of μ-, δ-, and κ-selective agonists (Zhou et al., 1998).

What are the mechanisms leading to antinociception following the activation of such neuronal opioid receptors? Opioids increase potassium and decrease calcium and sodium currents in the soma of dorsal root ganglion sensory neurons through interactions with G-proteins (G_i and/or G_o) (see references in Stein, 1995; Stein et al., 1997; Gavériaux-Ruff and Kieffer, Chap. 1 this volume). Provided that these events are similar throughout the neuron, they may underlie the following observations: Opioids attenuate the excitability of the peripheral nociceptive terminal and the propagation of action potentials (Russell et al., 1987; Andreev et al., 1994). Similar to their effects at the soma and at central terminals (Cesselin et al., Chap. 4 this volume), opioids inhibit the (calcium-dependent) release of excitatory proinflammatory compounds (e.g., substance P) from peripheral sensory nerve endings (Brodin et al., 1983; Yaksh, 1988). In addition, morphine has been shown to inhibit the transmitter release from sympathetic varicosities and the antidromic vasodilatation evoked by stimulation of C-fibers. The latter mechanisms may also account for opioid anti-inflammatory and antiarthritic actions (see references in Barber and Gottschlich, 1992; Stein et al., 1997).

Inflammation and Peripheral Opioid Receptors

Peripheral antinociceptive effects of exogenous opioids are enhanced under inflammatory conditions (for review, see Stein, 1993). One possible underlying mechanism for the increased efficacy of agonists is an up-regulation – that is, an increased number of receptors. Opioid receptors are synthesized in the dorsal root ganglion (Mansour et al., 1994; Schäfer et al., 1995). Axonal transport is responsible for delivering macromolecules from the cell body to nerve terminals. After the induction of peripheral inflammation, the axonal transport of opioid receptors in fibers of the sciatic nerve is greatly enhanced (Hassan et al., 1993; Jeanjean et al., 1995). Subsequently, the density of opioid receptors on cutaneous nerve fibers in the inflamed tissue increases, and this increase is abolished by ligating the sciatic nerve (Hassan et al., 1993). These findings indicate that inflammation enhances the peripherally directed axonal transport of opioid receptors, which leads to an increase in their number (up-regulation) on peripheral nerve terminals (Fig. 5.1).

In addition, pre-existent, but possibly inactive, neuronal opioid receptors may undergo changes owing to the specific milieu (e.g., low pH) of inflamed tissue and thus be rendered active. Indeed, low pH increases opioid agonist efficacy in vitro by altering the interaction of opioid receptors with G-proteins in neuronal membranes (Selley et al., 1993). Furthermore, the ability of opioids to decrease the excitability of primary afferent neurons (via inhibition of adenylyl cyclase and subsequent inhibition of cation currents) is much more pronounced when neuronal cyclic AMP levels are increased, a common scenario in inflammation (Ingram and Williams, 1994).

Finally, opioid agonists have easier access to neuronal opioid receptors because inflammation entails a disruption of the perineurium (a normally rather impermeable barrier sheath encasing peripheral nerve fibers) (Antonijevic et al., 1995) and because the number of peripheral sensory nerve terminals is increased in inflamed tissue, a phenomenon known as "sprouting" (Hassan et al., 1992).

Apart from the involvement of primary afferent neurons, evidence suggests that opioid receptors on sympathetic postganglionic neurons may contribute to peripheral opioid antinociception (Taiwo and Levine, 1991). In addition, opioid binding sites and the expression of opioid receptor transcripts have been conclusively demonstrated in immune cells (Gavériaux et al., 1995). Opioid-mediated modulation of the proliferation of these cells and of several of their functions (e.g., chemotaxis, superoxide production, and mast cell degranulation) has been reported (Sibinga and Goldstein, 1988; Bryant and Holaday, 1993). These immunomodulatory actions can be stimulatory as well as inhibitory and have been ascribed to the activation of opioid receptors on these cells. However, the significance of those effects with regard to nociception has not yet been investigated.

In summary, the available evidence indicates that opioid receptors on peripheral terminals of primary afferent nerves can mediate potent antinociceptive effects. Activation of these receptors inhibits excitability, action potential propagation, and release of excitatory proinflammatory neuropeptides. These phenomena are analogous to those occurring after activation of presynaptic opioid receptors on central sensory nerve terminals in the dorsal spinal cord (Cesselin et al., Chap. 4 this volume). The analogy to the situation in the spinal cord raises questions as to the origin and location of the endogenous agents activating this system in peripheral tissues.

Peripheral Endogenous Opioid Peptides

Opioid peptides are the natural ligands at opioid receptors. Three families of these peptides are well characterized in the central nervous and neuroendocrine systems. Each family derives from a distinct gene and precursor protein, namely, pro-opiomelanocortin (POMC), proenkephalin (PENK), and prodynorphin. Appropriate processing yields their respective major representative opioid peptides β-endorphin (β-END), enkephalin (ENK), and dynorphin (DYN). Each peptide exhibits different affinities and selectivities for the three opioid receptor types, μ, δ, and κ (Roques, Noble, and Fournié-Zaluski, Chap. 2 this volume).

Immune Cells

Initial studies in search of opioid peptides in the vicinity of the peripheral receptors produced evidence for immunoreactive β-END and ENK within immune cells in inflamed subcutaneous tissue (Weihe et al., 1988; Stein et al., 1990). However, the issue of whether immune cells are capable of synthesizing opioid peptides – that is, whether the genes of precursor peptides are expressed and appropriately translated – has been a subject of controversy (Sibinga and Goldstein, 1988; Sharp and Linner, 1993; Sharp and Yaksh, 1997). Blalock and Smith (1980) were the first to demonstrate POMC-derived peptides in immunocytes. Since then, POMC-related opioid peptides have been found in normal immune cells of different species, including humans (Stein et al., 1997). To determine whether these immune-competent cells synthesize POMC, rather than simply absorb related peptides from plasma, messenger ribonucleic acid (mRNA)-encoding POMC was sought and was demonstrated in many of these studies (Stein et al., 1997). Some of those cells, mostly from normal organisms, contain POMC mRNA molecules that are about 200–400 nucleotides shorter than the full-length POMC mRNA (c. 1,200 nucleotides) found in the pituitary and hypothalamus (the classical loci for production of POMC-derived peptides) (Stein et al., 1997). This finding has raised doubts about whether this shortened mRNA species is translated into functional POMC protein. However, as pointed out in a recent editorial (Sharp and Linner, 1993), the situation is apparently very different under pathologic conditions. For example, elevated levels of splenic POMC mRNA and β-END have been reported in polyarthritic rats, and virus-infected or tumor-derived immune cells were found to express a full-length POMC mRNA transcript (Stein et al., 1997).

Proenkephalin-derived opioid peptides have been detected in human and rodent immune cells (reviewed in Weisinger, 1995). Upon in vitro stimulation or under pathologic conditions these cells express enhanced levels of PENK mRNA, probably as a result of the induction of transcription factors (e.g., NF-κB) and the subsequent activation of the preproenkephalin promoter (Weisinger, 1995). In subpopulations of these cells this mRNA is highly homologous to brain PENK mRNA, abundant and apparently translated, because immunoreactive ENK is present and/or released (Zurawski et al., 1986; Weisinger, 1995). The appropriate enzymes necessary for post-translational processing of POMC and PENK have also been identified in immune cells. In addition, extracellular processing may be involved in generating opioid-active PENK products (see references in Stein et al., 1997).

In summary, a growing body of evidence indicates that immune cells produce both POMC- and PENK-derived opioid peptides (Fig. 5.1), but that the specific conditions of the local microenvironment may be of crucial importance for the characteristics and release of these peptides (Sharp and Linner, 1993; Sharp and Yaksh, 1997). Studies in a rat model of unilateral localized paw inflammation have yielded evidence consistent with this notion. Persistent inflammation is a pathophysiologic in vivo stimulus for the immune system and represents a condition that is closer to the clinical setting than some of the early in vitro studies. In this model mRNAs encoding POMC and PENK and their respective opioid peptide products β-END and ME are found in inflamed but not in noninflamed tissue (Przewlocki et al., 1992). Histomorphologic (Weihe et al., 1988; Stein et al., 1990) and double-staining procedures (Przewlocki et al., 1992; Cabot et al., 1997) have identified the opioid-containing cells as lymphocytes (predominantly memory T-cells) and monocytic cells. Small amounts of DYN are also detectable (Hassan et al., 1992). These findings indicate that local signals stimulate the synthesis of opioid peptides in different types of inflammatory cells at the site of tissue injury. Recent findings in synovial tissue from patients with arthritis confirm this notion (see "Clinical Implications" later in this chapter).

Other Sources

The classical loci for opioids in the periphery are the adrenals and the pituitary, but these have been excluded as sources of opioid ligands at peripheral receptors (Parsons et al., 1990). Opioid peptides have also been detected in sensory ganglia (Botticelli et al., 1981) and in peripheral terminals of sensory nerves (Weihe et al., 1985; Hassan et al., 1992). Interestingly, Frank and Sudha (1987) have proposed opioid receptors located on the inner surface of the cell membranes of peripheral nerve fibers where opioids produced within the neuron may modulate the excitability of its own axon. These findings suggest an "autoregulatory" role of nociceptor-derived opioid peptides, but to date direct functional evidence is lacking.

Interaction of Immune-Derived Opioids and Peripheral Opioid Receptors

Initial studies examining the interaction of peripheral opioid receptors and opioid peptides have used a model of stress (cold-water swim) to activate endogenous opioid systems (Stein et al., 1990). Following the cold-water swim, nociceptive thresholds increase selectively in inflamed tissue, and this effect is mediated by peripheral opioid receptors (Parsons et al., 1990; Stein et al., 1990). Moreover, this effect is abolished by antibodies against opioid peptides and by immunosuppression (Stein, Gramsch, and Herz, 1990; Stein, Hassan et al., 1990; Przewlocki et al., 1992). Together, these findings suggest that peripheral opioid receptors can mediate local antinociception following their activation by opioids released from immune cells during stress.

The identification of the exact mechanisms and stimuli for opioid secretion within inflamed tissue has only recently begun. Corticotropin-releasing factor (CRF) is a major physiologic secretagogue for opioid peptides in the pituitary (Fig. 5.1). Its releasing effects are potentiated by interleukin-1 (IL-1), and IL-1 (and other cytokines) can stimulate β-END release directly (see references in Stein et al., 1997). Receptors for each of these agents are present on immune cells and are up-regulated within inflamed tissue (Fig. 5.1) (Mousa et al., 1996). In cultured leukocytes, both CRF and IL-1 can stimulate release of β-END (Heijnen et al., 1991). In vivo, the local application of small, systemically inactive doses of CRF, IL-1, and other cytokines produces potent antinociceptive effects in inflamed but not in noninflamed tissue (Czlonkowski et al., 1993; Schäfer et al., 1994). These effects are reversible by immunosuppression, by passive immunization with antibodies against opioid peptides, and by opioid antagonists. Furthermore, short-term incubation with CRF or IL-1 can release β-END in immune cell suspensions prepared from lymph nodes in vitro (Schäfer et al., 1994; Cabot et al., 1997). This release is specific to CRF and IL-1 receptors, is calcium dependent, and is mimicked by elevated extracellular concentrations of potassium. This finding is consistent with a regulated pathway of release from secretory vesicles, as in neurons and endocrine cells (Cabot et al., 1997). In summary, these findings indicate that CRF and cytokines can cause secretion of opioids from immune cells, which subsequently activate opioid receptors on sensory nerves to inhibit nociception. The most important endogenous secretagogue appears to be locally produced CRF, because endogenous (stress-induced) analgesia in inflamed tissue is abolished when the synthesis of CRF in inflamed tissue is blocked by antisense oligodeoxynucleotides or when antagonists and antibodies against CRF are administered locally (Schäfer et al., 1996).

A final important aspect is the pharmacokinetics of this interaction. How do immune cell-derived opioid peptides reach their receptors on sensory neurons? This question is not trivial because, under normal circumstances, tight intercellular contacts at the innermost layer of the perineurium act as a diffusion barrier for high molecular weight or hydrophilic substances such as peptides. This barrier preserves homeostasis in the endoneurial tissue embedding peripheral neurons and continues up to the peripheral endings of afferent somatic and autonomic nerve fibers (Olsson, 1990). An exception is noncorpuscular nerve endings, a subgroup of somatic afferents, which terminate either within the perineurium or lack the perineurium at their very tips. Opioid receptors are located not only at the tips of afferent nerve terminals but also more proximally along the axon (Frank, 1985; Stein et al., 1990; Hassan et al., 1993). These loci are clearly ensheathed by perineurium (Olsson, 1990) and are potential sites of opioid action. Inflammatory conditions entail a deficiency of the perineurial barrier and/or an enhanced permeability of endoneurial capillaries. A similar leakage can be produced experimentally by the extraneural application of hyperosmolar solutions (Olsson, 1990) Recent studies have shown that peripheral opioid analgesia and perineurial disruption coincide during very early stages of an inflammatory reaction and that both can be induced by increasing the osmolarity in normal subcutaneous tissue (Antonijevic, 1995). Moreover, inflammatory or artificial disruption of the perineurium greatly facilitates the passage of opioid peptides and other macromolecules to sensory neurons (Antonijevic, 1995). These observations indicate an unrestricted transperineurial passage of peptides in inflammation, which is integral for the direct communication of immune cell–derived endogenous opioid peptides with sensory nerves.

Clinical Implications

Exogenous Opioids

Are peripheral opioid mechanisms of significance in the clinical setting? A growing body of literature concerns the analgesic efficacy of exogenous opioids outside the central nervous system (reviewed in Stein, 1995; Viel et al., 1996; Kalso et al., 1997; Stein et al., 1997). To test opioid actions in the vicinity of peripheral sensory nerve terminals, many studies have examined the intra-articular application of small doses (0.5–6 mg) of morphine during knee surgery (reviewed in Stein et al., 1997; Kalso et al., 1997). The effects on postoperative pain were evaluated by various direct (visual analog scale, numerical rating scale, verbal scales) or indirect (supplemental analgesic consumption, time to first supplemental analgesic requirement) parameters. The great majority of these trials have reported significant analgesic effects demonstrated by at least one of the measures just mentioned. These effects were shown to be opioid receptor specific (Stein et al., 1991), of similar potency to those of conventional local anesthetics (Khoury et al., 1992), and surprisingly long lasting (Khoury, Chen et al., 1992; Stein, Helmke et al., 1996; Likar, Schäfer et al., 1997). To confirm a peripheral site of action, equal doses of morphine were administered systemically as a control (Stein et al., 1991) or plasma levels of morphine were measured (Stein et al., 1997). The former were ineffective, and the latter were found to be much lower than those generally accepted as necessary for central analgesic actions. The reasons for the long duration of these peripheral opioid actions are unclear at present, but may include a low blood flow to the knee joint, morphine's low lipid solubility and its consequent slow absorption into the circulation, opioid anti-inflammatory actions (Barber and Gottschlich, 1992), or pre-emption of central sensitization (Woolf and Bromley, Chap. 11 this volume).

Other modes of peripheral opioid administration studied include the perineural (e.g., in ankle or axillary blocks) (Viel et al., 1996), intraperitoneal, and interpleural routes (Schulte-Steinberg et al., 1995). Although the number of studies is still small, most of the results are encouraging (Viel et al., 1996). Reasons for the lack of peripheral analgesia in some studies may be that, in contrast to receptors at the nerve terminals, proximal axonal opioid receptors are "in transit" (Hassan et al., 1993) and not integrated into the neuronal membrane (i.e., nonfunctional), or that opioid receptors are not easily accessible in noninflamed tissue because the perineurium is intact (see "Inflammation and Peripheral Opioid Receptors" earlier in this chapter).

Endogenous Opioids

Opioid receptors are present on peripheral terminals of nerve fibers in human synovia (Stein et al., 1996). The fact that intra-articular naloxone antagonizes the effect of locally applied morphine (Stein et al., 1991) indicates that these receptors are capable of mediating analgesia in humans. In search of the endogenous ligands, we examined inflamed synovial tissue from patients undergoing arthroscopic knee surgery. We found opioid peptides (mainly β-END and ME) in synovial lining cells and in immune cells such as lymphocytes, macrophages, and mast cells (Stein et al., 1993; Stein et al., 1996). We examined the interaction of synovial opioids with peripheral opioid receptors in patients undergoing knee surgery. Blocking of intra-articular receptors by the local administration of the antagonist naloxone resulted in significantly increased postoperative pain. This pain-enhancing effect was demonstrated by subjective measures as well as by increased supplemental analgesic requirements (Stein et al., 1993). Taken together, these findings suggest that in a stressful (e.g., postoperative) situation, opioids are tonically released from inflamed tissue and activate peripheral opioid receptors to attenuate clinical pain.

Interestingly, these endogenous opioids do not interfere with exogenous morphine – that is, intra-articular morphine is an equally potent analgesic in patients with and without opioid-producing inflammatory synovial cells (Stein et al., 1996). This finding suggests that, in contrast to the rapid development of tolerance in the central nervous system (Cox, Chap. 6 this volume), the immune cell–derived opioids do not produce cross-tolerance to morphine at peripheral opioid receptors. This finding is at variance with animal experiments that have used exogenous agonists to produce tolerance at peripheral opioid receptors in noninflamed tissue (Aley et al., 1995). This inconsistency raises questions as to whether tolerance development is different at central versus peripheral opioid receptors and in inflamed versus noninflamed tissue. Clarification of these issues is important for the use of peripherally acting opioids to treat chronic pain in arthritis and other inflammatory conditions (Stein et al., 1996; Likar et al., 1997).

Summary

Many experimental and clinical trials have demonstrated the analgesic efficacy of small, systemically inactive doses of exogenous opioids administered in the vicinity of peripheral nerve terminals. Opioid receptors are present on those nerve terminals, and endogenous opioid peptides are detectable in inflamed tissue of animals and humans. These peptides are found in cells of the immune system and produce endogenous inhibition of pain. Thus, it appears that peripheral opioid receptors can modulate sensory nerve impulses in a way similar to that of spinal presynaptic opioid receptors.

Melzack and Wall (1965) originally proposed that activation of the first central transmission cells in the dorsal horn marks the beginning of the sequence of intrinsic antinociceptive activities that occur when the body sustains damage. Evidently, this is only one possible mechanism. Intrinsic pain inhibition can be achieved even earlier through the attenuation of afferent sensory nerve activity at the peripheral end by immune-derived opioid peptides. Thus, the selection and filtering of incoming information is not restricted to the brain and spinal cord but also occurs in the periphery through an interaction of the immune and sensory nervous systems.

These findings have several interesting implications: (1) The local application not only of exogenous opioids but also of enzyme inhibitors preventing the degradation of endogenous opioid peptides (Roques et al., Chap. 2 this volume) provides a new perspective for pain management by producing analgesia without central side effects such as dysphoria, respiratory depression, sedation, nausea, or addiction. (2) The fact that such local opioid actions are particularly prominent in inflamed tissue is possibly an advantage considering that the most subacute or chronic painful conditions are associated with inflammation (e.g., postoperative pain, cancer pain, arthritis). (3) In addition to their immunologic functions, immunocytes are involved in intrinsic mechanisms of pain inhibition. This finding provides new insights into pain associated with a compromised immune system, as in AIDS or cancer. Furthermore, the activation of opioid production and release from immune cells may be a novel approach to the development of peripherally acting analgesics.

REFERENCES

Aley, K.O., Green, P.G., and Levine, J.D. (1995). Opioid and adenosine peripheral antinociception are subject to tolerance and withdrawal. *J. Neurosci.* **15**(12), 8031–8038.

Andreev, N., Urban, L., and Dray, A. (1994). Opioids suppress spontaneous activity of polymodal nociceptors in rat paw skin induced by ultraviolet irradiation. *Neuroscience.* **58,** 793–798.

Antonijevic, I., Mousa, S.A., Schäfer, M., and Stein, C. (1995). Perineurial defect and peripheral opioid analgesia in inflammation. *J. Neurosci.* **15**(1), 165–172.

Barber, A., and Gottschlich, R. (1992). Opioid agonists and antagonists: An evaluation of their peripheral actions in inflammation. *Med. Res. Rev.* **12,** 525–562.

Bartho, L., Stein, C., and Herz, A. (1990). Involvement of capsaicin-sensitive neurones in hyperalgesia and enhanced opioid antinociception in inflammation. *Naunyn Schmiedeberg's Arch. Pharmacol.* **342,** 666–670.

Blalock, J.E., and Smith, E.M. (1980). Human leukocyte interferon: Structural and biological relatedness to adrenocortical hormone and endorphins. *Proc. Natl. Acad. Sci. U.S.A.* **77,** 5972–5974.

Botticelli, L.J., Cox, B.M., and Goldstein, A. (1981). Immunoreactive dynorphin in mammalian spinal cord and dorsal root ganglia. *Proc. Natl. Acad. Sci. U.S.A.* **78,** 7783–7786.

Brodin, E., Gazelius, B., Panopoulos, P., and Olgart, L. (1983). Morphine inhibits substance P release from peripheral sensory nerve endings. *Acta Physiol. Scand.* **117,** 567–570.

Bryant, H.U., and Holaday, J.W. (1993). Opioids in immunologic processes. In *Opioids II: Handbook of experimental pharmacology,* vol 104/II, ed. A. Herz. Berlin: Springer-Verlag, pp. 551–570.

Cabot, P.J., Carter, L., Gaiddon, C., et al. (1997). Immune cell-derived β-endorphin: Production, release and control of inflammatory pain in rats. *J. Clin. Invest.* **100,** 142–148.

Chang, A.-C., Cowan, A., Takemori, A.E., and Portoghese, P.S. (1996). Aspartic acid conjugates of 2-(3,4-Dichlorophenyl)-N-methyl-N-[(1S)-1-(3-aminophenyl)-2-(1-pyrrolidinyl)ethyl]acetamide: κ Opioid receptor agonists with limited access to the central nervous system. *J. Med. Chem.* **39,** 4478–4482.

Czlonkowski, A., Stein, C., and Herz, A. (1993). Peripheral mechanisms of opioid antinociception in inflammation: Involvement of cytokines. *Eur. J. Pharmacol.* **242,** 229–235.

Frank, G.B. (1985). Stereospecific opioid receptors on excitable cell membranes. *Can. J. Physiol. Pharmacol.* **63,** 1023–1032.

Frank, G.B., and Sudha, T.S. (1987). Effects of enkephalin, applied intracellularly, on action potentials in vertebrate A and C nerve fibre axons. *Neuropharmacology.* **26,** 61–66.

Gavériaux, C., Peluso, J., Simonin, F., Laforet, J., and Kieffer, B. (1995). Identification of κ- and δ-opioid receptor transcripts in immune cells. *FEBS Lett.* **369,** 272–276.

Hassan, A.H.S., Ableitner, A., Stein, C., and Herz, A. (1993). Inflammation of the rat paw enhances axonal transport of opioid receptors in the sciatic nerve and increases their density in the inflamed tissue. *Neuroscience.* **55,** 185–195.

Hassan, A.H.S., Przewlocki, R., Herz, A., and Stein, C. (1992). Dynorphin, a preferential ligand for kappa-opioid receptors, is present in nerve fibers and immune cells within inflamed tissue of the rat. *Neurosci. Lett.* **140,** 85–88.

Heijnen, C.J., Kavelaars, A., Ballieux, R.E. (1991). β-Endorphin: Cytokine and neuropeptide. *Immunol. Rev.* **119,** 41–63.

Ingram, S.L., and Williams, J.T. (1994). Opioid inhibition of Ih via adenylyl cyclase. *Neuron.* **13,** 179–186.

Jeanjean, A.P., Moussaoui, S.M., Maloteaux, J.-M., and Laduron, P.M. (1995). Interleukin-1β induces long-term increase of axonally transported opiate receptors and substance P. *Neuroscience.* **68**(1), 151–157.

Ji, R.-R., Zhang, Q., Law, P.-Y., Low, H.H., Elde, R., and Hökfelt, T. (1995). Expression of μ-, δ-, and κ-opioid receptor-like immunoreactivities in rat dorsal root ganglia after carrageenan-induced inflammation. *J. Neurosci.* **15**(12), 8156–8166.

Kalso, E., Tramer, M.R., Carroll, D., McQuay, H.J., and Moore, R.A. (1997). Pain relief from intra-articular morphine after knee surgery: A qualitative systematic review. *Pain.* **71,** 127–134.

Khoury, G.F., Chen, A.C.N., Garland, D.E., and Stein, C. (1992). Intraarticular morphine, bupivacaine and morphine/bupivacaine for pain control after knee videoarthroscopy. *Anesthesiology.* *77,* 263–266.

LaMotte, C., Pert, C.B., and Snyder, S.H. (1976). Opiate receptor binding in primate spinal cord: Distribution and changes after dorsal root section. *Brain Res.* **112,** 407–412.

Likar, R., Schäfer, M., Paulak, F., et al. (1997). Intraarticular morphine analgesia in chronic pain patients with osteoarthritis. *Anesth. Analg.* **84,** 1313–1317.

Mansour, A., Fox, C.A., Thompson, R.C., Akil, H., and Watson, S.J. (1994). Mu-opioid receptor mRNA expression in the rat CNS: Comparison to mu-receptor binding. *Brain Res.* **643,** 245–265.

Melzack, R., and Wall, P.D. (1965). Pain mechanisms: A new theory. *Science.* **150,** 971–973.

Mousa, S.A., Schäfer, M., Mitchell, W.M., Hassan, A.H.S., and Stein, C. (1996). Local upregulation of corticotropin-releasing hormone and interleukin-1 receptors in rats with painful hindlimb inflammation. *Eur. J. Pharmacol.* **311,** 221–231.

Olsson, Y. (1990). Microenvironment of the peripheral nervous system under normal and pathological conditions. *Crit. Rev. Neurobiol.* **5**(3), 265–311.

Parsons, C.G., Czlonkowski, A., Stein, C., and Herz, A. (1990). Peripheral opioid receptors mediating antinociception in inflammation. Activation by endogenous opioids and role of the pituitary-adrenal axis. *Pain.* **41,** 81–93.

Przewlocki, R., Hassan, A.H.S., Lason, W., Epplen, C., Herz, A., and Stein, C. (1992). Gene expression and localization of opioid peptides in immune cells of inflamed tissue. Functional role in antinociception. *Neuroscience.* **48,** 491–500.

Russell, N.J.W., Schaible, H.G., and Schmidt, R.F. (1987). Opiates inhibit the discharges of fine afferent units from inflamed knee joint of the cat. *Neurosci. Lett.* **76,** 107–112.

Schäfer, M., Carter, L., and Stein, C. (1994). Interleukin-1β and corticotropin-releasing-factor inhibit pain by releasing opioids from immune cells in inflamed tissue. *Proc. Natl. Acad. Sci. U.S.A.* **91,** 4219–4223.

Schäfer, M., Imai, Y., Uhl, G.R., and Stein, C. (1995). Inflammation enhances peripheral μ-opioid receptor-mediated analgesia, but not μ-opioid receptor transcription in dorsal root ganglia. *Eur. J. Pharmacol.* **279,** 165–169.

Schäfer, M., Mousa, S.A., Zhang, Q., Carter, L., and Stein, C. (1996). Expression of corticotropin-releasing factor in inflamed tissue is required for intrinsic peripheral opioid analgesia. *Proc. Natl. Acad. Sci. U.S.A.* **93,** 6096–6100.

Schulte-Steinberg, H., Weninger, E., Jokisch, D., et al. (1995). Intraperitoneal versus interpleural morphine or bupivacaine for pain after laparoscopic cholecystectomy. *Anesthesiology.* **82,** 634–640.

Selley, D.E., Breivogel, C.S., and Childers, S.R. (1993). Modification of G protein-coupled functions by low pH pretreatment of membranes from NG108–15 cells: Increase in opioid agonist efficacy by decreased inactivation of G proteins. *Mol. Pharmacol.* **44,** 731–741.

Sharp, B., and Linner, K. (1993). Editorial: What do we know about the expression of pro-opiomelanocortin transcripts and related peptides in lymphoid tissue? *Endocrinology.* **133**(5), 1921A–1921B.

Sharp, B., and Yaksh, T. (1997). Pain killers of the immune system. *Nature Medicine.* **3**(8), 831–832.

Sibinga, N.E.S., and Goldstein, A. (1988). Opioid peptides and opioid receptors in cells of the immune system. *Annu. Rev. Immunol.* **6,** 219–249.

Stein, A., Helmke, K., Szopko, C., Stein, C., and Yassouridis, A. (1996). Intraartikuläre Morphin- versus Steroidapplikation bei Gonarthrose und Arthritis im akut schmerzhaften Gelenk [letter]. *Dtsch. Med. Wschr.* **8,** 255.

Stein, C. (1993). Peripheral mechanisms of opioid analgesia. *Anesth. Analg.* **76,** 182–191.

Stein, C. (1995). The control of pain in peripheral tissue by opioids. *N. Engl. J. Med.* **332**(25), 1685–1690.

Stein, C., Comisel, K., Haimerl, E., et al. (1991). Analgesic effect of intraarticular morphine after arthroscopic knee surgery. *N. Engl. J. Med.* **325,** 1123–1126.

Stein, C., Gramsch, C., and Herz, A. (1990). Intrinsic mechanisms of antinociception in inflammation. Local opioid receptors and β-endorphin. *J. Neurosci.* **10,** 1292–1298.

Stein, C., Hassan, A.H.S., Lehrberger, K., Giefing, J., and Yassouridis, A. (1993). Local analgesic effect of endogenous opioid peptides. *Lancet.* **342,** 321–324.

Stein, C., Hassan, A.H.S., Przewlocki, R., Gramsch, C., Peter, K., and Herz, A. (1990). Opioids from immunocytes interact with receptors on sensory nerves to inhibit nociception in inflammation. *Proc. Natl. Acad. Sci. U.S.A.* **87,** 5935–5939.

Stein, C., Pflüger, M., Yassouridis, A., et al. (1996). No tolerance to peripheral morphine analgesia in presence of opioid expression in inflamed synovia. *J. Clin. Invest.* **98,** 793–799.

Stein, C., Schäfer, M., Cabot, P.J., et al. (1997). Peripheral opioid analgesia. *Pain Rev.* **4,** 171–185.

Taiwo, Y.O., and Levine, J.D. (1991). Kappa- and delta-opioids block sympathetically dependent hyperalgesia. *J. Neurosci.* **11,** 928–932.

Viel, E.J., Bruelle, P., Lalourcey, L., and Eledjam, J.J. (1996). Perineural administration of opioids in combination with local anaesthetics. In *Highlights in pain therapy and regional anaesthesia V,* ed. A. Van Zundert. Barcelona: Permanyer, pp. 235–240.

Weihe, E., Hartschuh, W., and Weber, E. (1985). Prodynorphin opioid peptides in small somatosensory primary afferents of guinea pig. *Neurosci. Lett.* **58,** 347–352.

Weihe, E., Nohr, D., Millan, M.J., et al. (1998). Peptide neuroanatomy of adjuvant-induced arthritic inflammation in rat. *Agents and Actions.* **25,** 255–259.

Weisinger, G. (1995). The transcriptional regulation of the preproenkephalin gene. *Biochem. J.* **307,** 617–629.

Yaksh, T.L. (1988). Substance P release from knee joint afferent terminals: Modulation by opioids. *Brain Res.* **458,** 319–324.

Zhang, Q., Schäfer, M., and Stein, C. (1996). Effect of capsaicin on the expression of cloned opioid receptors in dorsal root ganglia. *Soc. Neurosci. Abstr.* **22/3**(3), 2004.

Zhou, L., Zhang, Q., Stein, C., and Schäfer, M. (in press). Contribution of opioid receptors on primary afferent versus sympathetic neurons to peripheral opioid analgesia. *J. Pharmacol. Exp. Ther.*

Zurawski, G., Benedik, M., Kamp, B.J., Abrams, J.S., Zurawski, S.M., and Lee, F.D. (1986). Activation of mouse T-helper cells induces abundant preproenkephalin mRNA synthesis. *Science* **232,** 772–775.

CHAPTER SIX

Mechanisms of Tolerance

BRIAN M. COX

Introduction

Accumulating evidence indicates that many neurons or neuronal systems adapt to chronic receptor activation by the expression of compensating mechanisms. These compensating mechanisms can take the form of a reduced sensitivity of the receptor through which the agonist acts (homologous desensitization), a reduced sensitivity of co-expressed receptors that serve similar functional roles (heterologous desensitization), and a change in the functions of effector systems to compensate for the persistent activation of one class of receptors. Each of these mechanisms has been observed in some circumstances following chronic exposure of cells or whole animals to morphine and other opiate drugs. All these processes may play a role in opiate drug tolerance, but their relative contributions will probably vary in different situations. Furthermore, the physiologic environment in which opiate drugs act may vary with time in ways that will influence the sensitivity of the system to opiates.

Altered Drug Metabolism in Opiate Tolerance

Chronic exposure to drugs like alcohol (ethanol) or barbiturates may lead to an increased metabolism of the drug and thus to a reduced pharmacologic effect, but there is little evidence of drug-induced changes in the metabolism of morphine and related drugs of sufficient magnitude to account for the level of tolerance that can be observed during chronic morphine treatment. Morphine is partially metabolized to an active metabolite, morphine-6-glucuronide, and this metabolite may contribute in part to the analgesic actions of morphine in vivo (Paul et al., 1989). To date there are no reports that the 6-glucuronidation of morphine is modified in morphine tolerance, but to the extent that the 6-glucuronide is more potent than morphine itself as an analgesic, some changes in the analgesic actions of morphine might be induced by alterations in the extent of its glucuronidation in the 6 position. It should be noted that the other glucuronidation products of morphine, morphine 3-glucuronide and morphine 3,6 diglucuronide, are not analgesic since they can no longer interact with

Christoph Stein, ed., *Opioids in Pain Control: Basic and Clinical Aspects*. Printed in the United States of

opioid receptors. These 3-glucuronide products are the primary metabolites of morphine in humans.

Noxious Stimulus Intensity and Opioid Tolerance

Opiate drugs are used therapeutically to treat conditions in which moderate or severe pain occurs. The pathologic processes underlying the pain are often progressing conditions, and the patient may also be receiving treatments designed to reverse the pathology causing pain. Thus, the level of activation of nociceptor neurons as a result of the pathology is potentially variable; that is, the stimulus for which the pain-relieving drug is given is not constant. The stimulus may increase and decrease during the course of one day or over periods of many months. Such changes in noxious stimulus intensity provide a moving baseline against which the effectiveness of analgesic drugs must be evaluated. Some patients show no apparent tolerance to moderate doses of morphine over significant periods of time; others report a declining level of relief from pain during opiate therapy over a relatively short time period (Foley, 1991; and see review by Colpaert, 1996, for a discussion of opioid tolerance in animal models of chronic pain). In such cases it is difficult to discern the factors involved in the loss of sensitivity to the drug. Reduced drug effect might result from a tolerance to the drug induced by prior drug treatment, but it might equally result from a progression in the pain-inducing pathology. Therefore, very careful attention to the progression of the disease is required to determine the extent to which tolerance to opiates occurs in the clinical environment.

Studies in healthy laboratory animals using an experimentally controlled acute noxious stimulus to assess the antinociceptive effects of drugs are less likely to be influenced by changes in the intensity of the noxious stimulus, but they may not provide good models of clinical conditions for which the drugs are ultimately intended. In recent years, the use of neuronal cell preparations in culture has been valuable in exposing potential adaptive responses to chronic drug administration at a molecular and cellular level, but such studies are even further removed from the clinical environment. Ultimately, the results of studies using each type of approach must be employed to understand the range of adaptive changes induced by chronic exposure to opiate drugs.

The following sections summarize current knowledge concerning the major adaptive processes induced by chronic opiate drug exposure.

Homologous Tolerance: Changes in Opioid Receptor Function and Amount

Several lines of evidence suggest that under certain circumstances impaired function of the receptor through which the tolerance-inducing drug produces an initial effect is a major component of opioid tolerance. In vivo studies of tolerance to the analgesic effects of morphine in rats, in which very high degrees of tolerance were generated by the use of a progressive regimen of multiple morphine pellet implantations, yielded morphine dose-response curves that were progressively shifted to the right, and with higher doses the maximum obtainable response was reduced (Bläsig et al., 1979). This pattern of dose-response curve shifts suggests a progressive loss of functional receptors similar to the effects of irreversible inactivation of receptors by alkylating agents. These and other studies from this time period suggested that chronic exposure to an opiate agonist in some way selectively impaired the function of the receptor through which the acute effects of the drug were mediated.

In parallel with these in vivo and isolated tissue studies, a cell line expressing opiate receptors became available. The NG 108–15 neuroblastoma X glioma hybrid cell developed by Sharma, Nirenberg, and Klee (1975) selectively expresses the δ class of opioid receptor. Activation of this receptor inhibits the activity of the enzyme adenylate cyclase. Morphine is not a potent agonist at this receptor type, but chronic exposure of NG 108–15 cells to a high concentration of morphine was shown to induce a loss of sensitivity to opiates. Perhaps more significantly, an increase in the activity of adenylyl cyclase was noted after removal of morphine from the system (Sharma, Klee, and Nirenberg, 1975). Mechanisms associated with the loss of opioid sensitivity in NG 108–15 cells were explored in more detail by Law et al. (1982). They used metabolically stable enkephalin analogs or the potent opiate drug etorphine as agonists to induce tolerance, since, unlike morphine, these agents behaved as full agonists at the δ receptors in NG 108–15 cells. Chronic exposure of NG 108–15 cells to etorphine led to a profound loss of opioid inhibition of adenylyl cyclase. Law et al. (1982) showed that at least two mechanisms were implicated in this effect. Loss of the ability of the agonist-occupied receptor to activate the inhibitory guanine nucleotide-binding transduction protein G_i, and thus to inhibit adenylyl cyclase, occurred within an hour of agonist exposure, at a time when the number of receptors that could be detected on the cell surface was not reduced. Only after longer exposure to a full agonist, was there also a significant reduction in the number of receptors that could be occupied by opiate receptor ligands. Thus, two processes were identified: an initial loss of receptor function (called desensitization) and a later loss of receptor protein from the cell surface (described as receptor down-regulation). Subsequent studies have demonstrated similar adaptive effects in μ-type opioid receptors in pituitary tumor cells in culture (Puttfarcken et al., 1989) and in human neuroblastoma SHSY5Y cells (Prather et al., 1994). The cloning of the δ, μ, and κ classes of opioid receptors eventually made it possible to transfect these receptors into cells not normally expressing them. Receptor desensitization and down-regulation have now been observed with each type of cloned opioid receptor after chronic agonist exposure (Blake et al., 1997; Chakrabarti et al., 1997; Kavoor et al., 1997).

The mechanism underlying the loss of opioid receptor function has been further studied by several groups. An initial event appears to be an uncoupling of the receptor from its associated GTP-binding protein (G-protein)–mediated transduction pathway (Law et al., 1982, Puttfarcken et al., 1989). Agonist occupation of an opioid receptor reduces the affinity for GDP of receptor-associated G-protein molecules, permitting endogenous GTP to bind to the transiently unoccupied nucleotide-binding site on the G-protein. This process can be studied by observing the opioid agonist–induced stimulation of binding of a labeled GTP analog, ^{35}S[GTPγS] (Traynor and Nahorski, 1995; Selley et al., 1997). Tolerance to the stimulation of ^{35}S[GTPγS] binding by both μ and δ receptors develops rapidly, indicating that an early adaptive response to chronic agonist exposure occurs in the interaction of the receptor and associated G-proteins (Breivogel et al., 1997; Elliott, Guo, and Traynor, 1997). These results are fully consistent with the earlier proposals by Law et al. (1982) and Puttfarcken et al. (1989) that the first event in opioid-agonist induced loss of opioid sensitivity is a functional uncoupling of the agonist-occupied receptor from its transduction system.

Functional uncoupling is followed fairly rapidly by a relocation of the receptor from the plasma membrane. Sternini et al. (1996), in studies of the opiate-sensitive myenteric plexus neurons of guinea pig, have shown that administration of etorphine for 30 minutes or longer resulted in the relocation of μ opioid receptor protein from the plasma membrane to intracellular cytoplasmic vesicles, suggesting that etorphine induced a translocation of the receptor protein to the interior of the cell. This effect was prevented or reversed by prior or subsequent administration of the opiate antagonist naloxone, indicating that receptor occupation by etorphine was required. Morphine did not itself induce internalization, but was able to reduce etorphine-induced internalization. The mechanism of internalization is still being studied; initial results suggest a role for receptor phosphorylation. Studies on cloned δ receptors stably expressed in 293 human embryonic kidney cells indicate that agonist-induced δ-receptor desensitization is associated with a threefold increase in receptor phosphorylation (Pei et al., 1995). Delta receptors in these cells can be phosphorylated by protein kinase C (PKC) and by β-adrenergic receptor kinase (β-ARK). Down-regulation of PKC did not reduce opiate agonist-induced phosphorylation of δ receptors, but co-expression of a dominant negative mutant form of β-ARK significanly reduced agonist-dependent phosphorylation, suggesting that β-ARK was critically involved in δ receptor desensitization in these cells (Pei et al., 1995). Recently, Kavoor et al. (1997) used reconstitution experiments in *Xenopus* oocytes to show that β-ARK and β-arrestin are critical factors in the agonist-induced down-regulation of μ and δ opioid receptors expressed in this system. Finally, Trapaidze et al. (1996) have reported that a C-terminal region of the δ opioid receptor sequence containing several Ser and Thr phosphorylation sites is critical for agonist-induced receptor internalization. They also found that δ receptor internalization is much reduced by agents that block the formation of clathrin-coated pits in the cell membrane, suggesting that opioid receptor internalization is mediated via the well-defined clathrin-dependent endocytotic pathway. These results suggest that opioid receptors behave like other G-protein–coupled receptors in their response to chronic agonist exposure

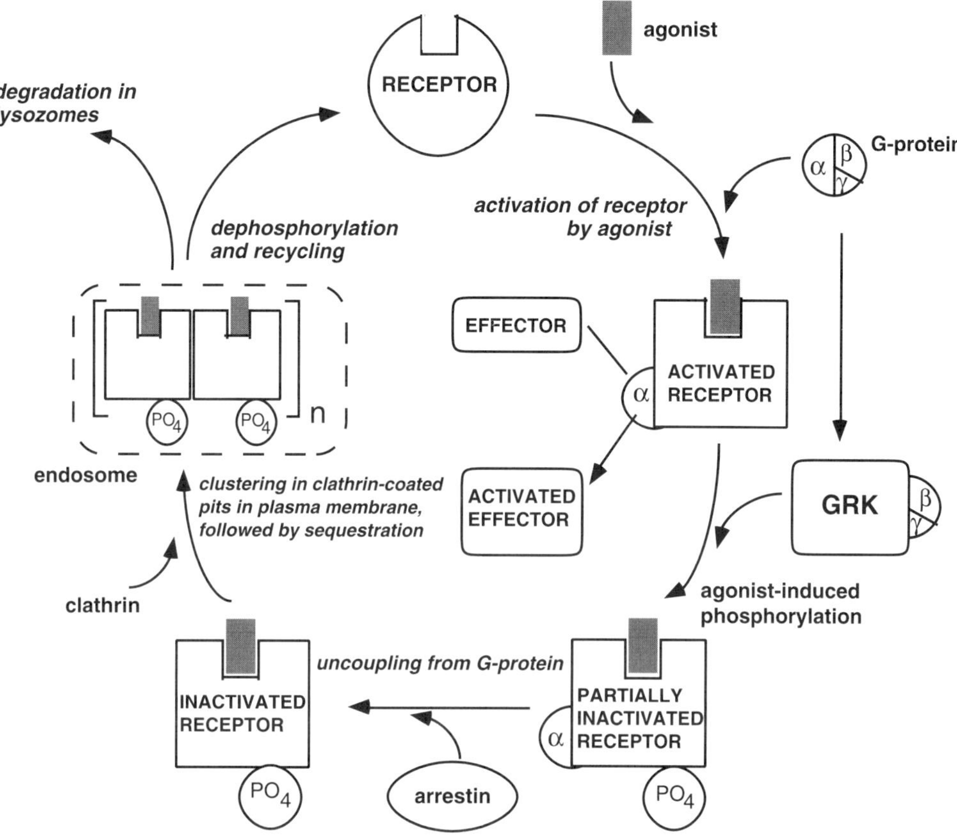

Figure 6.1. A schematic representation of the steps presumed to be involved in homologous desensitization of opioid receptors and in receptor internalization and down-regulation, based on the model developed by Lefkowitz and colleagues (Inglese et al., 1993) for β-adrenoceptor desensitization (see Chuang et al., 1996, for a brief review). Receptors occupied by opioid agonist interact with G-proteins to activate their effector system(s). At the same time, an associated G-protein–coupled receptor kinase (GRK) is activated, probably by the liberated G-protein βγ subunits; this enzyme preferentially phosphorylates agonist-occupied G-protein–coupled receptors, leading to a partial but not complete loss of receptor-mediated activation of G-protein. However, the phosphorylated receptor can now bind arrestin, which results in complete inactivation of the receptor, and leads to receptor clustering and internalization. Internalized receptors are recycled after dephosphorylation (with no resulting reduction in receptor number) or are degraded in lysozomes (receptor own-regulation; i.e., a reduction in the number of receptors expressed by the cell).

and suggest that the processes of desensitization and down-regulation are similar to those originally proposed for β-adrenergic receptors (see review by Chuang et al., 1996). A schematic outlining the mechanism by which homologous desensitization and down-regulation of opioid receptors might occur is presented in Figure 6.1.

It should be noted, however, that it has been difficult to demonstrate μ receptor down-regulation in vivo following chronic morphine treatments inducing significant tolerance. In a few studies using very intense chronic morphine treatments, a modest degree of receptor down-regulation has been observed (e.g., Werling et al., 1989). However, others have found that morphine treatment regimens inducing significant tolerance do not reduce the number of μ receptors in brain (e.g., Dum et al., 1979) or in guinea pig myenteric plexus neurons (Sternini et al., 1996). A chronic morphine treatment inducing significant tolerance and physical dependence has also been shown not to alter the levels of μ or δ receptor mRNAs in selected regions of rat brain (Buzas et al., 1996). These results make it likely that other processes play a more important role in tolerance to morphine in vivo. Whereas more efficacious agents at μ receptors (e.g., etorphine, opioid peptides) can induce μ receptor down-regulation, this is probably not critical to the occurrence of loss of opioid effect after chronic agonist treatments. Delta opioid receptor down-regulation may occur more readily in vivo than μ receptor down-regulation. Several years ago, Steece et al. (1986) reported a reduction in δ receptor binding after repeated intraventricular injections of Met-enkephalin, and Tao et al. (1988) reported a down-regulation of δ receptors in rat forebrain structures after chronic intraventricular administration of a synthetic enkephalin analog. However, intepretation of these results is complicated by the use of labeled agonists to measure receptor number, since uncoupled receptors that are still present in the membrane display very low affinity for agonists. Recently Narita et al. (1997) noted that recovery of the spinal antinociceptive actions of δ_2 opioid agonists after chronic exposure to the same agonists is significantly delayed if the mice are treated with an antisense oligonucleotide to δ receptor mRNA, suggesting that recovery from this type of tolerance requires the synthesis of new δ receptors.

Overall, these studies suggest that a loss of the ability of agonist-occupied receptor to activate G proteins is an important early event in opiate tolerance. Full agonists may, in addition, cause removal of the receptor from the cell surface, but by this time opioid sensitivity has already been substantially lost.

Efficacy and Tolerance

The degree of observed tolerance after a chronic opiate drug treatment is related to the efficiency of receptor activation both of the drug used to induce tolerance and the agent used to determine the sensitivity to the opiate drug after treatment. It is now well established that in most experimental situations a greater degree of tolerance is observed if opiate sensitivity is evaluated with a partial agonist (e.g., morphine) than with a full agonist (e.g., the very potent opiates etorphine or sufentanil) (Saeki and Yaksh, 1993). This is fully understandable in the light of the evidence discussed earlier that chronic opiate receptor activation results in a reduction in the number of functional receptors, both as a result of desensitization (uncoupling) of receptors and of receptor down-regulation. Since partial agonists must occupy a greater fraction of the available pool of functional receptors than full agonists to activate an equivalent number of receptors (and thus to induce a response of similar magnitude), a reduction in the number of functional receptors results in a greater increase in the required fractional occupancy for partial agonists than for full agonists. Experimental studies suggest that a chronic treatment with a partial agonist will also induce more tolerance than chronic treatment with a full agonist when dosage regimens initially producing equivalent analgesia are used, irrespective of whether the opioid sensitivity is determined with a full or partial agonist (Saeki and Yaksh, 1993). It should be pointed out, however, that chronic treatments with full agonists can result in a substantial reduction in opioid receptor numbers (particularly at δ-type receptors), whereas partial agonists generally do not significantly reduce the number of receptors during an in vivo chronic exposure (e.g., Sternini et al., 1996). Thus, when a high-dose regimen of opiate full agonist is used, receptor down-regulation may play a significant role in the level of observed tolerance; recovery of analgesic responsiveness will in part be dependent on the synthesis of new receptor protein. In contrast, chronic treatment with a partial opioid agonist is unlikely to induce down-regulation; recovery of opioid sensitivity will now require reversal of the desensitization process (perhaps by dephosphorylation). This process may occur more rapidly than synthesis of new receptors.

Heterologous Tolerance

Early studies using the guinea pig ileum preparation (summarized by Johnson and Flemming, 1989) demonstrated that opiate drugs induce a heterologous form of tolerance in the guinea pig myenteric plexus. Tolerance to morphine was accompanied by tolerance to other inhibitory agents, although there was often supersensitivity to stimulatory agents. Recent studies have confirmed that heterologous tolerance is also induced in the central nervous system by chronic opiate treatment (Table 6.1). Thus, Nestby et al. (1995) observed that morphine treatment can result in loss of function at dopamine D_2 receptors in rat striatum. This result was confirmed by Noble and Cox (1997), who showed that chronic morphine treatment (morphine is predominantly a μ receptor agonist) also desensitized δ opioid receptors in rat striatum. These studies analyzed neural systems not obviously involved in pain regulation, but heterologous tolerance is also clearly manifest in pain pathways. A recent very complete study by Aley and Levine (1997) reported that bidirectional cross tolerance is observed between μ–opioid, α_2-adrenergic, and A_1-adenosine receptors in primary afferent neurons. Heterologous tolerance is probably a common consequence of sustained or repeated activation of opioid receptors. However, activation of nonopioid receptors in opioid receptor–expressing neurons may also lead to a loss of function of co-expressed opioid receptors.

Several mechanisms have been proposed to account for opioid-induced heterologous tolerance. In the examples just noted, the bidirectional tolerance among δ and dopamine D_2 receptors in striato-pallidal neurons (Noble and Cox, 1997), or among the μ, α_2, and A_1 receptors in primary afferent neurons (Aley and Levine, 1997), the

Table 6.1. *Recently Reported Examples of Heterologous Tolerance Induced by Chronic Opioid Exposure*

Heterologous Adaptations	System	References
Intermittent morphine treatment induces dopamine D_2 receptor desensitization	Rat striatum	Nestby et al., 1995
Delta opioid receptor agonists induce desensitization of D_2 receptors	SK-N-BE human neuroblastoma cells	Namir et al., 1997
Chronic morphine treatment induces δ opioid and D_2 receptor desensitization	Rat caudate-putamen and nucleus accumbens	Noble and Cox, 1997
Bidirectional cross tolerance among μ, α_2, and A_1 receptors mediating antinociceptive responses	Rat spinal cord	Aley and Levine, 1997

affected receptors all utilize the guanine nucleotide-binding proteins G_i and or G_o in their transduction pathway. It remains to be determined whether a common pool of G-proteins is available to each of these co-localized receptors, or whether each receptor interacts with a unique group of closely associated G-proteins. Whatever the local stochiometry, it is possible that G-protein receptor–coupled kinases (GRKs; i.e., enzymes like β-ARK that preferentially phosphorylate agonist-occupied G-protein–coupled receptors), activated by chronic activation of one receptor type, rapidly desensitize adjacent heterologous receptors (Fig. 6.2). It is not clear whether this requires agonist occupation of the heterologous receptor. It is very likely that at any particular time in vivo a fraction of heterologous co-expressed receptors is occupied by endogenous ligands as a result of a low tonic release of endogenous agonists. However, it is also possible that under some circumstances GRKs can phosphorylate receptors not occupied by agonists. A basal level of G-protein activation in the absence of agonists has been observed with some of these receptor types, as indicated by the ability of selected antagonists to induce a reduction of basal GTPase activity below "baseline" levels in the absence of agonist; that is, the antagonist behaves as an inverse agonist (Costa et al., 1989). This suggests that even in the absence of agonist these receptor types may transiently adopt a conformation which can activate G-proteins. In this transient conformation, these receptors may become substrates for GRKs.

G-protein–coupled receptors may also be desensitized by heterologous receptor-mediated activation of protein kinase A (PKA), PKC, or calmodulin-dependent protein kinases (Mestek et al., 1995; Pei et al., 1995; Fig. 6.2). Since opiates do not usually activate PKC or other kinases, this is not likely to be the major mechanism by which opiate drugs induce heterologous desensitization, but agonists at other receptors might desensitize opioid receptors by this mechanism.

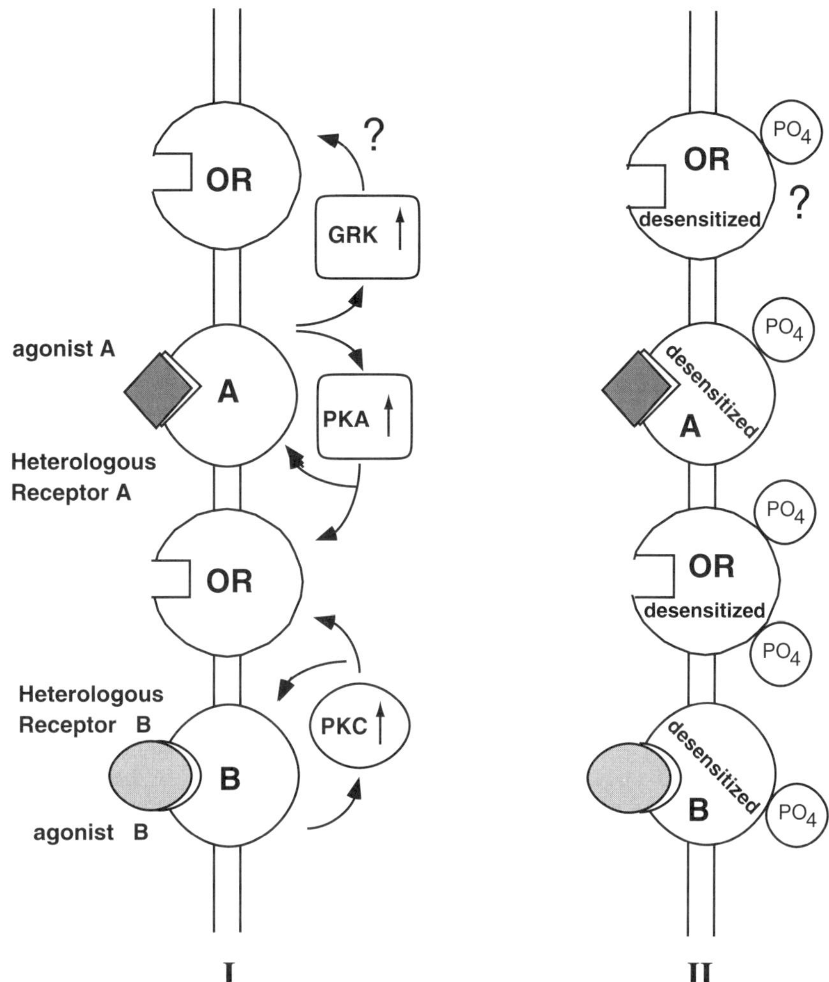

Figure 6.2. Potential roles of kinases in heterologous receptor desensitization. Opioid receptors have been shown to be less efficient at activating transduction systems after phosphorylation by PKA or PKC (Pei et al., 1995; Chuang et al., 1996). Thus, in principle, activation of receptors activating PKA or PKC (column 1) can desensitize opioid receptors expressed in the same cells by phosphorylation of the receptor (column 2). Opioid-receptor activation usually inhibits PKA activity and probably does not change PKC activity. It is unlikely, therefore, that activation of PKA or PKC activation plays any role in homologous desensitization. However, these enzymes might modify opioid-receptor function if they are activated through heterologous receptors (receptors A or B). Heterologous desensitization also results from activation of nonopioid G-protein–coupled inhibitory receptors (Noble and Cox, 1997). It is possible (although not yet demonstrated) that G-protein–coupled receptor kinases (GRK), hyperactivated through heterologous receptors, might under some circumstances phosphorylate and desensitize opioid receptors even though the opioid receptors are not occupied by agonist (e.g., if at any given time a fraction of nonoccupied receptors are transiently in the agonist-occupied conformation). Alternatively, heterologous desensitization of opioid receptors might occur if a heterologously induced elevation of GRK activity coincides with a low tonic level of receptor occupation by endogenous opioids. (Abbreviations: GRK = G-protein–coupled receptor kinase; OR = opioid receptor; PKA = protein kinase A; PKC = protein kinase C.)

Opioid agonists usually inhibit adenylyl cyclase activity and thus will reduce PKA activation, making it unlikely that PKA is involved in opioid-induced heterologous desensitization. However, some forms of adenylyl cyclase can be activated by opioids. Recent studies by Avidor-Reiss et al. (1997) have shown that adenylyl cyclase types II, III, and VII can be stimulated by opioids. It is thus possible that in neurons expressing these forms of adenylyl cyclase, activation of opioid receptors might lead to a PKA-mediated heterologous desensitization of all co-expressed receptor forms that are sensitive to PKA-mediated phosphorylation. It remains to be determined if these opiate-activated adenylyl cyclases are expressed in neurons also expressing opioid receptors. Withdrawal from chronic exposure to opioids has also been shown to induce a superactivation of those adenylyl cyclase forms that are inhibited by opioids; types I, V, VI, and VIII (Sharma, Klee, and Nirenberg, 1975; Avidor-Reiss et al.,1997). The mechanism of this superactivation is still unknown. However, adenylyl cyclase superactivation, with concomitant activation of PKA and induction of PKA-mediated heterologous receptor desensitization, may well occur during opiate withdrawal. The importance of the specific effector system coupled to opioid receptors in the degree of heterologous tolerance expressed as a result of chronic opiate treatment is indicated by the observation by Kaneko et al. (1997) that in *Xenopus* oocytes expressing μ and κ opioid receptors regulating N-type calcium channels, activation of either receptor type leads to a heterologous tolerance at both opioid receptors, with the extent of desensitization being critically dependent on the specific isoform of calcium channel expressed in the oocyte.

PKA activation or inhibition may also have indirect effects on receptor expression. Thus, in NG 108–15 cells, PKA activation has been shown to reduce the levels of mRNA for δ opioid receptors, leading to a reduction in the level of receptor protein by about 50% (Buzas et al., 1996). Although the mechanisms underlying this action are not understood, it is probable that expression of the δ receptor gene is in part under the control (direct or indirect) of PKA-regulated transcription factors. There are other examples of heterologous regulation of the expression of receptor mRNAs. Alvaro et al. (1996) have shown that morphine treatment down-regulates the expression of melanocortin-4 (MCR-4) receptors in striatum and periaqueductal gray regions of rat brain. They suggest that since α-MSH, an endogenous ligand for MCR-4 receptors, antagonizes the development of morphine tolerance, the down-regulation of MCR-4 receptors may play a role in opioid tolerance. Alterations in gene expression as a consequence of sustained opioid exposure are discussed further in the next section.

The importance of the neural context in which receptor activation occurs in determining whether heterologous desensitization results from chronic drug treatment is suggested by recent studies by Noble and Cox (1997). Chronic morphine treatment of rats induced a heterologous desensitization of dopamine D_2 and δ opioid receptors in striato-pallidal neurons, but in the same animals did not induce μ receptor tolerance in the striato-nigral pathway. It is possible that tolerance was not evoked in the striato-nigral pathway because the morphine treatment induced a coincident-sustained activation of these neurons through dopamine D_1 receptors. A hypothetical explanation of the different consequences of chronic morphine treatment on the striato-nigral and striato-pallidal pathways is presented in Figure 6.3. This study suggests that the extent of heterologous tolerance is determined by the overall pattern of receptor and second messenger systems activated within a neuronal pathway; transynaptic activity is clearly an important determinant of the extent of desensitization in in vivo systems. It is likely that more instances of heterologous receptor tolerance during chronic opiate exposure will be identified in the future in view of the numerous mechanisms that may result in reduced function of heterologous receptors.

Postreceptor Adaptations

Although homologous and heterologous desensitization contributes to tolerance to the actions of opiate drugs, the role of receptor desensitization in the expression of dependence on opiate drugs (in which the continued activation of opioid receptors by an agonist is required to prevent the onset of withdrawal symptoms) is not clear. The most probable explanation of opiate withdrawal is that neurons adapt to sustained opioid receptor activation by a series of compensatory changes altering the activity both of systems directly affected by the acute actions of the opiate drug and of systems that can produce effects which oppose the acute actions of the opiate. To the extent that the compensatory adaptation directly opposes the acute actions of opiate receptor activation, a tolerance to opiate drug action will be observed. When the opiate drug is withdrawn, these adaptive responses will decay to the basal state; but if the adaptive response in a system opposing opiate acute effects persists beyond the duration of acute action of the residual opiate drug, the compensatory response will be observed as a hyperactivity of the affected system. This hyperactivity is manifested as a withdrawal or abstinence symptom. The intensity of the withdrawal syndrome will be related to the extent of adaptive changes induced by the opiate drug treatment; its duration will be affected principally by the rate at which the altered process reverts to its baseline state after drug withdrawal. If the adaptation involves the increased expression of a functional protein, its reversion to the baseline level will be at a rate determined by the degradation or inactivation of the induced protein. However, this rate of recovery from dependence will also be influenced by the rate of removal of the tolerance-inducing drug if the rate of elimination of this drug is comparable to or slower than the rate of recovery of the adaptive responses induced by the drug treatment. In fact, it appears that there are numerous adaptive responses, and the relative importance of each may vary under different conditions and in different neuronal populations. The rate of recovery from the dependent state is therefore probably determined by a weighted average of the decay rates for many adaptive processes as well as by the rate of removal of the drug from the body. A

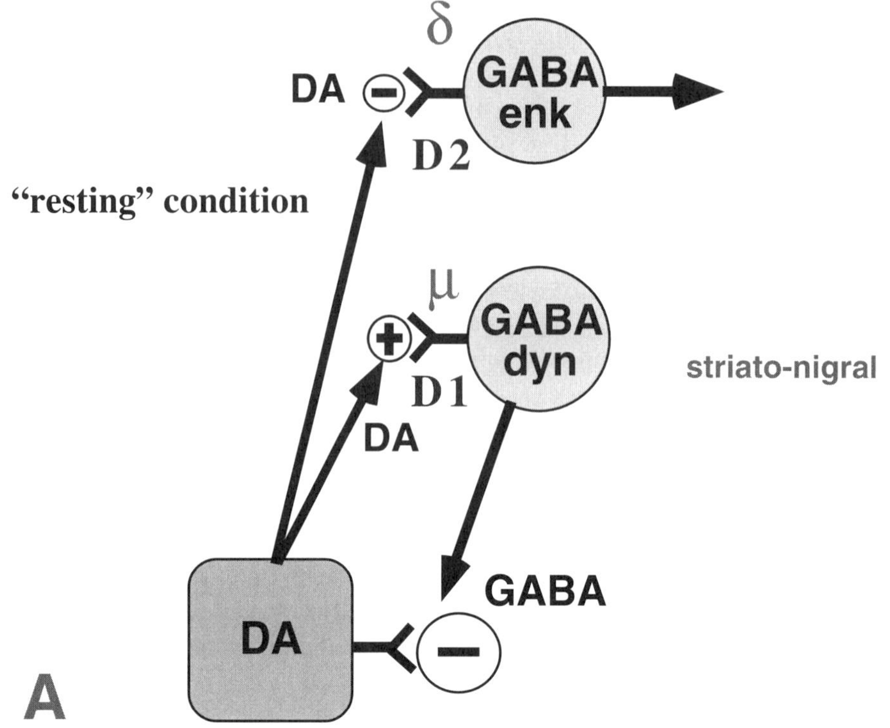
striato-pallidal
δ
DA
GABA
enk
D2
"resting" condition
μ
GABA
dyn
striato-nigral
D1
DA
GABA
DA
A

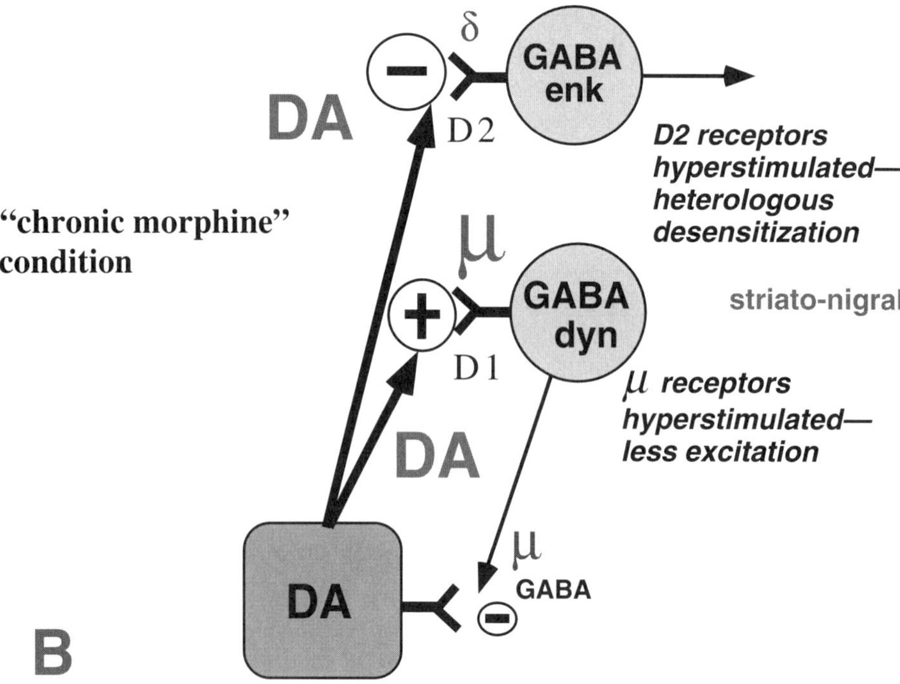
striato-pallidal
δ
GABA
enk
DA
D2
D2 receptors
hyperstimulated—
heterologous
desensitization
"chronic morphine"
condition
μ
GABA
dyn
striato-nigral
D1
μ receptors
hyperstimulated—
less excitation
DA
μ
GABA
DA
B

summary of the kinetics of the immediate and longer-term adaptive processes induced by chronic treatments is shown in Figure 6.4.

Specific adaptive processes are only slowly being identified. One of the first adaptations to be noted was the observation that chronic morphine exposure induces superactivation of adenylyl cyclase (Sharma, Klee, and Nirenberg, 1975; Avidor-Reiss et al., 1996). This adaptation both reduces the sensitivity to opiate drug-mediated inhibition of adenylyl cyclase and renders cAMP-regulated intracellular systems hyperactive when the opiate drug is withdrawn. In this example, the adaptive response clearly occurs in the neural population that also expresses the opioid receptor. The phenomenon was first observed in a homogeneous population of neuroblastoma-glioma hybrid cells (Sharma, Klee, and Nirenberg, 1975), although it has also been observed in discrete brain nuclei after chronic opiate treatment (reviewed by Nestler, 1996). Another example in which the adaptation appears to be in the opiate-sensitive neuron is the apparent change in Na^+/K^+ ATPase activity in myenteric neurons induced by morphine treatment (Johnson and Flemming, 1989). With reduced electrogenic pumping by the enzyme, a modest increase in intracellular sodium leads to a slight reduction in membrane potential and thus to reduced sensitivity to hyperpolarizing agents (heterologous tolerance) and increased sensitivity to depolarizing stimuli (manifest as withdrawal contractions when the opiate drug is withdrawn). In other cases in which opiate-induced adaptive responses have been observed, it may not be

---

Opposite

Figure 6.3. Hypothetical mechanism underlying the heterologous desensitization of dopamine D_2 and δ opioid receptors in caudate-putamen by chronic morphine treatment. Chronic treatment of rats with morphine induces a heterologous desensitization of δ opioid and dopamine D_2 receptors regulating adenylyl cyclase in rat caudate-putamen; μ opioid receptors inhibiting adenylyl cyclase in the caudate-putamen are not desensitized (Noble and Cox, 1997). Previous studies have suggested that the μ receptors and dopamine D_1 receptors are located on striato-nigral neurons, whereas δ and dopamine D_2 receptors are located on striato-pallidal neurons. Under baseline "resting" conditions (Fig. 6.3a), it is suggested that the output of the striato-pallidal neurons is regulated by the striato-nigral feedback loop in which dppamine (DA) release leads to an increase in firing of the inhibitory striato-nigral neurons, in turn inhibiting firing in the DA neurons. During chronic morphine exposure (Fig. 6.3b), morphine inhibits the firing of the striato-nigral neurons by activating μ opioid receptors both on the cell soma and on the terminals. This disinhibits the DA neurons, leading to increased firing and increased release of DA. The increased level of DA does not excite the striato-nigral neurons since they are inhibited by the morphine treatment, but provides a strong inhibitory stimulus through dopamine D_2 receptors to the striato-pallidal pathway. The reduced firing in this pathway is proposed to result in a compensatory heterologous desensitization of the inhibitory receptors, dopamine D_2 and δ opioid, expressed in these cells.

It is not clear whether the failure to observe desensitization of the striato-nigral μ receptors is because these desensitize less readily than δ receptors (although μ receptor desensitization was observed in other brain regions in the same animals (Noble and Cox, 1996) or because desensitization occurs less readily in neurons receiving a strong activating stimulus, in this case through dopamine D_1 receptors. (Abbreviations: DA = dopamine; δ = delta opioid receptor; dyn = dynorphin; enk = enkephalin; GABA = γ-aminobutyric acid; μ = μ opioid receptor.)

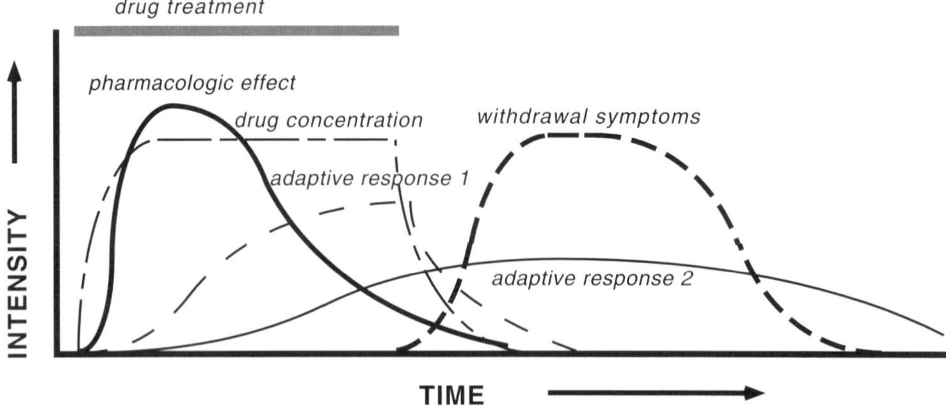

Figure 6.4. Kinetics of chronic drug action: a hypothetical representation of the relative time courses of events induced by chronic drug administration. A drug treatment (indicated by the hatched horizontal bar) leads to a rise in the blood concentration of the drug to an equilibrium level. The concentration declines when drug administration is terminated. The rates of rise and decline in drug concentration are largely determined by the elimination rate for the drug. The elevated drug concentration induces a pharmacologic effect indicated by the solid line. The magnitude of this effect is initially related to the drug concentration, but at later time points the pharmacologic effect is attenuated as a result of an adaptive change (adaptive response 1), which in this example has a time constant similar to that of the drug elimination rate. Adaptive response 1 might represent the onset and decay of receptor desensitization, a process limiting the magnitude of drug effect. A second series of adaptive responses is also assumed to be induced by the drug action (adaptive response 2). These adaptations have a significantly longer time constant; thus, the changed physiology induced by these events significantly exceeds the duration of drug action and the time during which active drug is present. Adaptive response 2 in this diagram might reflect the time course of production of transcription factors, including the chronic FRAs (Nye and Nestler, 1996). If adaptive response 2 leads to a physiologic response opposing the initial drug action, this process will contribute to the observed degree of drug tolerance and in addition will result in the appearance of withdrawal symptoms as the drug concentration and initial pharmacologic effect decline.

possible to determine whether this effect occurs in the neuron regulated by opiates or is a trans-synaptically mediated regulation of other neurons in the pathway.

Altered Functions of GABA and Glutamatergic Systems

Some recently identified examples of altered expression of specific genes or proteins and of functional adaptations in neural responsiveness after chronic opiate drug treatments are listed in Table 6.2. In various studies, altered expression or function of neurotransmitter receptors, of specific ion channel isoforms, of intracellular regulatory enzymes (e.g., adenylyl cyclase, nitric oxide synthase), and of proteins involved in the mechanisms of transmitter release have all been observed. In some cases the functional significance of the specific changes in protein or gene expression are not entirely clear, although it appears that most alterations in gene expression have the

Table 6.2. *Adaptations in Neural Systems Induced by Chronic Morphine Treatments*

Adaptation	Location	References
Analgesic synergism between spinal and supraspinally administered opiates is lost after chronic treatment	Spinal/supraspinal interactions (rat)	Kolesnikov et al., 1996
Enhanced expression of some potassium channel isoforms	Motor neurons of spinal cord	Matus-Leibovitch et al., 1996
Increased probability of GABA release in opiate withdrawal	VTA	Bonci and Williams, 1997
Opiate tolerance is reduced by nitric oxide synthase inhibitors	Site of action not defined	Elliott et al., 1994
Chronic morphine down-regulates the mRNA for melanocortin-4 receptors	Rat striatum and PAG	Alvaro et al., 1996
Superactivation of adenylyl cyclase isoforms; mechanism unknown	Transfected COS-7 cells	Avidor-Reiss et al., 1996
Increased expression of synapsin 1 mRNA	Locus coeruleus, amygdala, dorsal horn of spinal cord	Matus-Liebovitch et al., 1995
Intermittent morphine up-regulates GluR1 levels	VTA	Fitzgerald et al., 1996
Viral vector-mediated GluR1 expression sensitizes rats to morphine	VTA	Carlezon et al., 1996
Opiate tolerance is reduced by antagonists acting at NMDA and metabotropic glutamate receptors	Site of action not defined	Trujillo and Akil, 1991; Elliott et al., 1994; Fundyatus et al., 1997a, 1997b

functional consequence of reducing cellular sensitivity to the acute actions of opiates. For example, the increased probability of GABA release in the ventral tegmental area (VTA) after chronic morphine treatment observed by Bonci and Williams (1997) is directly opposed to the acute actions of opiates in directly inhibiting GABA release in this brain structure. However, the induced adaptations may also have other functions. Thus, a recent study suggests that a morphine-induced increase in GluR1 receptor subunit expression in VTA is responsible for the sensitization to the locomotor and behaviorally reinforcing actions of opiates, which probably plays an important role in maintaining self-administration of opiate drugs in dependent subjects (Carlezon et al., 1997). These two examples also indicate that multiple adaptations may occur within a single brain structure – in this case the VTA. It should also be noted that other drugs or treatments (including cocaine and stress) leading to behavioral sensitization also induce GluR1 receptor expression in VTA (Fitzgerald et al., 1996). An experimentally induced increase in GluR2 receptor subunits did not have the same sensitizing action (Carlezon et al., 1997). Either GluR1 or GluR2 subunits can form AMPA-type glutamate receptors; however, receptors formed from both GluR1 and GluR2 subunits are largely impermeable to calcium, whereas receptors comprised exclusively of GluR1 subunits permit the passage of this ion. It remains to be determined whether an increase in calcium flux through newly expressed GluR1-type AMPA receptors can fully account for sensitization to opiates and cocaine in the VTA.

Other studies have suggested different roles for NMDA and metabotropic glutamate receptors in opiate tolerance. Thus, analgesic tolerance can be reduced or reversed by treatment with NMDA or metabotropic glutamate receptor antagonists (Trujilo and Akil, 1991; Elliott et al., 1994; Fundyatus and Coderre, 1997; Fundyatus, Ritchie, and Coderre, 1997) and enhanced activity at NMDA receptors has been implicated in the enhanced nociceptive responsiveness induced in spinal cord by chronic sensory activation (a phenomenon described as "wind-up"; Chapman, Haley, and Dickenson, 1994). Further studies will be needed to determine the relative contributions of altered expression or function of the various types of glutamate receptors as a result of chronic opioid treatment. In addition, it seems likely that many further examples of post receptor adaptations induced by chronic morphine administration will be identified in the future.

Antiopiate Systems

It has long been known that activation of certain physiologic systems may antagonize the acute actions of opiates; this in part explains the significance of enhanced activity at glutamate receptors in opiate tolerance. Other neurotransmitters and neuromodulators may also play a role in systems antagonistic to opiate actions; examples include mammalian analogs of the moluscan peptide FMRFamide, including neuropeptide FF (Devillers et al., 1995); CCK (Nichols et al., 1996); dynorphin (Holmes and Fujimoto, 1993); and orphanin FQ (Mogil et al., 1996). Possible roles in opiate tolerance for endogenous peptides related to melanocyte inhibitory factor (e.g., Tyr-Pro-Leu-Gly-NH_2, Tyr-Pro-Trp-Gly-NH_2) that may exhibit partial agonist activity at some types of opiate receptors have also been proposed (Zadina et al., 1995). Several of these neuropeptides have been shown to antagonize opiate drug actions during acute drug administration, and in some cases there is evidence to suggest their release is facilitated by acute opiate administration. Increased expression of CCK mRNA during chronic morphine treatment has been reported (Ding and Bayer, 1993). It remains to be demonstrated, however, that increased expression of one or more of these endogenous antiopiate peptides plays a role in the reduced sensitivity to opiate drugs induced by chronic opiate treatment. But in view of the wide range of changes in gene expression induced by chronic opiate drug exposure, it is quite feasible that the expression of some of these peptides might be increased in discrete systems.

Table 6.3. *Adaptations in Transcriptional Regulators and Second Messenger Systems Induced by Chronic Morphine Treatments*

Adaptation	System	References
Increase in levels of Fos-related antigens	Striatum, nucleus accumbens, other brain regions	Nye and Nester, 1996
Increased levels of ERKs-1 and -2 without change in MEK activity	Locus coeruleus, caudate-putamen	Ortiz et al., 1995
Increased ERK and tyrosine hydroxylase activity; effects inhibited by BDNF and glutamate receptor antagonists	VTA	Berhow et al., 1996
Decreased CREB immunoreactivity	Nucleus accumbens	Widnall et al., 1996
Mice with mutations in the α and δ isoforms of CREB show reduced opiate withdrawal symptoms	Genetic alteration expressed in all systems	Maldonado et al., 1996

Mechanisms of Postreceptor Adaptation

The mechanisms by which the various adaptations to long-term opiate drug exposure are induced also remain to be clarified in detail. At this time it is clear that chronic drug administration leads to significant changes in the level of transcription of many genes coding for critical functional proteins both in neurons directly sensitive to opiates and in neurons synaptically connected to opiate-regulated neurons. Factors regulating the altered expression of functional proteins include both short- and long-term transcriptional regulators (Table 6.3). The later manifestations of opiate withdrawal may be related in particular to the induction by chronic morphine treatment of transcriptional regulators related to the immediate early gene c-Fos. Consistent with its primary role in activating the expression of other functional proteins, c-Fos itself displays a rapid turnover. However, chronic morphine also induces Fos-related proteins with much longer half-lives. These regulators are known as chronic Fos-related antigens, or chronic-FRAs (Nye and Nestler, 1996), and several of these display half-lives measured in days. It is likely that the chronic FRAs serve as inducers of expression of functional proteins that mediate neuronal hyperactivity during opiate withdrawal. Other long-term transcriptional regulators associated with chronic opiate drug treatments will probably be identified in the future. Eventually, it may be possible to link the increased expression of specific proteins with individual symptoms of opiate dependence or withdrawal. It is unlikely that all neurons will respond to chronic opiate treatments in the same way; the patterns of altered gene expression will be influenced by the specific phenotypes of each opiate-regulated neuron and the phenotypes of the neurons with which they are synaptically linked.

Summary

Opiate tolerance is a very complex phenomenon. Chronic opiate exposure leads to adaptations at the receptor level in processes mediating the acute actions of opiates, as well as to adaptations in the regulation in the longer term of the function of neural systems whose activity is modified by opiate drug actions. The relative importance of each adaptive response will vary in different systems, and these changes are imposed on functional pathways whose baseline levels of activity are themselves subject to regulation by physiologic and pathologic processes that may be independent of the actions of opiate drugs. However, as more is learned of the processes underlying adaptation to opiate drug exposure, it is likely that it will become possible to use pharmacologic approaches to modify both the development of opiate drug tolerance and dependence and the expression of specific withdrawal symptoms.

ACKNOWLEDGMENTS

The author thanks Dr. Charles Chavkin and Dr. Florence Noble for giving permission to cite work in press and Dr. James Zadina for his helpful comments on the potential roles of antiopiate peptides in opiate tolerance. Work from the author's laboratory was supported by grants from the National Institute on Drug Abuse. The opinions and assertions contained in this chapter represent the private views of the author. They should not be construed as representing the opinions of the Uniformed Services University or the U.S. Department of Defense.

REFERENCES

Aley, K.O., and Levine, J.D. (1997). Multiple receptors involved in peripheral α_2, μ, and A_1 antinociception, tolerance and withdrawal. *J. Neurosci.* **17,** 735–744.

Alvaro, J.D., Tatro, J.B., Quillan, J.M., Fogliano, M., Eisenhard, M., Lerner, M.R., Nestler, E.J., and Duman, R.S. (1996). Morphine down-regulates melanocortin-4 receptor expression in brain regions that mediate opiate action. *Mol. Pharmacol.* **50,** 583–591.

Ammer, H., and Schulz, R. (1997). Chronic morphine treatment increases stimulatory β-2 adrenoceptor signaling in A431 cells stably expressing the mu opioid receptor. *J. Pharmacol. Exp. Ther.* **280,** 512–520.

Avidor-Reiss, T., Nevo, I., Levy, R., Pfeuffer, T., and Vogel, Z. (1996). Chronic opioid treatment induces adenylyl cyclase V superactivation: Involvement of $G_{\beta\gamma}$. *J. Biol. Chem.* **271**(21), 309–312.

Avidor-Reiss, T., Nevo, I., Saya, D., Bayewitch, M., and Vogel, Z. (1997). Chronic opioid treatment induces adenylyl cyclase V superactivation. *J. Biol. Chem.* **271,** 21309–21315.

Berhow, M.T., Hiroi, N., and Nestler, E.J. (1996). Regulation of ERK (extracellular signal regulated kinase), part of the neurotrophin signal transduction cascade, in the rat mesolimbic dopaminergic system by chronic exposure to morphine or cocaine. *J. Neurosci.* **16,** 3026–3034.

Blake, A.D., Bot, G., Freeman, J.C., and Reisine, T. (1997). Differential opioid agonist regulation of the mouse mu opioid receptor. *J. Biol. Chem.* **272,** 782–790.

Bläsig, J., Meyer, G., Höllt, V., Hengstenburg, J., Dum, J., and Herz, A. (1979). Non-competitive nature of the antagonistic mechanism responsible for tolerance development to opiate analgesia. *Neuropharmacology.* **18,** 473–481.

Bonci, A., and Williams, J.T. (1997). Increased probability of GABA release during withdrawal from morphine. *J. Neurosci.* **17,** 796–803.

Breivogel, C.S,. Selley, D.E., and Childers, S.R. (1997). Acute and chronic effects of opioids on delta and mu receptor activation of G proteins in NG 108–15 and SK-N-SH cell membranes. *J. Neurochem.* **68,** 1462–1472.

Buzas, B., Rosenberger, J., and Cox, B.M. (1996). Mu and delta opioid receptor gene expression after chronic treatment with opioid agonist. *Neuroreport.* **7,** 1505–1508.

Carlezon, W.A. Jr., Boundy, V.A., Haile, C.N., Lane, S.B., Kalb, R.G., Neve, R.L., and Nestler, E.J. (1997). Sensitization to morphine induced by viral-mediated gene transfer. *Science.* **277,** 812–814.

Chakarabarti, S., Yang, W., Law, P.Y., and Loh, H.H. (1997). The mu-opioid receptor downregulates differently from the delta-opioid receptor: Requirement of a high affinity receptor/G protein complex formation, *Mol. Pharmacol.* **52,** 105–113.

Chapman, V., Haley, J.E., and Dickenson, A.H. (1994). Electrophysiologic analysis of preemptive effects of spinal opioids on N-methyl-D-aspartate receptor mediated events. *Anesthesiology.* **81,** 1429–1435.

Chuang, T.T., Iacovelli, L., Sallese, M., and De Blasi, A. (1996). G protein-coupled receptors: Heterologous regulation of homologous desensitization and its implications. *Trends Pharmacol. Sci.* **17,** 416–421.

Colpaert, F.C. (1996). System theory of pain and of opiate analgesia: No tolerance to opiates. *Pharmacol Rev.* **48,** 355–402.

Costa, M., Lang, J., Gless, C., and Herz, A. (1989). Spontaneous association between opioid receptors and GTP-binding regulatory proteins in native membranes: Specific regulation by antagonists and sodium ions. *Mol. Pharmacol.* **37,** 383–394.

Devillers, J.P., Boisserie, F., Laulin, J.P., Larcher, A., and Simonnet, G. (1995). Simultaneous activation of spinal antiopioid system (neuropeptide FF) and pain facilitatory circuitry by stimulation of opioid receptors in rats. *Brain Res.* **700,** 173–181.

Ding, X.Z., and Bayer, B.M. (1993). Increases of CCK mRNA and peptide in different brain areas following acute and chronic administration of morphine. *Brain Res.* **625,** 139–144.

Dum, J., Meyer, G., Höllt, V., and Herz, A. (1979). In vivo opiate binding unchanged in tolerant/dependent mice. *Eur. J. Pharmacol.* **548,** 453–460.

Elliott, J., Guo, L., and Traynor, J.R. (1977). Tolerance to mu-opioid agonists in human neuroblastoma SH-SY5Y cells as determined by changes in guanosine-5′-O-(3-[^{35}S]-thio)triphosphate binding. *Brit. J. Pharmacol.* **121,** 1422–1428.

Elliott, K., Minami, N., Kolesnikov, Y.A., Pasternak, G.W., and Inturrisi, C.E. (1994). The NMDA receptor antagonists, LY274614 and MK801, and the nitric oxide synthase inhibitor, NG-nitro-L-arginine, attenuate analgesic tolerance to the mu-opioid morphine but not to kappa opioids. *Pain.* **56,** 69–75.

Fitzgerald, L.W., Ortiz, J., Hamandani, A.G., and Nestler, E.J. (1996). Drugs of abuse and stress increase the expression of GluR1 and NMDAR1 glutamate receptor subunits in the rat ventral tegmental area: Common adaptations among cross-sensitizing agents. *J. Neurosci.* **16,** 274–282.

Foley, K.M. (1991). Clinical tolerance to opioids. In *Towards a new pharmacotherapy of pain,* A.I. Basbaum and J.-M. Besson, eds. Chichester, U.K.: John Wiley, pp 181–203.

Fundyatus, M., and Coderre, T.J. (1997). Attenuation of precipitated morphine withdrawal symptoms by acute i.c.v. administration of a group II mGluR antagonist. *Brit. J. Pharmacol.* **121,** 511–514.

Fundyatus, M., Ritchie, J., and Coderre, T.J. (1997). Attenuation of morphine withdrawal symptoms by subtype – selective metabotropic glutamate receptor antagonists. *Brit. J. Pharmacol.* **120b,** 1015–1020.

Johnson, S.M., and Flemming, W.W. (1989). Mechanisms of cellular adaptative sensitivity changes: Applications to opioid tolerance and dependence. *Pharmacol. Rev.* **41,** 435–488.

Holmes, B.B., and Fujimoto, J.M. (1993). Inhibiting a spinal dynorphin A component enhances intrathecal morphine antinociception in mice. *Anesth. and Analg.* **77,** 1166–1173.

Inglese, J., Freedman, N.J., Kock, J., and Lefkowitz, R.J. (1993). Structure and mechanism of the G protein-coupled receptor kinase. *J. Biol. Chem.* **268**(23), 738.

Kaneko, S., Yada, N., Fukuda, K., Kikuwaka, M., Akaike, K., and Satoh, M. (1997). Inhibition of Ca^{2+} channel current by mu and kappa opioid receptors co-expressed in *Xenopus* oocytes: Desensitization dependence on Ca^{2+} channels α_1 subunits. *Brit. J. Pharmacol.* **121,** 806–812.

Kovoor, A., Nappey, V., Kieffer, B., and Chavkin, C. (1997). Mu and delta opioid receptors are differentially desensitized by the co-expression of β-adrenergic receptor kinase 2 and β-arrestin 2 in *Xenopus* oocytes. *J. Biol. Chem.* **272,** 27,605–27,611.

Kolesnikov, Y.A., Jain, S., Wilson, R., and Pasternak, G.W. (1996). Peripheral morphine analgesia: Synergy with central sites and a target of morphine tolerance. *J. Pharmacol. Exp. Ther.* **279,** 502–506.

Law, P.Y., Hom, D.S., and Loh, H.H. (1982). Loss of opiate receptor activity in neuroblastoma X glioma NG 108–15 hybrid cells after chronic opiate treatment: A multistep process. *Mol. Pharmacol.* **22,** 1–4.

Maldonado, R., Blendy, J.A., Tzavara, E., Gass, P., Roques, B.P., Hanoune, J., and Schutz, G. (1996). Reduction of morphine abstinence in mice with a mutation in the gene encoding CREB. *Science.* **273,** 657–659

Matus-Leibovitch, N., Ezra-Macabee, V., Saya, D., Attali, B., Avidor-Reiss, T., Barg, J., and Vogel, Z. (1995). Increased expression of synapsin I mRNA in defined areas of the rat central nervous system following chronic morphine treatment. *Mol. Brain Res.* **34,** 221–230.

Matus-Leibovitch, N., Vogel, Z., Ezra-Macabee, V., Etkin, S., Nevo, I., and Attali, B. (1996). Chronic morphine treatment enhances the expression of Kv1.5 and Kv1.6 voltage-gated K^+ channels in rat spinal cord. *Mol. Brain Res.* **40,** 261–270.

Mestek, A., Hurley, J.H., Bye, L.S., Campbell, A.D., Chen, Y., Tian, M., Liu, J., Schulman, H., and Yu, L. (1995). The human μ opioid receptor: Modulation of functional desensitization by calcium/calmodulin-dependent protein kinase and protein kinase C. *J. Neurosci.* **15,** 2396–2406.

Mogil, J.S., Grisel, J.E., Zhangs, G., Belknap, J.K., and Grandy, D.K. (1996). Functional antagonism of mu-, delta-, and kappa-opioid antinociception by orphanin FQ. *Neurosci. Lett.* **214,** 131–134.

Namir, N., Polastron, J., Allouche, S., Hasbi, A., and Jauzac, P. (1997). The delta-opioid receptor in NK-N-BE human neuroblastoma cell line undergoes heterologous desensitization. *J. Neurochem.* **68,** 1764–1772.

Narita, M., Mizoguchi, H., Kampine, J.P., and Tseng, L.F. (1997). The effect of pretreatment with the delta-2-opioid receptor antisense oligonucleotide on the recovery from antinociceptive tolerance to delta-2 opioid receptor agonist in the mouse spinal cord. *Brit. J. Pharmacol.* **120,** 587–592.

Nestby, P., Tjon, G.H.K., Visser, D.T.M., Drukarch, B., Leysen, J.E., Mukler, A.H., and Schoffelmeer, A.N.M. (1995). Intermittent morphine treatment causes long-term desensitization of functional dopamine D_2 receptors in rat striatum. *Eur. J. Pharmacol.* **294,** 771–777.

Nestler, E.J. (1996). Under seige: The brain on opiates. *Neuron* **16,** 897–900.

Nichols, M.L., Bian, D., Ossipov, M.H., Malan, T.P., and Porreca, F. (1996). Antiallodynic effects of a CCKB antagonist in rats with nerve ligation inury: Role of endogenous enkephalins. *Neurosci. Lett.* **215,** 161–164.

Noble, F., and Cox, B.M. (1996). Differential desensitization of mu and delta opioid receptors in selected neural pathways following chronic morphine treatment. *Brit. J. Pharmacol.* **117,** 161–169.

Noble, F., and Cox, B.M. (1997). The role of dopaminergic systems in opioid receptor desensitization in nucleus accumbens and caudate-putamen of rat following chronic morphine treatment. *J. Pharmacol. Exp. Ther.* **283,** 557–565.

Nye, H.E., and Nestler, E.J. (1996). Induction of chronic Fos-related antigens in rat brain by chronic morphine administration. *Mol. Pharmacol.* **49,** 636–645.

Ortiz, J., Harris, H.W., Guitart, X., Terwilliger, R.Z., Haycock, J.W., and Nestler, E.J. (1995). Extracellular signal-regulated protein kinases (ERKs) and ERK kinase (MEK) in brain: Regional distribution and regulation by chronic morphine. *J. Neurosci.* **15,** 1285–1297.

Paul, D., Standifer, K.M., Interissi, C.E., and Pasternak, G.W. (1989). Pharmacological characterization of morphine-6β-glucuronide, a very potent morphine metabolite. *J. Pharmacol. Exp. Ther.* **251,** 477–483.

Pei, G., Keiffer, B.L., Lefkowitz, R.J., and Freedman, N.J. (1995). Agonist-dependent phosphorylation of the mouse delta-opioid receptor: Involvement of G protein-coupled receptor kinases but not protein kinase C. *Mol. Pharmacol.* **48,** 173–177.

Prather, P.L., Tsai, A.W., and Law, P.Y. (1994). Mu and delta opioid receptor desenstization in undifferentiated human neuroblastoma SHSY5Y cells. *J. Pharmacol. Exp. Ther.* **270,** 177–184.

Puttfarcken, P.S., Werling, L.L., and Cox, B.M. (1989). Effects of chronic morphine exposure on opioid inhibition of adenylyl cyclase in 7315c cell membranes: A useful model for the study of tolerance at mu opioid receptors. *Mol. Pharmacol.* **33,** 520–527.

Saeki, S., and Yaksh, T.L. (1993). Suppression of nociceptive responses by spinal mu opioid agonists: Effects of stimulus intensity and agonist efficacy. *Anesth. and Analg.* **77,** 265–274.

Selley, D.E., Sim, L.J., Xiao, R., Liu, Q., and Childers, S.R. (1997). Mu-opioid receptor-stimulated guanosine-5′-O-(γ-thio)-triphosphate binding in rat thalamus and cultures cell lines: Signal transduction mechanisms underlyng agonist afficacy. *Mol. Pharmacol.* **51,** 87–96.

Sharma, S.K., Klee, W.A., and Nirenberg, M. (1975). Dual regulation of adenylate cyclase accounts for narcotic tolerance and dependence. *Proc. Natl. Acad. Sci. U.S.A.* **72,** 3092–3096.

Sharma, S.K., Nirenberg, M., and Klee, W.A. (1975). Morphine receptors as regulators of adenylate cyclase activity. *Proc. Natl. Acad. Sci. U.S.A.* **72,** 590–594.

Steece, K.A., DeLeon-Jones, F.A., Meyerson, L.R., Lee, J.M., Fields, J.Z., and Ritzman, R.F. (1986). In vivo down-regulation of rat striatal opioid receptors by chronic enkephalin. *Brain Res. Bull.* **17,** 255–257.

Sternini, C., Spann, M., Anton, B., Keith, D.E. Jr., Bunnett, N.W., von Zastrow, M., Evans,

C., and Brecha, N.C. (1996). Agonist-selective endocytosis of mu opioid receptor by neurons in vivo. *Proc. Natl. Acad. Sci. U.S.A.* **93,** 9241–9246.

Tao, P.-L., Chang, L.-R., Law, P.Y., and Loh, H.H. (1988). Decrease in delta receptor density in rat brain after chronic [D-Ala^2, D-Leu^5]enkephalin treatment. *Brain Res.* **462,** 313–320.

Trapaidze, N., Keith, D.E., Cvejic, S., Evans, C.J., and Devi, L.A. (1996). Sequestration of the delta opioid receptor: Role of the C terminus in agonist-mediated internalization. *J. Biol. Chem.* **46,** 29279–29285.

Traynor, J.R., and Nahorski, S.R. (1995). Modulation by mu-opioid agonists of guanosine-5′-O-(3-[35S]thio)triphosphate binding to membranes from human neuroblastoma SH-SY5Y cells. *Mol. Pharmacol.* **47,** 848–854.

Trujillo, K., and Akil, H. (1991). Inhibition of morphine tolerance and dependence by the NMDA receptor antagonist MK801. *Science.* **251,** 85–87.

Werling, L.L., McMahon, P.N., and Cox, B.M. (1989). Selective changes in mu receptor properties induced by chronic morphine exposure. *Proc. Natl. Acad. Sci. U.S.A.* **86,** 6393–6397.

Widnell, K.L., Self, D.W., Lane, S.B., Russell, D.S., Vaidya, V.A., Miserendino, M.J., Rubin, C.S., and Duman, R.S. (1996). Regulation of CREB expression: In vivo evidence for a functional role in morphine action in the nucleus accumbens. *J. Pharmacol. Exp. Ther.* **276,** 306–315.

Zadina, J.E., Kastin, A.J., Harrison, L.M., Ge, L.-J., and Chang, S.L. (1995). Opiate receptor changes after chronic exposure to agonists and antagonists. *Ann. N.Y. Acad. Sci.* **757,** 353–360.

CHAPTER SEVEN

Opioid–Nonopioid Interactions

ZSUZSANNA WIESENFELD-HALLIN AND XIAO-JUN XU

Introduction

The antinociceptive and/or analgesic effect of opioids is subjected to bidirectional modulation by a range of neuroactive nonopioid substances. In some cases the interaction between opioids and antiopioids is purely pharmacologic, whereas in other cases the interactions may have important physiologic significance. Antiopioids not only modulate antinociception induced by exogenously administered opioids but may also be involved in the development of opioid tolerance, dependence, and opioid insensitivity in neuropathic pain.

Several types of interactions between opioids and nonopioids have been described: (1) Synergistic antinociception between opioids and nonopioids that have antinociceptive properties. The best described interaction is between spinally administered opioids and α-2 adrenoceptor agonists, which cause enhanced antinociception. (2) Potentiation of opioid-induced antinociception by other inhibitory substances that are not antinociceptive by themselves. (3) Antagonism of the effects of opioids by antiopioid endogenous peptides. (4) Opioid-induced increases in activation of N-methyl-D-aspartate (NMDA) receptors for glutamate, which curtail the effects of opioids.

The concept that there exist endogenous antiopioids has been suggested for some time (see Cesselin, 1995, for review). The original concept referred primarily to peptides, including cholecystokinin (CCK), FMRFamide-related peptides, and melanocyte inhibiting-factor (MIF)-related peptides (Faris et al., 1983; Kastin et al., 1984; Yang et al., 1985). Recent data suggest that endogenous antiopioids may also include glutamate acting on NMDA receptors (Mao et al., 1995a). In this chapter, we focus on the endogenous antiopioids and discuss the possible involvement of these systems in modulating opioid analgesia in normal and pathologic conditions.

Cholecystokinin and Opioid Analgesia

Overview

Cholecystokinin (CCK) belongs to the gastrin family of peptides. In the nervous system it is mainly present in the form of the C-terminal octapeptide CCK-8. CCK has

Christoph Stein, ed., *Opioids in Pain Control: Basic and Clinical Aspects.* Printed in the United States of America.

been visualized in sensory neurons in guinea pig and monkeys, but not in rats (Seroogy et al., 1990; Verge et al., 1993), whereas in the spinal cord, CCK-mRNA and CCK-like (CCK-LI) immunoreactivity has been observed in a substantial number of dorsal horn neurons and in dense networks of fibers across many species (Williams et al., 1987; Verge et al., 1993; Zhang et al., 1995). CCK-LI and mRNA expression has also been described in many supraspinal areas related to nociceptive transmission (Williams et al., 1987). In general, there is an overlap in the anatomic distribution of CCK, opioids, and their receptors in the spinal cord and brain, which may underlie the documented interaction betweeen the opioid and CCK systems.

CCK receptors are heterogeneous, with receptors predominantly located in the periphery differing from those in the central nervous system (CNS). Moran et al. (1986) termed the peripheral type the CCK-A receptor in order to distinguish it from the classical brain (type B) receptor, which is identical to the gastrin receptor in the periphery. However, it is now known that even the peripheral type CCK-A receptor is present to a limited extent in the CNS, particularly in primates (Hill et al., 1990). Receptor-binding sites for CCK have been visualized in areas throughout the spinal dorsal horn, with the highest density in the superficial laminae. In the rat, receptors are A- and B-type, whereas in primates, the majority of receptors are the A-type (Hill et al., 1990; Ghilarde et al., 1992; Mercer and Beart, 1997). It has been suggested that a substantial portion of the CCK-binding sites in the superficial dorsal horn arise from small-diameter primary sensory neurons, since neonatal capsaicin treatment reduced CCK binding (Ghilarde et al., 1992). Although the binding sites in rat DRG have been reported to be of low density, and in situ hybridization studies indicated that only about 4% of rat DRG neurons synthesize CCK-B receptor mRNA, up to 90% of DRG cells in the rabbit and 20% in the monkey express CCK-binding sites (Ghilarde et al., 1992; Zhang et al., 1993). Interestingly, in all species examined, the receptors in DRG cells appeared to be the B-type (Ghilarde et al., 1992).

Modulation of Opioid-Mediated Analgesia by CCK

Faris et al.(1983) were the first to demonstrate that systemically administered CCK attenuated morphine-induced antinociception, and a large body of literature supports this observation. Thus, upon local, systemic, intrathecal (IT), or intracerebral injection, CCK reduces the effect of exogenous opioids as tested in behavioral and electrophysiologic studies (see Cesselin, 1995; and Wiesenfeld-Hallin and Xu, 1996, for a review). CCK also blocks the antinociceptive effect of endogenous opioids produced by electroacupuncture or electric shocks (Watkins et al., 1985; Han et al., 1986). CCK interacts with opioids at multiple sites, including periphery, spinal cord, and brain. Among the three types of opioid receptors, it appeares that μ and κ receptor-mediated analgesia is antagonized by CCK, whereas δ opioids are less influenced (Magnuson et al., 1990; Wang et al., 1990).

There is a tonic antagonism by CCK of opioid-induced analgesia because blockade of endogenous CCK results in an enhancement of opioid-induced antinociception. This finding has been confirmed with several highly potent and specific CCK receptor antagonists, as well as with CCK-B receptor antisense oligonucleotides (see Cesselin, 1995; and Wiesenfeld-Hallin and Xu, 1996, for a review). Comparison of the potency of these drugs indicates that the CCK-B receptor is responsible for the interaction between the CCK and opioid systems in rodents. The antinociceptive effect of endogenously released opioids following the administration of endopeptidases or electroacupuncture is also potentiated by CCK-B receptor antagonists (Noble et al., 1995).

The mechanism by which CCK antagonizes opioid analgesia is not fully understood. Clearly, the blockade of morphine analgesia by CCK is not due to a direct hyperalgesic effect of CCK because CCK does not alter the baseline pain threshold. The majority of receptor binding studies fail to show an affinity of CCK for opioid receptors (cf. Wang and Han, 1989). However, one study indicates that binding of CCK-8 to the CCK receptor reduces the binding affinity of μ receptor ligands (Wang and Han, 1989). There is also evidence that the CCK may counteract intracellular events subsequent to opioid receptor activation (Wang et al., 1992). If such interaction occurs in cells that have both opioid and CCK receptors, the result will be decreased opioid-induced analgesia. This hypothesis is supported by the similar distribution of opioid and CCK receptors in a number of CNS areas important for opioid analgesia. Another hypothesis concerning the mechanism of CCK-induced antagonism of opioid analgesia was suggested by Watkins's group (Wiertelak et al., 1992). They found that CCK is the mediator for conditioned antianalgesia, a behavioral procedure related to safety signals with reduced analgesia induced by morphine.

CCK antagonists are not analgesic on their own in most behavioral and electrophysiologic studies, indicating that there is no significant tonic inhibition by CCK of the effects of endogenous opioids. However, increased stimulation of opioid receptors by either exogenously administered opioids or by increased endogenous release may stimulate the release of CCK, which in turn reduces and curtails the action of opioids. Some experimental evidence supports this hypothesis. Several groups have reported increased release of CCK-LI from the spinal cord after morphine treatment in vivo and in vitro (Tang et al., 1984; Benoliel et al., 1991; Zhou et al., 1993). Acute morphine treatment may also increase CCK gene expression and tissue content of CCK in several brain regions and in the spinal cord (Ding and Beyer, 1993).

CCK and Opioid Tolerance

Repeated and chronic administration of opiates induces a gradual reduction in the ability of opiates to induce analgesia, a condition known as tolerance. Because CCK is a potent antagonist of opiate analgesia and is widely distributed, it is possible that endogenous CCK may be involved in the development of tolerance. Studies of tolerance with CCK receptor antagonists have shown that this is indeed the case. Thus, both the weak, nonspecific antagonist proglumide and the more recently developed potent antagonists L-365,260 and CI-988 were found both to prevent (where antagonists were applied chronically together with morphine) and to reverse (where antagonists were applied acutely in already tolerant animals) tolerance (see Cesselin, 1995; and Wiesenfeld-Hallin and Xu, 1996, for review). Interestingly, the symptoms of physical dependence induced by chronic morphine were not prevented by CCK-B receptor antagonists, nor did CCK precipitate withdrawal symptoms, indicating a CCK-independent mechanism for opioid dependence (Dourish et al., 1990; Xu et al., 1992).

The mechanism for the prevention and reversal of morphine tolerance by CCK antagonists has been addressed. Repeated administration of morphine causes tolerance and induces up-regulation of CCK mRNA in the spinal cord and in discrete brain areas, which is accompanied by increased CCK content in brain and spinal cord (Ding and Beyer, 1993; Zhou et al., 1994). Thus, opiate tolerance may be related to an up-regulation of endogenous CCK, inducing greater blockade of opiate analgesia, hence causing tolerance. Blockade of the action of the up-regulated CCK system by receptor antagonists restores some of the analgesic effect of the opioid, resulting in the reversal of morphine tolerance (Hoffmann and Wiesenfeld-Hallin, 1995). Up-regulation of the CCK system may require chronic stimulation of CCK receptors by repeated opiate administration because CCK antagonists also prevent morphine tolerance.

CCK and Opioid Sensitivity

The analgesic effects of morphine vary in different clinical pain states. Neuropathic pain, involving injury to the nervous system, usually responds poorly to opiates (Arnér and Meyerson, 1993). This finding is supported by experimental evidence indicating that morphine causes less spinal antinociception after peripheral nerve injury in rats (Xu and Weisenfeld-Hallin, 1993; Lee et al., 1995; Mao et al., 1995b; Ossipov et al., 1995). The mechanism(s) for a lack (or reduced) effect of morphine in neuropathic pain is unclear, but may have some features in common with morphine tolerance – that is, under both circumstances morphine fails to elicit analgesia. Thus, it is possible that CCK may be involved in both phenomena. Peripheral axotomy caused a dramatic up-regulation of CCK and CCK-B receptor mRNA in rat DRG cells (Verge et al., 1993; Xu et al., 1993; Zhang et al., 1993). Electrophysiologic and behavioral experiments have verifed the implications of this plasticity in morphine-induced antinociception (or the lack of it). Systemic morphine-induced reduced antinociception in axotomized rats compared to normals, and addition of the CCK-B receptor antagonist CI-988 strongly potentiated the effect of morphine (Xu et al., 1994). Furthermore, chronic IT morphine did not block autotomy behavior, a sign of neuropathic pain in rats, after peripheral nerve section. However, the combination of

CI-988 plus morphine significantly suppressed autotomy (Xu et al., 1993). These data indicate that in the rat opioid insensitivity after nerve injury may be related to enhanced activity in the endogenous CCK system. These initial findings have been supported by recent behavioral data using rat models of peripheral nerve injury where CCK-B receptor antagonists were found to exert an antinociceptive effect and to restore the effect of opioids in alleviating neuropathic pain-related behaviors (Nichols et al., 1995; Yamamoto and Nozakitaguchi, 1995).

Control over the degree of sensitivity to opioids by CCK is also observed in animal models of inflammation, although it is the opposite of that observed following nerve injury. Inflammation enhances the antinociceptive effect of opiates in animals, and during carrageenan-induced inflammation exogenous CCK is still able to attenuate the antinociceptive effect of morphine, indicating that the mechanism by which CCK reduces the action of morphine is still intact. However, during inflammation CCK receptor antagonists no longer enhance the antinociceptive effect of morphine (Stanfa and Dickenson, 1993). Thus, a decrease in the availability of CCK within the spinal cord following inflammation, either due to decreased release of CCK or reduced concentration of this peptide within the dorsal horn, may underlie the lack of effect of the CCK antagonists.

Neuropeptide FF and Opioid Analgesia

Overview

The octapeptide Phe-Leu-Phe-Gln-Pro-Gln-Arg-Phe-NH_2 (neuropeptide FF, NPFF, or F8Fa) is the mammalian counterpart of the invertebrate tetrapeptide Phe-Met-Arg-Phe-NH_2 (FMRFamide). First isolated from bovine brain using antibodies directed against FMRFamide (Yang et al., 1985), the presence of NPFF has been established in the CNS in numerous species, including humans (Majane et al., 1988; Lee et al., 1995). Cells containing neuropeptide FF can be visualized in laminae I–IV and X of the spinal cord. In addition, networks of fibers and terminals containing NPFF-LI are present throughout the spinal cord, including superficial laminae of the dorsal horn (Kivipelto and Panula, 1991). It has been suggested that the NPFF-LI in the spinal cord is of intrinsic spinal origin. In the brain, NPFF-containing cells are located primarily within two areas: the medial hypothalamus and the nucleus tractus solitarius (Lee et al., 1995).

There are high-affinity binding sites for neuropeptide FF in the CNS, probably representing neuropeptide FF receptors. Although it has not been cloned, there is evidence indicating that the neuropeptide FF receptor is G-protein coupled (Payza and Yang, 1993). Autoradiographic work has shown that receptors for NPFF are located in the superficial laminae of the spinal dorsal horn and in numerous brain structures (Allard et al., 1992).

NPFF and Opioid Analgesia: Tolerance and Dependence

Yang et al. (1985) were the first to report that intracerebroventricularly (ICV) administered NPFF caused hyperalgesia and antagonized morphine-induced antinociception. This initial finding has been supported by other studies that used both behavioral and electrophysiologic techniques at spinal and supraspinal levels (see Cesselin, 1995, for review). One interesting feature of the antiopioid effect of NPFF is its extremely short duration of action, indicating very rapid enzymatic degradation of this peptide.

Unlike CCK, there are no high-affinity nonpeptide receptor antagonists for NPFF available, which has hampered the elucidation of the role of endogenous NPFF in modulating opioid antinociception. In the studies addressing this question, either neuropeptide FF antiserum or peptidergic analogs have been used. There are problems associated with these approaches, and it has been difficult to draw firm conclusions from these studies since results have been inconsistent.

It is unclear whether endogenous NPFF inhibits opioid-induced analgesia tonically, as is the case for CCK. Although some studies reported that ICV-administered NPFF antiserum potentiated morphine-induced antinociception (see Cesselin, 1995, for review), others found that neither NPFF antiserum nor Desamino YFLFQPQRamide (an NPFF analog) influenced acute morphine-induced antinociception (Lake et al., 1991, 1992). More consistent results have been reported concerning the role of NPFF in morphine tolerance. Several reports indicated that the antinociceptive effect of morphine can be restored in morphine-tolerant animals with either NPFF antiserum or analog (see Cesselin, 1995, for review).

In contrast to CCK, which plays no role in morphine dependence, NPFF may be a factor in the physical dependence associated with opioids. Thus, ICV NPFF precipitated opioid abstinence (Malin et al., 1990), whereas an NPFF analog attenuated naloxone-precipitated withdrawal in morphine-dependent rats (Malin et al., 1991).

In conclusion, although it is clear that exogenously administered NFFF antagonizes opioid-induced analgesia, firm evidence for an endogenous role of this peptide as a modulator of opioid systems is lacking and awaits the development of specific high-affinity nonpeptide antagonists of NPFF receptors.

Other Endogenous Antiopioid Peptides

In addition to CCK and NPFF, a large number of peptides have been reported to antagonize opioid-induced analgesia upon exogenous administration. These include angiotensin II, MIF, TRH, calcitonin, somatostatin, and ACTH (see Cesselin, 1995). However, for most of the peptides the interaction has been established only at the pharmacologic level. As described earlier, the mechanism by which CCK antagonizes opioid analgesia may involve interaction at the second messenger level. Thus, it is not surprising that other peptides may have opioid-blocking effects since they may have similar effects on second messengers. However, for these peptides to interact with opioids physiologically requires the presence of the antiopioid peptides and opioids, as well as their receptors, in the same neural tissues. Moreover, opioids should be able to modulate the release and production of these peptides upon acute and chronic administration. Finally, it needs to be established whether blockade of the receptors for these peptides influences opioid analgesia, tolerance, and dependence. In this sense, only CCK and probably NPFF can be defined as endogenous antiopioid peptides, whereas solid evidence for a role of the other peptides is lacking.

The Role of NMDA Receptor Activation in Opioid Analgesia and Tolerance

The NMDA Receptor and Acute Opioid Tolerance/Dependence

Opioid antagonists are able to elicit withdrawal symptoms after the administration of a single dose of opioid agonist, which has been termed acute dependence and/or tolerance (Ziegelgänsberger and Tölle, 1993). It has been hypothesized that even a single opioid administration elicits adaptive changes in the nervous system, leading to an attenuation of the effect of the opioid. These adaptive changes persist when the antinociceptive and other depressive effects of opioids are reversed, resulting in hyperexcitability and withdrawal. Activation of NMDA receptors constitutes an important step in these adaptive changes (Ziegelgänsberger and Tölle, 1993; Mao et al., 1995a). Iontophoretically applied opioids, in addition to a blockade of glutamate-induced responses in dorsal horn neurons, paradoxically enhanced the response to glutamate upon washout (Ziegelgänsberger and Tulloch, 1979). The enhancement of NMDA receptor-mediated neuronal responses by opiates has also been reported in other CNS areas (see Ziegelgänsberger and Tölle, 1993, for review). In particular, intracellular studies conducted on dorsal horn neurons in vitro indicated an enhanced NMDA-evoked response by μ opioid agonists (Chen and Huang, 1991; Rusin and Randic, 1991).

Enhancement of Acute Morphine Antinociception by NMDA Receptor Antagonists

Activation of NMDA receptors following opioid treatment may reduce the magnitude and duration of opioid-induced antinociception. Thus, blockade of NMDA receptors may be expected to acutely enhance opioid-induced antinociception. Surprisingly, however, no such interaction was observed in the majority of earlier studies examining the acute interaction between morphine and NMDA antagonists (Trujillo and Akil, 1991; Tiseo and Inturrisi, 1993; Elliott, Hynansky, and Inturrisi, 1994; Elliott, Minami et al., 1994). In these studies it was found that NMDA antagonists co-administered with morphine reduced the development of tolerance (see next section), but the design of the studies was not optimal for observing an acute interaction between the co-administered drugs. Even in studies in which such potentiation was noted, the significance of the results was overlooked (Ben-Eliyahu et al., 1992). This finding has contributed to some of the recent discussion concerning whether or not NMDA receptor antagonists reverse morphine tolerance (see next section). We have recently examined this issue and found a significant potentiation and prolongation of systemic morphine-induced antinociception by NMDA antagonists in rats. The potentiation can be observed with both the noncompetitive antagonists dextromethorphan and MK-801, as well as with the competitive antagonist CGS 19755 (Grass et al., 1996; Hoffmann and Wiesenfeld-Hallin, 1996). Thus, our data indicate an intense potentiation of opioid-induced antinociception by NMDA antagonists, which are supported by several behavioral and electrophysiologic studies (Chapman and Dickenson, 1992; Bell and Belgian, 1995; Mao et al., 1996).

The NMDA Receptor and Opioid Tolerance

Co-administration of different classes of NMDA antagonists prevent or reduce morphine tolerance (Marek et al., 1991; Trujillo and Akil, 1991; Ben Eliyahu et al., 1992; Tiseo and Inturrisi, 1993; Elliott, Hynansky, and Inturrisi, 1994; Elliott, Minami et al., 1994; Lutfy et al., 1995; Mao et al., 1996). It has been proposed that acute enhancement of NMDA receptor activity by opioids may lead to persistent changes in the states of NMDA receptors following chronic opioid administration, possibly involving the production of nitric oxide and/or activation of protein kinase C. Such changes in NMDA receptors increase excitatory transmission in the nervous system and lead to opioid tolerance (see Mao et al., 1995a, for review). It has been further suggested that in opiate tolerance the administration of NMDA antagonists could re-establish the antinociceptive effect of opioids (Tiseo and Inturrisi, 1993; Elliott, Hynansky, and Inturrisi, 1994; Elliott, Minami et al., 1994; Shimoyama et al., 1996). The interpretation of the results from these studies is based on the assumption that there is no acute potentiation of opioid antinociception by NMDA antagonists. This notion is, however, not supported by other data (see earlier). Therefore, it is possible that the apparent reversal of tolerance may result from the potentiation of the residual effect of the opioid by the NMDA antagonists rather than from a genuine reversal of tolerance.

Summary

As discussed in this chapter, endogenous antiopioid mechanisms, particularly peptides (CCK, NPFF) and excitatory amino acids acting on NMDA receptors, may have a role in mediating the magnitude of opioid analgesia and the development of tolerance and opioid insensitivity observed in some pain states. Thus, blockade of endogenous antiopioid mechanisms may have potential clinical applications in pain management. Combinations of blockers of the endogenous antiopioid systems with opioids may reduce the required analgesic dose of the opioid. This would not only lead to fewer and weaker side effects, but might also delay the development of tolerance because of low-level stimulation of opioid receptors. Furthermore, in opioid-insensitive pain states, antagonists of the endogenous antiopioid systems may be analgesic or may reinstate the analgesic effect of opioids. These concepts need to be vigorously tested in clinical studies with clinically available antagonists of the anti-opioid systems.

REFERENCES

Allard, M., Zajac, J.M., and Simonnet, G. (1992). Autoradiographic distribution of receptors to FLFQPQRFamide, a morphine-modulating peptide, in rat central nervous system. *Neuroscience.* **49,** 101–116.

Arnér, S., and Meyerson, B. (1993). Opioids in neuropathic pain. *Pain Dig.* **3,** 15–22.

Bell, J.A., and Beglan, C.L. (1995). MK-801 blocks the expression but not the development of tolerance to morphine in the isolated spinal cord of the neonatal rat. *Eur. J. Pharmacol.* **294,** 289–296.

Ben-Eliyahu, S., Marek, P., Vaccarino, A.L., Mogil, J.S., Sternberg, W.F., and Liebeskind, J.C. (1992). The NMDA receptor antagonist MK-801 prevents long-lasting non-associative morphine tolerance in the rat. *Brain Res.* **575,** 304–308.

Benoliel, J.J., Bourgoin, S., Mauborgne, A., Legrand, J.C., Hamon, M., and Cesselin, F. (1991). Differential inhibitory/stimulatory modulation of spinal CCK release by mu and delta opioid agonists, and selective blockade of mu-dependent inhibition by kappa receptor stimulation. *Neurosci. Lett.* **124,** 204–207.

Cesselin, F. (1995). Opioid and anti-opioid peptides. *Fundam. Clin. Pharmacol.* **9,** 409–433.

Chapman, V., and Dickenson, A.H. (1992). The combination of NMDA antagonism and morphine produces profound antinociception in the rat dorsal horn. *Brain Res.* **573,** 321–323.

Chen, L., and Huang, L.Y. (1991). Substained potentiation of NMDA receptor-mediated glutamate responses through activation of protein-kinase C by a μ-opioid. *Neuron.* **7,** 319–326.

Ding, X.Z., and Bayer, B.M. (1993). Increases of CCK mRNA and peptide in different brain areas following acute and chronic administration of morphine. *Brain Res.* **625,** 139–144.

Dourish, C.T., O'Neill, M.F., Coughlan, J., Kitchener, S.J., Hawley, D., and Iversen, S.D. (1990). The selective CCK-B receptor antagonist L-365,260 enhances morphine analgesia and prevents morphine tolerance in the rat. *Eur. J. Pharmacol.* **176,** 35–44.

Elliott, K., Hynansky, A., and Inturrisi, C.E. (1994). Dextromethorphan attenuates and reverses analgesic tolerance to morphine. *Pain.* **59,** 361–368.

Elliott, K., Minami, N., Kolesnikov, Y.A., Pasternak, G.W., and Inturrisi, C.E. (1994). The NMDA receptor antagonists, LY274614 and MK-801, and the nitric oxide synthase inhibitor, NG-nitro-L-arginine, attenuate analgesic tolerance to the mu-opioid morphine but not to kappa opioids. *Pain.* **56,** 69–75.

Faris, P.L., Komisaruk, B.R., Watkins, L.R., and Mayer, D.J. (1983). Evidence for the neuropeptide cholecystokinin as an antagonist of opiate analgesia. *Science.* **219,** 310–312.

Ghilardi, J.R., Allen, C.J., Vigna, S.R., McVey, D.C., and Mantyh, P.W. (1992). Trigeminal and dorsal root ganglion neurons express CCK receptor binding sites in the rat, rabbit and monkey: Possible site of opiate-CCK analgesic interactions. *J. Neurosci.* **12,** 4854–4866.

Grass, S., Hoffmann, O., Xu, X.-J., and Wiesenfeld-Hallin, Z. (1996). N-methyl-D-aspartate receptor antagonists potentiate morphine's antinociceptive effect in the rat. *Acta Physiol. Scand.* **158,** 269–273.

Han, J.S., Ding, X.Z., and Fan, S.G. (1986). Cholecystokinin octapeptide (CCK-8): Antagonism to electroacupuncture analgesia and a possible role in electroacupuncture tolerance. *Pain.* **27,** 101–115.

Hill, D.R., Shaw, T.M., Graham, W., and Woodruff, G.N. (1990). Autoradiographical detection of cholecystokinin-A receptors in primate brain using 125I-bolton hunter CCK-8 and 3H-MK-329. *J. Neurosci.* **10,** 1070–1081.

Hoffmann, O., and Wiesenfeld-Hallin, Z. (1995). The CCK-B receptor antagonist Cl 988 reverses tolerance to morphine in rats. *Neuroreport.* **5,** 2565–2568.

Hoffmann, O., and Wiesenfeld-Hallin, Z. (1996). Dextromethorphan potentiates morphine antinociception, but does not reverse tolerance in rats. *Neuroreport.* **7,** 838–840.

Kastin, A.J., Stephens, E., Ehrensing, R.H., and Fischman, A.J. (1984). Tyr-MIF-I acts as an opiate antagonist in the tail flick test. *Pharmacol. Biochem. Behav.* **21,** 937–941.

Kivipelto, L., and Panula, P. (1991). Origin and distribution of neuropeptide FF-like immunoreactivity in the spinal cord of rats. *J. Comp. Neurol.* **307,** 107–119.

Lake, J.R., Hammond, M.V., Shaddox, B.C., Hunsicker, L.M., Yang, H.Y., and Malin, D.H. (1991). IgG from neuropeptide FF antiserum reverses morphine tolerance in the rat. *Neurosci. Lett.* **132,** 29–32.

Lake, J.R., Hebert, K.M., Payza, K., et al. (1992). Analog of neuropeptide FF attenuates morphine tolerance. *Neurosci. Lett.* **146,** 203–206.

Lee, C.H., Wasowicz, K., Brown, R., Majane, E.A., Yang, H.Y.T., and Panula, P. (1995). Distribution and characterization of neuropeptide FF-like immunoreactivity in the rat nervous system with a monoclonal antibody. *Eur. J. Neurosci.* **7,** 1339–1348.

Lee, Y.-W., Chaplan, S.R., and Yaksh, T.L. (1995). Systemic and supraspinal, but not spinal, opiates suppress allodynia in a rat neuropathic pain model. *Neurosci. Lett.* **186,** 111–114.

Lutfy, K., Shen, K.Z., Kwon, I.S., et al. (1995). Blockade of morphine tolerance by ACEA-1328, a novel NMDA receptor/glycine site antagonist. *Eur. J. Pharmacol.* **273,** 187–189.

Magnuson, D.S., Sullivan, A.F., Simonnet, G., Roques, B.P., and Dickenson, A.H. (1990). Differential interactions of cholecystokinin and FLFQPQRF-NH2 with mu and delta opioid antinociception in the rat spinal cord. *Neuropeptides.* **16,** 213–218.

Majane, E.A., Casanova, M.F., and Yang, H.Y.T. (1988). Biochemical characterization of FMRF-NH2-like peptides in the spinal cord of various mammalian species using specific radioimmunoassays. *Peptides.* **8,** 1137–1144.

Malin, D.H., Lake, J.R., Fowler, D.E., et al. (1990). FMRF-NH2-like mammalian peptide precipitates morphine abstinence syndrome. *Peptides.* **11,** 277–280.

Malin, D.H., Lake, J.R., Levva, J.E., et al. (1991). Analog of neuropeptide FF attenuates morphine abstinence syndrome. *Peptides.* **12,** 1011–1014.

Mao, J., Price, D.D., Caruso, F.S., and Mayer, D.J. (1996). Oral administration of dextromethorphan prevents the development of morphine tolerance and dependence in rats. *Pain.* **67,** 361–368.

Mao, J., Price, D.D., and Mayer, D.J. (1995a). Mechanisms of hyperalgesia and morphine tolerance: A current view of their possible interactions. *Pain.* **62,** 259–274.

Mao, J., Price, D.D., and Mayer, D.J. (1995b). Experimental mononeuropathy reduces the antinociceptive effects of morphine: Implications for common intracellular mechanisms involved in morphine tolerance and neuropathic pain. *Pain.* **61,** 353–364.

Marek, P., Ben-Eliyahu, S., Gold, M., and Liebeskind, J.C. (1991). Excitatory amino acid antagonists (kynurenic acid and MK-801) attenuate the development of morphine tolerance in the rat. *Brain Res.* **547,** 77–81.

Mercer, L.D., and Beart, P.M. (1997). Histochemistry in rat brain and spinal cord with an antibody direction at the cholecystokinin A receptor. *Neurosci. Lett.* **225,** 97–100.

Moran, T., Robinson, P., Goldrich, M.S., and McHugh, P. (1986). Two brain cholecystokinin receptors: Implications for behavioural actions. *Brain Res.* **362,** 175–179.

Nichols, M.L., Bian, D., Ossipov, M.H., Lai, J., and Porreca, F. (1995). Regulation of morphine antiallodynic efficacy by cholecystokinin in a model of neuropathic pain in rats. *J. Pharmacol. Exp. Ther.* **275,** 1399–1345.

Noble, F., Blommaert, A., Fournié-Zaluski, M.C., and Roques, B.P. (1995). A selective CCK-B receptor antagonist potentiates mu- but not delta-opioid receptor-mediated antinociception in the formalin test. *Eur. J. Pharmacol.* **273,** 145–151.

Ossipov, M.H., Lopez, Y., Nichols, M.L., Bian, D., and Porreca, F. (1995). Inhibition by spinal morphine of the tail-flick response is attenuated in rats with nerve ligation injury. *Neurosci. Lett.* **199,** 83–86.

Payza, K., and Yang, H.Y. (1993). Modulation of neuropeptide FF receptors by guanine nucleotides and cations in membranes of rat brain and spinal cord. *J. Neurochem.* **60,** 1894–1899.

Rusin, K.I., and Randic, M. (1991). Modulation of NMDA-induced currents by mu-opioid receptor agonist DAGO in acutely isolated rat spinal dorsal horn neurons. *Neurosci. Lett.* **124,** 208–212.

Seroogy, K.B., Mohapatra, N.K., Lund, P.K., Réthelyi, M., McGehee, D.S., and Perl, ER. (1990). Species-specific expression of cholecystokinin messenger RNA in rodent dorsal root ganglia. *Mol. Brain Res.* **7,** 171–176.

Shimoyama, N., Shimoyama, M., Inturrisi, C.E., and Elliott, K.J. (1996). Ketamine attenuates and reverses morphine tolerance in rodents. *Anesthesiology.* **85,** 1357–1366.

Stanfa, L.C., and Dickenson, A.H. (1993). Cholecystokinin as a factor in the enhanced potency of spinal morphine following carrageenin inflammation. *Br. J. Pharmacol.* **108,** 967–973.

Tang, J., Chou, J., Iadarola, M., Yang, H.Y., and Costa, E. (1984). Proglumide prevents and curtails acute tolerance to morphine in rats. *Neuropharmacology.* **23,** 715–718.

Tiseo, P.J., and Inturrisi, C.E. (1993). Attenuation and reversal of morphine tolerance by the competitive N-methyl-D-aspartate receptor antagonist LY274614. *J. Pharmacol. Exp. Ther.* **264,** 1090–1096.

Trujillo, K.A., and Akil, H. (1991). Inhibition of morphine tolerance and dependence by the NMDA receptor antagonist MK-801. *Science.* **251,** 85–87.

Verge, V.M.K., Wiesenfeld-Hallin, Z., and Hökfelt, T. (1993). Cholecystokinin in mammalian primary sensory neurons and spinal cord: In situ hybridization studies in rat and monkey. *Eur. J. Neurosci.* **5,** 240–250.

Wang, X.J., and Han, J.S. (1989). Modification by cholecystokinin octapeptide of the binding of μ-, δ- and κ-opioid receptors. *J. Neurochem.* **55,** 1379–1382.

Wang, X.J., Wang, X.H., and Han, J.S. (1990). Cholecystokinin octapeptide antagonized opioid analgesia mediated by μ- and κ- but not δ-receptor in rat spinal cord. *Brain Res.* **523,** 5–10.

Wang, J.F., Ren, M.F., and Han, J.S. (1992). Mobilization of calcium from intracellular stores is one of the mechanisms underlying the antiopioid effect of cholecystokinin octapeptide. *Peptides.* **13,** 947–951.

Watkins, L.R., Kinscheck, I.B., Kaufman, E.F., Miller, J., Frenk, H., and Mayer, D.J. (1985). Cholecystokinin antagonists selectively potentiate analgesia induced by endogenous opiates. *Brain Res.* **327,** 181–190.

Wiertelak, E.P., Maier, S.F., and Watkins, L.R. (1992). Cholecystokinin antianalgesia: Safety cues abolish morphine analgesia. *Science.* **256,** 830–833.

Wiesenfeld-Hallin Z., and Xu, X.-J. (1996). The role of cholecystokinin in nociception, neuropathic pain and opiate tolerance. *Regul. Pept.* **65,** 23–28.

Williams, R.G., Dimaline, R., Varro, A., Isetta, A.M., Trizio, D., and Dockray, G.J. (1987). Cholecystokinin octapeptide in rat central nervous system: Immunocytochemical studies using a monoclonal antibody that does not react with CGRP. *Neurochem. Int.* **11,** 433–442.

Xu, X.-J., Hökfelt, T., Hughes, J., and Wiesenfeld-Hallin, Z. (1994). The CCK-B antagonist CI988 enhances the reflex-depressive effect of morphine in axotomized rats. *Neuroreport.* **5,** 718–720.

Xu, X.-J., Puke, M.J.C., Verge, V.M.K., Wiesenfeld-Hallin, Z., Hughes, J., and Hökfelt, T. (1993). Up-regulation of cholecystokinin in primary sensory neurons is associated with morphine insensitivity in experimental neuropathic pain. *Neurosci. Lett.* **152,** 129–132.

Xu, X.-J., and Wiesenfeld-Hallin, Z. (1991). The threshold for the depressive effect of intrathecal morphine on the spinal nociceptive flexor reflex is increased during autotomy after sciatic nerve section in rats. *Pain.* **46,** 223–229.

Xu, X.-J., Wiesenfeld-Hallin, Z., Hughes, J., Horwell, D.C., and Hökfelt, T. (1992). CI988, a selective antagonist of cholecystokinin type-B receptor, prevents morphine tolerance in the rat. *Br. J. Pharmacol.* **105,** 591–596.

Yamamoto, T., and Nozakitaguchi, N. (1995). Role of cholecystokinin-B receptor in the maintenance of thermal hyperalgesia induced by unilateral constriction injury to the sciatic nerve in the rat. *Neurosci. Lett.* **202,** 89–92.

Yang, H.Y.T., Fratta, W., Majabe, E.A., and Costa, E. (1985). Isolation, sequencing, synthesis and pharmacological characterization of two brain neuropeptides that modulate the action of morphine. *Proc. Natl. Acad. Sci. U.S.A.* **82,** 7757–7761.

Zhang, X., Dagerlind, Å., Elde, R.P., et al. (1993). Marked increase in cholecystokinin B receptor messenger RNA levels in rat dorsal root ganglia after peripheral axotomy. *Neuroscience.* **57,** 227–233.

Zhang, X., Nicholas, A.P., and Hökfelt, T. (1995). Ultrastructural studies on peptides in the dorsal horn of the rat spinal cord. 2. Coexistence of galanin with other peptides in local neurons. *Neuroscience.* **64,** 875–891.

Zhou, Y., Sun, Y.H., Zhang, Z.W., and Han, J.S. (1993). Increased release of immunoreactive cholecystokinin octapeptide by morphine and potentiation of μ-opioid analgesia by CCKB receptor antagonist L365,260 in rat spinal cord. *Eur. J. Pharmacol.* **234,** 147–154.

Zhou, Y., Sun, Y.H., Zhang, Z.W., and Han, J.S. (1994). Accelerated expression of cholecystokinin gene in the brain of rats rendered tolerant to morphine. *Neuroreport.* **3,** 1121–1123.

Ziegelgänsberger, W., and Tölle, T.R. (1993). The pharmacology of pain signalling. *Curr. Opinion Neurobiol.* **3,** 611–618.

Zieglgänsberger, W., and Tulloch, I.F. (1979). The effects of methionine- and leucine-enkephalin on spinal neurones of the cat. *Brain Res.* **167,** 53–64.

CHAPTER EIGHT

Transplantation of Opioid-Producing Cells

JACQUELINE SAGEN

Sources of Opioid-Producing Cells

Adrenal Medulla

Chromaffin cells of the adrenal medulla produce and secrete a variety of neuroactive substances in addition to the traditionally recognized catecholamines. Most notably, these cells are a rich source of neuropeptides and neurotrophic factors (see Carmichael and Stoddard, 1993, and Unsicker, 1993, for reviews). Although several of these latter agents may be useful in pain control, the adrenal medulla has been well characterized as a rich source of opioid peptides (Viveros et al., 1979; Hexum et al., 1980; Lewis et al., 1980; Yang et al., 1980; Kilpatrick et al., 1982). These are primarily derived from the proenkephalin A precursor; thus, the active peptides are predominantly those of the enkephalin-containing family. In bovine adrenal gland, proenkephalin mRNA levels are 20–400 times higher than in the brain (Pittius et al., 1985). Levels of opioid peptide production in the adrenal medulla is species dependent to some extent, with high levels found in bovine, porcine, and canine glands and lower levels in rodents (Hexum et al., 1980; Yang et al., 1980). However, both proenkephalin mRNA and opioid peptide levels increase in the rat adrenal with denervation and with time in tissue culture, suggesting that environmental factors have a strong influence on opioid peptide production (Kilpatrick et al., 1984; Zhu et al., 1992).

In contrast to the CNS, where proenkephalin is processed nearly completely to the pentapeptides, Met^5-enkephalin and Leu^5-enkephalin, the adrenal medulla in addition processes this precursor to several small, intermediate, and larger peptides that may contain single or multiple encrypted pentapeptide sequences (Lewis et al., 1980; Stern et al., 1980; Liston et al., 1984; Wilson, 1991). Some of these have been tested for and demonstrate analgesic or opiate activity, including Met-enkephalin-Arg-Phe, Met-enkephalin-Arg-Gly-Leu, peptides E and F, BAM-12, BAM-18, BAM-20 and BAM-22 (Inturrisi et al., 1980; Mizuno et al., 1980; Höllt, Haarman et al., 1982; Höllt, Tulunay et al., 1982; Iadorola et al., 1986; Evans et al., 1988; Stevens et al., 1988). Interestingly, although the pentapeptides are thought to be fairly selective for δ opioid receptors, some of the intermediate- and larger-sized enkephalin-containing

Christoph Stein, ed., *Opioids in Pain Control: Basic and Clinical Aspects*. Printed in the United States of America.

peptides have significant activity at the μ site, and possibly at the κ site (Höllt, 1986; Evans et al., 1988). In addition, there is some evidence for a synergistic interaction between μ and δ opioid agonists in antinociception (Larson et al., 1980; Porreca et al., 1990), and agents having high affinity for both are among the most potent (Yaksh and Noueihed, 1985; Yaksh, 1987). Thus, adrenal medullary chromaffin cells are a potentially rich source of opioid peptides for pain control.

In addition to opioid peptides, the adrenal medulla also apparently contains "true opiates" (Goldstein et al., 1985; Donnerer et al., 1987; Hathaway and Epple, 1990). The opiate alkaloids morphine and codeine are enriched in the synaptosomal fraction as a sulfate conjugate and may be co-localized with catecholamines.

Another potential advantage of chromaffin cells as transplant donors for pain relief is the apparent antinociceptive synergism between opioid and α-adrenergic agonists (Yaksh and Reddy, 1981; Wilcox et al., 1987; Drasner and Fields, 1988; Sherman et al., 1988). Further, the co-administration of subeffective levels of these agents may produce potent analgesia while reducing the development of tolerance. Numerous studies have demonstrated that chromaffin cells co-release opioid peptides and catecholamines (Viveros et al., 1979; Livett et al., 1981; Chaminade et al., 1984; Nguyen and de Léon, 1987).

The majority of neural transplant studies for analgesia in animal models have utilized adrenal medullary tissue or isolated chromaffin cells as the opioid-producing cell source (Sagen, Pappas, and Perlow, 1986; Sagan, Pappas, and Pollard, 1986; Ginzburg and Seltzer, 1990; Pacheco-Cano et al., 1990; Ruz-Franzi and Gonzalez-Darder, 1991; Hama and Sagen, 1993, 1994a; Ortega-Alvaro et al., 1994; Wang and Sagen, 1994a, 1995; Yeomans et al., 1996; Yu et al., 1996; Siegan and Sagen, 1997). Both acute and chronic pain models have been explored (see later for a review of chronic pain studies). In our laboratory, acute analgesiometric tests have included the tail-flick, paw-pressure (Randall-Selitto test), and hot-plate responses (Sagen, Pappas, and Perlow, 1986; Sagen, Pappas, and Pollard, 1986; Sagen, Wang et al., 1993; Wang and Sagen, 1994a, 1994b). Adrenal medullary tissue for transplantation is dissected from the adrenal glands of adult donor rats (allografts) and implanted into the spinal subarachnoid space at L1–L2 via a laminectomy and slit in the dura (for details, see Czech and Sagen, 1995). Generally, medullary tissue from two adrenal glands has been used because this method has been found to produce reliable antinociception in several models, although a dose-response relationship has been found in acute analgesiometric tests when graft tissue amount is varied (Wang and Sagen, 1994a). In other studies, xenogeneic chromaffin cells obtained from bovine adrenal medullae were used, either as cell suspensions in immunosuppressed animals or in immunoisolatory polymer capsules (Sagen, Pappas, and Pollard, 1986; Sagen, Wang et al., 1993). These studies have revealed that there is little change in baseline nociceptive responses using acute noxious stimuli following adrenal medullary implantation. However, following the injection of low doses of nicotine (0.1 mg/kg, SC), antinociception is observed using all three acute stimuli (Sagen, Pappas, and Pollard, 1986;

Sagen, Wang et al., 1993; Wang and Sagen, 1994a). This most likely results from increased release from chromaffin cells following stimulation of cell surface nicotinic receptors. An example is shown in Figure 8.1A. Animals received either adrenal medullary allografts from two adrenal glands ($n = 5$) or equal volumes of control striated muscle tissue ($n = 5$). Baseline tail-flick latencies were determined one month following implantation, and animals were then injected with nicotine (0.1 mg/kg, SC) and tested again at 2, 10, 30, and 60 minutes. The results indicated that although baseline nociceptive responses were unaltered compared with controls, nicotine stimulation produced significant elevations in tail-flick latencies, peaking at 2 minutes following injection and diminishing toward baseline by 30 minutes. The magnitude and time course of this effect were similar to those found in previous studies (Sagen, Pappas, and Pollard, 1986; Wang and Sagen, 1994a).

Pituitary: Intermediate Lobe

Another potential source of opioid-producing cells is the intermediate lobe of the pituitary gland. Both the anterior and intermediate lobes of the pituitary gland synthesize peptides derived from another opioid precursor family, pro-opiomelanocortin (POMC). In the intermediate lobe in particular, more extensive processing occurs to form opiate-active peptide β-endorphin (Evans et al., 1981; Smyth, 1983). Preliminary findings in our laboratory have suggested that implantation of intermediate-lobe tissue in the spinal subarachnoid space can produce antinociception to acute noxious stimuli (Wang and Sagen, 1991). Figure 8.1B and C show examples. Animals were implanted either with intermediate-lobe tissue ($n = 8$) or control striated muscle tissue ($n = 9$) and tested 4–5 weeks postimplant. Similar to findings with adrenal medullary implants, baseline nociceptive thresholds were not altered. Since the secretion of POMC peptides from the intermediate lobe may be stimulated by either the hypothalamic peptide corticotropin-releasing factor (CRF) or serotonin (5-HT; Kraicer and Morris, 1976; Sakly et al., 1982; Randle et al., 1983; Vale et al., 1983; Palkovits et al., 1986; Saland et al., 1988), these agents were injected intrathecally in animals with implants.

The intrathecal injection of ovine CRF (20 μg), a dose that had no effect on control implanted animals, produced modest elevations in tail-flick latencies in animals with intermediate-lobe implants (Fig. 8.1B). This antinociception was apparent 5–30 minutes following intrathecal injection and tended toward baseline by 60 minutes. CRF itself has been reported by others to produce potent and long-lasting antinociception in the writhing assay when injected intrathecally, but does not alter tail-flick responses at doses up to 20 times higher (Song and Takemori, 1991). Thus, it is unlikely that effects of CRF independent of the transplants contributed to the observed antinociception. However, it has also been demonstrated that intrathecally injected CRF can significantly attenuate the antinociceptive action of morphine (Song and Takemori, 1991). This could potentially interfere with CRF-induced

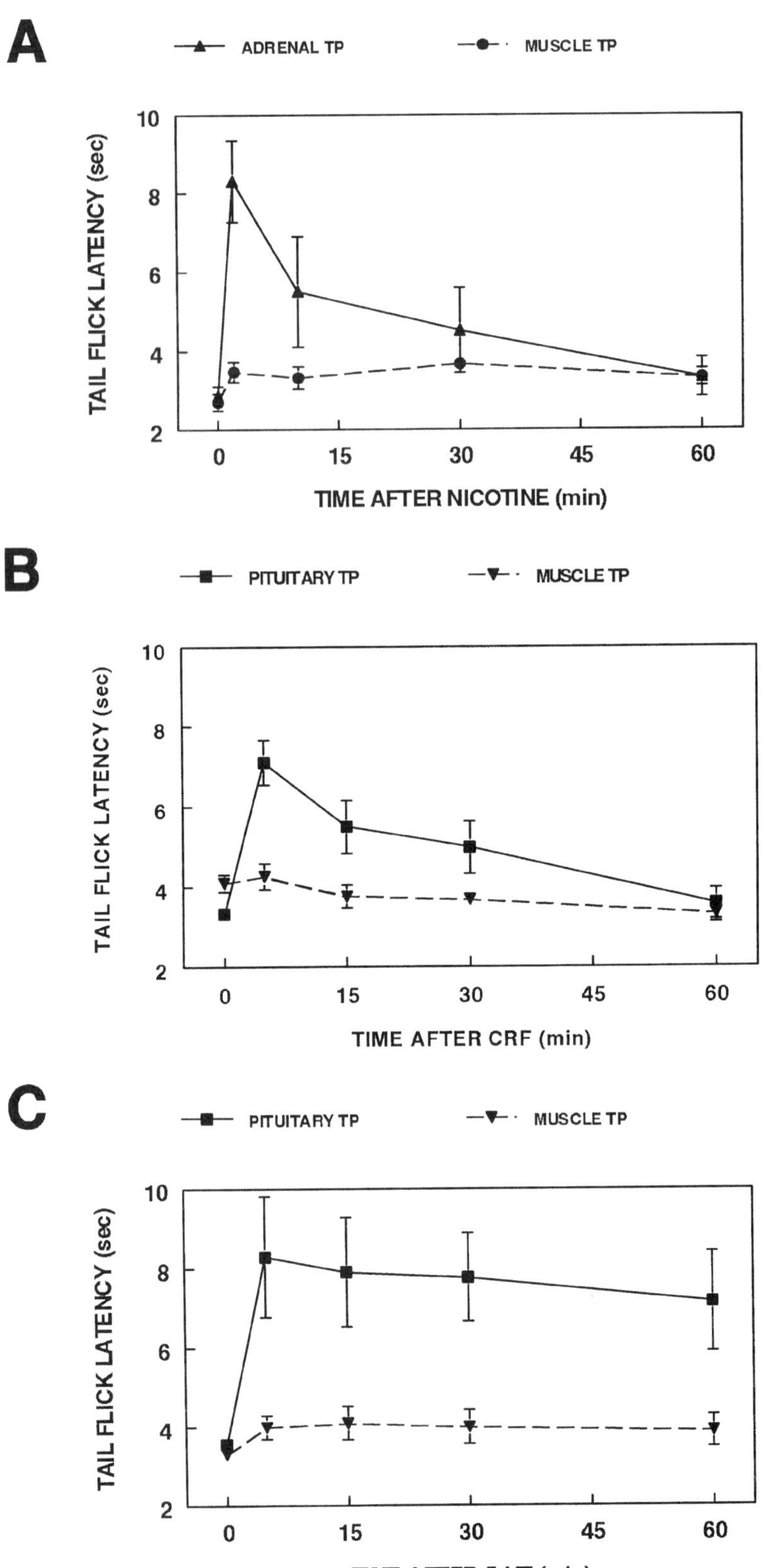
A
ADRENAL TP
MUSCLE TP
TAIL FLICK LATENCY (sec)
10
8
6
4
2
0
15
30
45
60
TIME AFTER NICOTINE (min)
B
PITUITARY TP
MUSCLE TP
TAIL FLICK LATENCY (sec)
10
8
6
4
2
0
15
30
45
60
TIME AFTER CRF (min)
C
PITUITARY TP
MUSCLE TP
TAIL FLICK LATENCY (sec)
10
8
6
4
2
0
15
30
45
60
TIME AFTER 5-HT (min)

antinociception in the current study since the implanted cells are likely to mediate their behavioral effects via CRF-stimulated release of β-endorphin. Preliminary results indicate that this antinociception is blocked by naloxone.

The intrathecal injection of 5-HT (creatine sulfate, 80 μg), which did not alter tail-flick latencies in animals with control transplants, produced significant and prolonged antinociception in animals with intermediate-lobe transplants, lasting over 60 minutes. Since 5-HT itself has antinociceptive activity at somewhat higher doses (Yaksh and Wilson, 1979; Kuraishi et al., 1985), it is possible that the latter antinociceptive effect of 5-HT in intermediate-lobe-implanted animals is mediated in part by direct effects of 5-HT itself. However, preliminary findings indicate that this prolonged analgesia can be prevented by naloxone pretreatment, suggesting a role for release of opioids from the implanted cells.

Tumor Cell Lines

Several cell lines have also been employed to deliver opioid peptides in cellular implantation studies for pain. In particular, AtT-20 cells, which were originally derived from a mouse anterior pituitary tumor, synthesize and secrete β-endorphin (Sabol, 1980; Hook et al., 1982). These cells have been implanted in mouse and rat spinal intrathecal space (Wu et al., 1993, 1994; Saitoh et al., 1995a). When implanted at lumbar levels, baseline pain responses to acute noxious stimuli (tail flick, hot plate) up to 21 days postimplantation were not altered, but intrathecally administered β-adrenergic agonist isoproterenol with a phosphodiesterase inhibitor, which is thought to increase β-endorphin release from the cells, produced antinociception (Wu et al., 1993, 1994). The antinociceptive effects of isoproterenol were dose related and naloxone reversible, and peaked at 5–10 minutes postinjection, returning toward baseline by 30 minutes. In another study, AtT-20 cells were immunologically isolated in polymer capsules and implanted in the spinal subarachnoid space at the atlanto-occipital junction (Saitoh et al., 1995a). In this study, baseline responses to acute noxious stimuli were elevated at 2 and 4 weeks postimplantation.

AtT-20 cells have also been transfected with the human proenkephalin gene and secrete enkephalin in addition to β-endorphin (Comb et al., 1985). These cells have also been utilized in neural transplantation studies demonstrating antinociceptive effects (Wu et al., 1993, 1994). Another β-endorphin-secreting cell line, a POMC

Opposite

Figure 8.1. Antinociceptive responses assessed by the tail-flick test in animals with either adrenal medullary or control striated muscle transplants (A: $n = 5$); pituitary intermediate-lobe or control striated muscle transplants (B and C: $n = 8–9$). Baseline nociceptive responses are indicated at time 0; responses following either nicotine (0.1 mg/kg, SC; A), CRF (20 μg, IT; B), or 5-HT (80 μg, IT; C) are shown up to 60 minutes postinjection. Points represent mean ± S.E.M. TP = transplant.

transfected mouse neuroblastoma line, Neuro2A, has also been implanted in immunoisolatory polymer capsules (Saitoh et al., 1995a, 1995b). These implants reduce pain sensitivity for at least one month following implantation. Finally, PC12 cells, derived from a rat adrenal medullary tumor, have been tested as potential cellular implants in pain studies. However, these cells do not normally produce high levels of opioid peptides. To increase Met-enkephalin production and release, PC12 cells were transfected with the human proenkephalin gene (Kim et al., 1996). These cells produced increased levels and secretion of Met-enkephalin, and preliminary findings indicate that implantation into the spinal subarachnoid space reduces nociceptive responses, in contrast to parent cell lines.

The Role of Opioid Peptides/Receptors in Adrenal Medullary Transplant-Induced Analgesia

Reversal by Opioid Antagonists

Evidence that antinociceptive effects of adrenal medullary implants are mediated in part by opioid peptides released from implanted chromaffin cells is derived mainly from antagonist studies. In acute pain models such as tail flick, paw pressure, and hot plate, analgesia following nicotine injection in implanted animals is attenuated by administration of the broad opiate antagonist naloxone (2 mg/kg, SC) when administered either prior to or just after nicotine (Sagen, Pappas, and Perlow, 1986; Sagen, Pappas, and Pollard, 1986; Sagen et al., 1993). This is most likely due to blockade of spinal opioid receptors, since naloxone administered intrathecally is equally effective in attenuating antinociception in adrenal medullary–implanted animals (Wang and Sagen, 1993). However, at least three opioid receptor types have been implicated in the production of antinociception at the spinal level. Although naloxone has been reported to have different relative affinities for the opiate receptor types, being the most potent in binding to the μ receptor, it also binds to the δ and κ receptors and blocks δ and κ agonist effects with sufficient potency that it is difficult to distinguish effects on opiate receptor types, even at low doses (Yaksh, 1987). Thus, in order to assess the role of opiate receptor types in the antinociception by adrenal medullary transplants, more specific opiate antagonists were used: the δ receptor antagonist naltrindole (NTI), the κ receptor antagonist nor-binaltorphimine (norBNI), and the μ receptor antagonist β-funaltrexamine (β-FNA). Intrathecal doses of drugs and the timing of peak antagonist activities were chosen based on studies from other laboratories demonstrating specific receptor antagonism using these agents (Adams et al., 1987; Russell et al., 1987; Takemori and Porteghese, 1987; Long et al., 1989; Mjander and Yaksh, 1991; Tiseo and Yaksh, 1993; Yu et al., 1995). For both NTI and norBNI, drug solutions were injected intrathecally 10 minutes prior to assessment of pain sensitivity and nicotine (0.1 mg/kg, SC) injection. However, since β-FNA must be administered at least 24 hours prior to testing in order to obtain a specific response (Takemori and Porteghese, 1987; Mjander and Yaksh, 1991), analgesiometric testing and response to nicotine took place 24 hours after the intrathecal β-FNA. In addition, as β-FNA is an irreversible μ antagonist, animals were tested with this agent last.

Results are shown in Figure 8.2 (Wang and Sagen, 1993). As assessed by the tail-flick test (Fig. 8.2A), all three agents produced a dose-dependent antagonism of the antinociceptive effects of nicotine in adrenal medullary–implanted animals (compared to saline vehicle). β-FNA and NTI were the most potent in producing this effect, whereas norBNI was considerably weaker in blocking the antinociception. As assessed by the hot plate (Fig. 8.2B), β-FNA was the most potent in blocking analgesia in adrenal medullary–implanted animals, followed by NTI. Again, norBNI produced only a modest attenuation of the analgesia even at the highest doses tested. Thus, both μ, and δ, and possibly κ, opioid receptors appear to be involved in mediating the analgesic effects of adrenal medullary implants. This finding is consistent with previous descriptions of adrenal opioid peptide activities at both μ and δ receptors (see earlier discussion). Interestingly, none of these specific antagonists completely reversed the tail-flick latencies to levels observed following naloxone injections (Sagen, Pappas, and Perlow, 1986; Sagen, Pappas, and Pollard, 1986; Sagen et al., 1993). This again suggests the possibility that multiple opioid receptors are involved in mediating the antinociceptive effects of the implants. Although antagonist combination studies are difficult due to potential interactions (e.g., β-FNA has been reported to reduce the potency of δ receptor antagonists), preliminary findings in our laboratory have indicated that combined administration of β-FNA, NTI, and norBNI at intermediate doses (10 nmol each) can completely reverse the antinociceptive effects of nicotine in adrenal medullary implanted animals.

Prolongation of Analgesia by Enkephalinase Inhibition

Additional evidence for the role of opioid peptides in the antinociceptive effects of adrenal medullary implants comes from studies utilizing enkephalinase inhibitors to reduce opioid peptide degradation (Sagen and Wang, 1990). The antinociception produced by adrenal medullary or chromaffin cell implants following nicotine stimulation is transient (e.g., see Fig. 8.1A), peaking at 2 minutes and rapidly recovering toward baseline. One possible explanation for this short duration is the rapid degradation of opioid peptides in the spinal subarachnoid space. Similarly, the direct injection of small opioid peptides into the rat CNS also produces a transient analgesia of similar duration (Yaksh et al., 1977; Inturrisi et al., 1980). At least three separate peptidases have been implicated in the rapid degradation of the enkephalins: an endopeptidase (enkephalinase A), which cleaves the Gly^3-Phe^4 bond; an aminopeptidase, which degrades the Tyr^1-Gly^2 bond; and a dipeptidylaminopeptidase, which cleaves the Gly^2-Gly^3 bond. Although specific inhibitors of these enzymes – for example, thiorphan, which inhibits the endopeptidase, or bestatin, which inhibits the

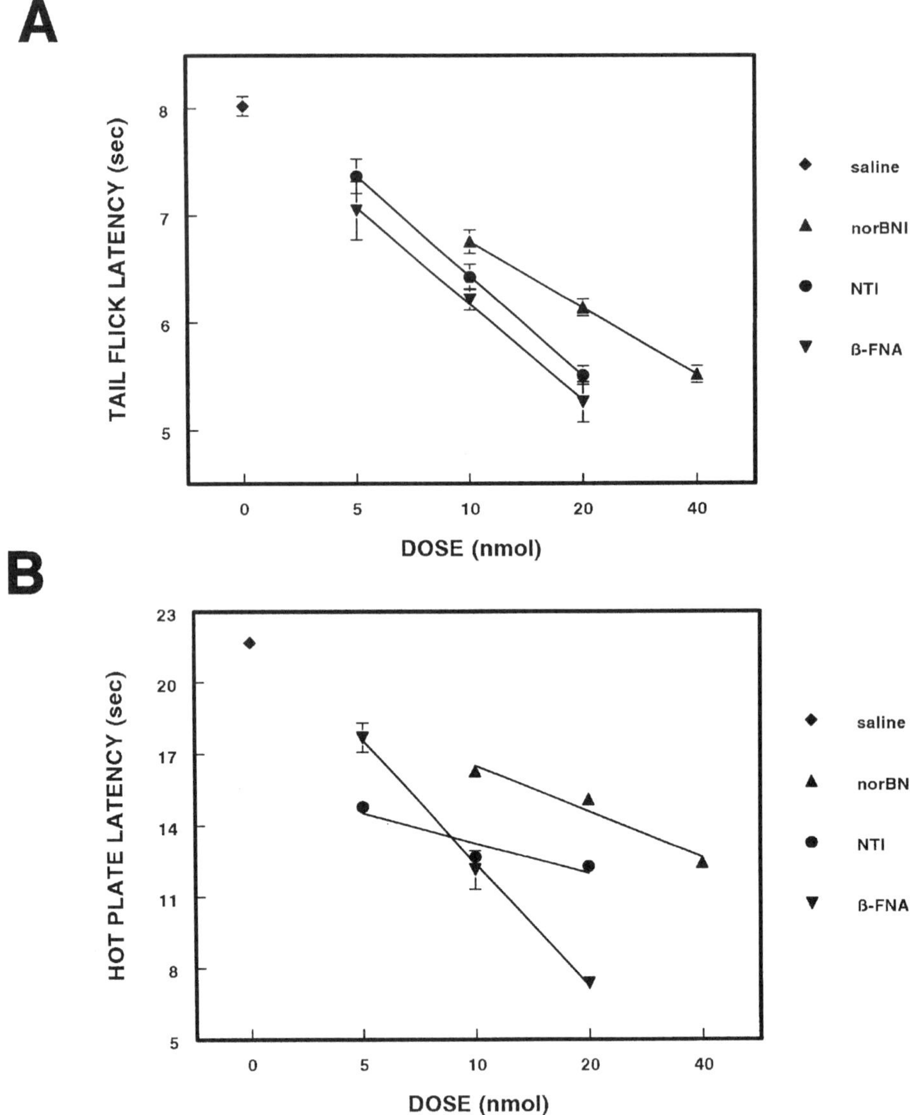

Figure 8.2. Antinociceptive responses to acute nicotine stimulation (0.1 mg/kg, SC) in animals with adrenal medullary implants following pretreatment with specific opiate antagonists: δ receptor antagonist naltrindole (NTI), κ receptor antagonist nor-binaltorphimine (norBNI), or μ receptor antagonist β-funaltrexamine (β-FNA). For comparison, responses in saline-pretreated animals are shown (diamond). *n* = 7–9 animals per group. Points represent mean ± S.E.M.

aminopeptidase – can potentiate and prolong the analgesic effects of opioid peptides, the inhibition of both or possibly of all three enzymes may produce the maximal effect (Yaksh and Harty, 1982; Fournié-Zaluski et al., 1984; Reggiani et al., 1984). Kelatorphan, a complete enkephalinase inhibitor that inhibits all three enzymes, produces potent analgesia when co-administered with opioid peptides (Fournié-Zaluski et al., 1984). When this agent is injected intrathecally into animals with adrenal medullary implants (50 μg, gift of B. Roques, Université René Descartes, Paris) 15 minutes prior to nicotine injection, prolonged elevations in tail-flick latencies, paw-pressure thresholds, and hot-plate latencies were obtained (Sagen and Wang, 1990). No significant effects were observed in control implanted animals. Although the peak antinociceptive responses were not increased, indicating no change in potency, this peak was maintained for nearly one hour following nicotine stimulation, compared to less than 10 minutes in the absence of kelatorphan. To confirm that this prolongation was opiate mediated, animals were pretreated with naloxone concurrently with kelatorphan. This completely eliminated antinociceptive activity in implanted animals. Similar findings were obtained in animals with implants of isolated suspensions of bovine chromaffin cells (Sagen and Wang, 1990).

Release of Opioid Peptides from Implanted Chromaffin Cells

Another piece of evidence supporting delivery of opioid peptides from implanted cells for pain control comes from release studies. In our laboratory, we have measured spinal CSF levels of Met-enkephalin in animals with adrenal medullary implants in the spinal subarachnoid space using push-pull superfusion (Sagen and Kemmler, 1989; Wang and Sagen, 1994a). Results of this study indicated that basal spinal CSF levels of Met-enkephalin were elevated at least twofold in animals with adrenal medullary implants, and this level was further increased by nicotine injections (Sagen and Kemmler, 1989). When the adrenal medullary content of the implant was altered by varying the amount of donor adrenal medullary tissue, CSF Met-enkephalin levels were increased in a dose-related fashion from 1 to 4 glands (Wang and Sagen, 1994a). Although similar spinal superfusion studies were not conducted in animals with isolated bovine chromaffin cell implants, release from these cells was measured from cells implanted into the periaqueductal gray (PAG) using a brain slice preparation (Ortega and Sagen, 1993). Basal Met-enkephalin release in superfusate samples was increased 8–10-fold above control PAG from animals with implants of approximately 100,000 bovine chromaffin cells up to 8 weeks following implantation. Further increases in Met-enkephalin content in the superfusates were obtained with nicotine stimulation in a dose-related fashion. Finally, in animals implanted with encapsulated bovine chromaffin cells in the spinal subarachnoid space, Met-enkephalin release from capsules retrieved at three months postimplantation was sustained and could be additionally stimulated by nicotine (Sagen et al., 1993).

Adrenal Medullary Implants in Chronic Pain

The studies just described suggest that adrenal medullary and chromaffin cell transplants in the spinal subarachnoid space produce antinociception to acute noxious stimuli, which is mediated, at least in part, by release of opioid peptides from the implanted cells. In contrast, the role of opioid peptides in alleviation of chronic pain is less clear. Using inflammatory pain models such as the adjuvant arthritis model, researchers observed that adrenal medullary implants attenuate indicators of chronic pain, such as body weight reduction and hyperventilation consequent to the inflammation (Sagen et al., 1990; Wang and Sagen, 1995). Unlike acute pain reduction, nicotinic stimulation was not necessary to achieve these results, suggesting that sufficient levels of pain-reducing neuroactive substances are released basally from the implants to reduce chronic pain. Similarly, reduction of pain behaviors in neuropathic pain models by adrenal medullary implants does not require nicotine (see later). In the adjuvant arthritis model, naloxone alone failed to reverse the attenuation in hyperventilation in adrenal medullary–implanted animals unless it was combined with α-adrenergic antagonist phentolamine (Wang and Sagen, 1995). In contrast, using another measure in this model, hypervocalization responses in closely grouped animals, it was found that increased vocalizations consequent to adjuvant arthritis are attenuated by adrenal medullary implants only after nicotine stimulation, and this can be blocked by naloxone pretreatment (Sagen et al., 1990). Interestingly, this hypervocalization response is thought to be a measure of acute pain in these animals resulting from stimulation of the inflamed paws (Colpaert, 1987); thus, these findings are consistent with previous findings in acute pain models.

Recent studies in our laboratory have also demonstrated that transplants of adrenal medullary tissue or isolated bovine chromaffin cells can reduce pain behaviors in a neuropathic pain model (Hama and Sagen, 1993, 1994a, 1994b; Hama et al., 1996; Siegan et al., 1996a; Ibuki et al., 1997). For these studies, neuropathic pain was induced by a unilateral chronic constriction injury of the sciatic nerve (Bennett and Xie, 1988). Behavioral assessments included tests for allodynia (cold and tactile) and hyperalgesia (mechanical and thermal). Results indicated that adrenal medullary implants substantially attenuate or completely reverse thermal hyperalgesia and cold allodynia and partially attenuate mechanical hyperalgesia and tactile allodynia by one week postimplantation until the end of the testing period when pain symptoms resolve, usually 6–10 weeks post–nerve injury. Some aspects of these beneficial effects of adrenal medullary implants are attenuated by the opiate antagonist naloxone, such as responses to noxious thermal stimuli. However, the role of opioid peptides provided by the implanted cells in reducing allodynia is unclear, since the process is not markedly reversed by naloxone. In addition, recent studies have revealed that adrenal medullary transplants in the spinal subarachnoid space can reduce pathologic changes in the spinal cord resulting from peripheral nerve injury, such as induction of nitric oxide synthase and cGMP and loss of inhibitory interneurons (Hama and Sagen, 1994b; Hama et al., 1996; Siegan et al., 1996a; Ibuki et al., 1997). These findings suggest the possibility that effects of adrenal medullary implants may be mediated by interference in the spinal hyperexcitability cascade thought to be involved in initiating and maintaining chronic pain. In support of these findings, recent studies in our laboratory have demonstrated that adrenal medullary implants can attenuate allodynia and hyperalgesia resulting from the direct intrathecal injection of NMDA, and this is not blocked by naloxone pretreatment (Siegan et al., 1995).

In order to clarify pharmacologic mechanisms of pain reduction by adrenal medullary implants, the formalin model was utilized, since this test is composed of an acute pain phase (within the first minute following formalin injection) and a more prolonged tonic phase (approximately 25–50 minutes postformalin) thought to be predictive of chronic pain initiation. In animals with adrenal medullary, but not control implants, both phases of the formalin response were significantly attenuated (Siegan and Sagen, 1997). However, when animals with adrenal medullary implants were pretreated with the opiate antagonist naloxone, only the first phase of the formalin response was restored, whereas the second phase remained suppressed (Fig. 8.3). These findings again suggest that attenuation of acute pain by adrenal medullary implants is opiate mediated, but question the role of opioid peptides in the attenuation of chronic pain responses by these implants.

It should be noted that other laboratories have reported a reversal of chronic pain responses by naloxone in animals with chromaffin cell implants. For example, chronic allodynia responses in animals with spinal ischemic injury are alleviated by intrathecal bovine chromaffin cell implants; this process is reversed by either naloxone or α-adrenergic antagonist phentolamine (Yu et al., 1996). In addition, Vaquero et al. (1991) found naloxone reversal of adrenal medullary implant suppression of formalin pain responses one hour following formalin injection. Thus, opioid peptides appear to contribute to chronic pain reduction by chromaffin cells implants, but additional mechanisms are likely to be involved. In addition to opioid peptides and catecholamines, these cells produce several other neuropeptides, including somatostatin, neuropeptide Y, VIP, and neurotensin, as well as a "cocktail" of neurotrophic factors and neuropeptides that may provide neurotrophic support, including basic fibroblast growth factor (β-FGF), transforming growth factors β (TGF-β), interleukin-1 (IL-1), and neurotrophin (NT)-4/5 (Unsicker, 1993; Unsicker et al., 1996). Chromaffin cells have also been reported to produce antioxidants such as ascorbate and NO scavenging heme proteins (Carmichael and Stoddard, 1993), which could potentially act via the NMDA-NO excitability cascade, as well as a novel peptide recently isolated from the adrenal medulla, histogranin, which modulates NMDA binding and reduces the convulsive activity of NMDA (Lemaire et al., 1993). Interestingly, preliminary findings in our laboratory have demonstrated that intrathecally injected histogranin attenuates the second, but not the first, phase of the formalin test (Siegan et al., 1996b).

Tolerance

One of the critical issues facing the successful utilization of cellular implantation for opioid delivery in pain is the potential for tolerance development with continued exposure to opioid peptides released from the cells. Our laboratory has addressed

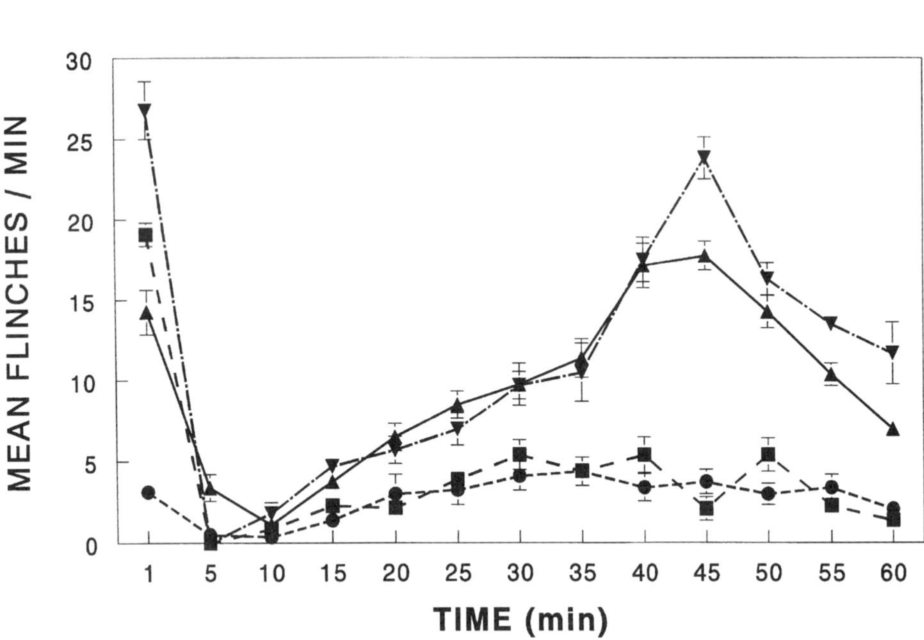

Figure 8.3. Biphasic formalin response in animals with either adrenal medullary (ADR) or control striated muscle (CON) transplants in the spinal subarachnoid space. In order to assess the contribution of opioid peptides, animals were pretreated with the opiate antagonist naloxone (NAL; 2.0 mg/kg, SC) or saline vehicle (SAL) prior to formalin injection. n = 6–8 animals per group. Points represent mean ± S.E.M. (Adapted from Siegan and Sagen, 1997.)

this issue in a number of ways. Early studies in our laboratory using acute pain models demonstrated that it was possible to repeatedly induce antinociception in adrenal medullary–implanted animals on a daily basis with nicotine injections (Wang and Sagen, 1994b). This finding is in contrast to the rapid tolerance development obtained with repeated systemic or intrathecal opioid administration in animal models (Yaksh et al., 1977). In addition to acute pain models, there was no evidence of decreasing analgesic potency following transplantation throughout the 7–10 week testing periods in the chronic arthritic or neuropathic pain models. Together, these studies suggest that there is limited analgesic tolerance development to opioids released from chromaffin cell implants. A possible explanation is that the cells release subeffective levels of opioid peptides and other pain-reducing neuroactive substances that synergize to produce antinociception at levels lower than those that would lead to tolerance. For example, co-administration of subeffective doses of opiates and α-adrenergic agents have been found to reduce tolerance development to these agents (Yaksh and Reddy, 1981). As another example, Wu et al. (1993, 1994) demonstrated that implanted AtT-20/hENK cells, which produce both β-endorphin and enkephalins, reduced the development of acute morphine tolerance, whereas

AtT-20 cells, which produce only β-endorphin, did not. These findings suggest that enkephalins can alter the development of opiate tolerance. Since chromaffin cells synthesize both μ- and δ-acting opioid peptides, as well as α-adrenergic agonists, it is likely that these agents synergize to produce antinociception and reduced tolerance development.

In addition to agents released from the transplanted cells, studies in our laboratory have addressed the issues of cross tolerance with exogenously administered opiates. In earlier studies, dose responsiveness to acute morphine injections was assessed in animals before and following transplantation of either adrenal medullary or control striated muscle tissue (Wang and Sagen, 1994b). Results demonstrated that rather than a rightward shift in the morphine dose-response curve as one might expect with chronic opioid exposure, the transplants actually potentiated the antinociceptive efficacy of morphine, as indicated by a leftward shift in the dose-response curves. Again, it is possible that agents released from the implanted cells provide additive analgesic substances when combined with exogenous morphine.

More recent studies have examined whether adrenal medullary implants alter the development of morphine tolerance or responses to morphine in animals made tolerant, using subcutaneously implanted morphine pellets (NIDA; 75 mg). In the first study, animals received either adrenal medullary or control striated muscle transplants two weeks prior to implantation of morphine or placebo pellets. Morphine dose-response curves to acute morphine injections were generated before transplant, following transplant, and one week following morphine pellet implantation when tolerance to morphine presumably has developed. Results revealed that in animals with control transplants, tolerance to acute morphine injections developed following pellet implantation, as indicated by a rightward shift in the morphine dose-response curve. In contrast, this rightward shift did not occur in animals with adrenal medullary implants, suggesting prevention of morphine tolerance by the transplants.

In a similar study to examine tolerance reversal, animals were first made tolerant to morphine by pellet implantation and later received adrenal medullary or striated muscle control implants. The results, shown in Figure 8.4, demonstrated that the adrenal medullary transplants could partially reverse the established morphine tolerance in these animals. In this study, responses to acute injections of 5 mg/kg morphine are shown in animals that have received either control or morphine pellets (SC) followed one week later by implantation of either adrenal medullary or control striated muscle tissue in the spinal subarachnoid space. Morphine pellets significantly reduced the antinociceptive response to acute morphine injection in animals with control implants, compared with responses in the presence of control pellets, as assessed by both tail-flick (Fig. 8.4A) and paw-pressure (Fig. 8.4B) tests. In contrast, significant morphine antinociception was still obtained in animals with adrenal medullary transplants and morphine pellets, compared with pellets alone prior to adrenal medullary transplants (not shown). However, tolerance was not completely reversed in these animals, since there was a decrement in the antinociceptive potency

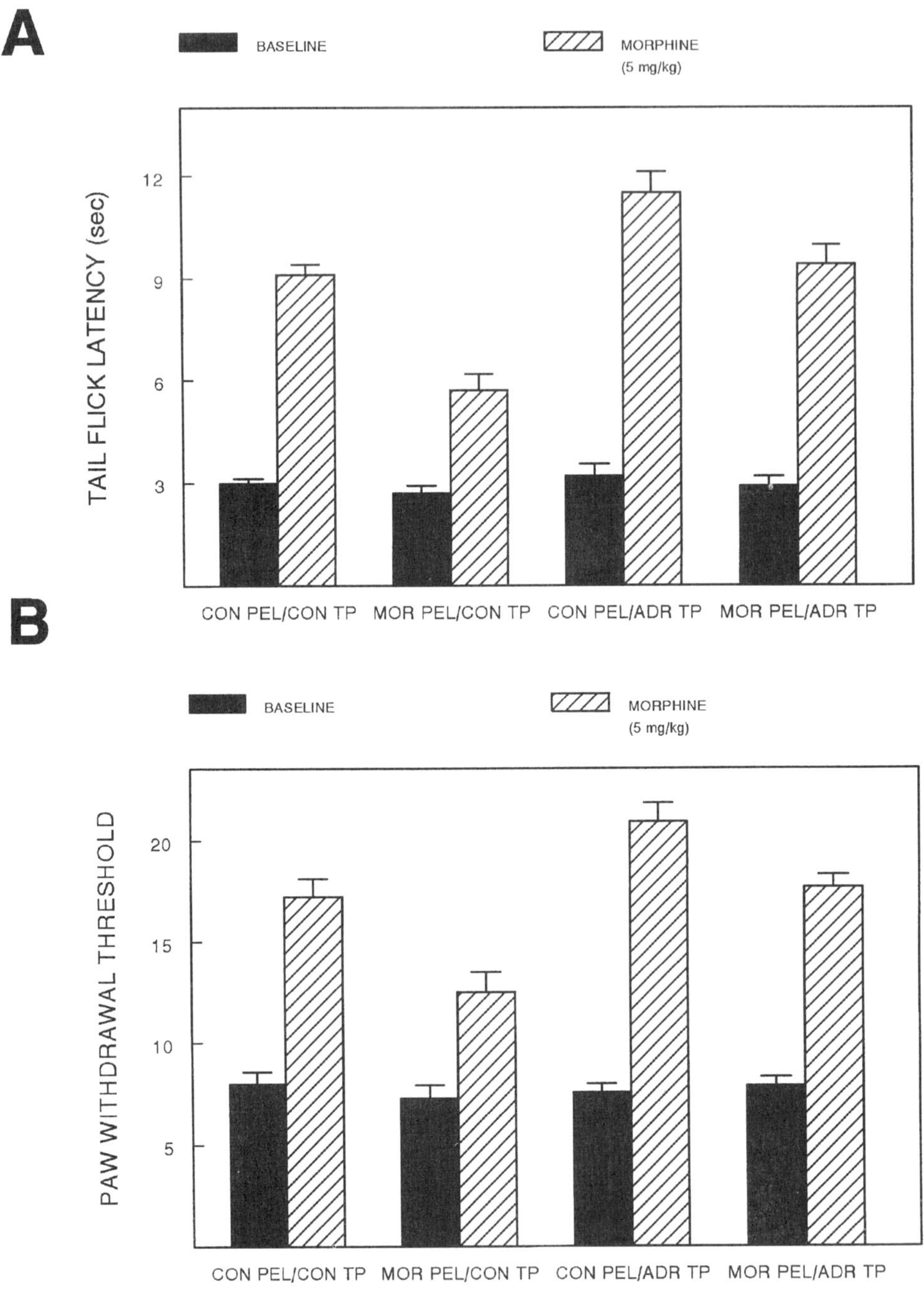

Figure 8.4. Assessment of reversal in morphine tolerance in animals implanted with either morphine pellets (MOR PEL; 75 mg, SC) or control pellets (CON PEL) one week prior to transplantation of adrenal medullary (ADR TP) or control striated muscle tissue (CON TP). Baseline pain sensitivity and responses to acute injections of morphine (5.0 mg/kg, SC) are shown 30 minutes following the injection. $n = 6$ animals per group. Bars represent mean ± S.E.M.

of morphine in these animals compared to animals with control pellets. The explanation for these findings that adrenal medullary transplants can prevent and partially reverse morphine tolerance is unclear, but recent findings in other laboratories have demonstrated prevention and possibly reversal of morphine tolerance with NMDA antagonists (Elliott et al., 1994; Mao et al., 1996), and the adrenal transplants may act via similar mechanisms.

Clinical Trials

As a result of the success of the preclinical work, limited clinical trials have been initiated at several centers. At the University of Illinois at Chicago, five patients with intractable pain secondary to nonresectable cancerous lesions were implanted with adrenal medullary allografts from human donor glands. Approval was obtained from the University of Illinois Internal Review Board (IRB) to obtain informed consent and enroll patients with prognoses of less than six months. Donor adrenal medullary tissue for implantation was obtained via the Regional Organ Donor Bank of Illinois, and adrenal glands were transported back to the laboratory, dissected, and maintained in explant culture for approximately 7 days to check for chromaffin cell viability. Tissue from approximately 2 adrenal medullae was implanted in the spinal lumbar cistern via lumbar puncture. Patients initially received cyclosporine (10 mg/kg/day) starting on the day prior to implant and were asked to continue this regimen for 2 weeks; however, most of them discontinued cyclosporine within the first week following implantation due to side effects such as nausea. Follow-up pain evaluations included pain scoring (visual analog scale), analgesic consumption, and CSF sampling. In this uncontrolled study, four of the patients reported significant pain reduction by one month postimplantation, with further improvement up to 8–10 weeks, when the patients were essentially pain free. Concomitant reduction in analgesic consumption was also noted. Pain reappeared in one of these patients after approximately 10 weeks. This patient was found to have some spinal cord compression due to metastasis in the vertebral column, unrelated to the implant, which may have interfered with CSF flow or implant viability. The rest remained pain free until death, two for nearly one year postimplantation. One of the latter patients reported improvements in physical activity and quality of life as a function of pain reduction. Details of this study have been reported in Winnie et al. (1993). It should be noted that a cautious interpretation of this data is warranted because the study was not placebo controlled.

A protocol similar to the one followed in Chicago was conducted by Lazorthes et al. (1995). The clinical trial involved eight patients suffering from intractable cancer pain. Consenting patients enrolled in the study had received inadequate pain control from oral morphine and were thus receiving opioids via implanted intrathecal pumps to maintain sufficient pain control before adrenal medullary implantation. Adrenal medullary tissue was prepared and implanted as above. A multidisciplinary pain evaluation demonstrated progressively decreased pain scores in six of the patients. Concomitant opioid analgesic intake was decreased in three of the patients and stabilized in three others. At another center, one patient with intractable pain was implanted with adrenal medullary tissue with "striking results" (Dr. R. Drucker-Colín, Universidad Nacional Autonoma de Mexico, personal communication). This patient showed gradual reduction in somatic pain VAS scores (from 10, most severe, prior to implantation), reaching zero by approximately 1 month post-transplantation and remaining at this level until death at 3 months. There was a concomitant reduction in analgesic intake.

Phase I clinical trials have been conducted at the University of Lausanne, Switzerland, to assess safety and preliminary efficacy utilizing encapsulated xenogeneic chromaffin cells from bovine adrenal glands (Aebischer et al., 1994). Approximately 2 million cells were loaded into the capsules, based on a linear scaling from animal results. Cell-loaded devices were tested for catecholamine output prior to implantation. In a preliminary report, three patients with terminal cancer pain were included. Of these, two patients markedly reduced opiate analgesic intake following implantation. CSF catecholamine levels were increased in two of the patients, and microscopic examination of retrieved devices revealed good cell viability and positive immunocytochemical staining for tyrosine hydroxylase. In a second report, seven patients with severe chronic pain inadequately managed with conventional therapies were enrolled. Of these, four patients who were originally receiving epidural morphine at the time of the implant decreased their analgesic usage during the study, with either a modest improvement or no worsening in pain ratings. Three of the other patients demonstrated improvements in McGill pain ratings, and two showed improved VAS scores. All devices were recovered after implant periods of 41 to 176 days. Post-retrieval histology revealed viable chromaffin cells with positive immunostaining for tyrosine hydroxylase and Met-enkephalin in 6 of 7 devices analyzed. A similar phase 1 clinical trial is nearing completion in the United States, and preliminary results have been recently reported (Burgess et al., 1996). Thus far, of 15 patients implanted, evidence of analgesic efficacy was indicated by reductions in VAS and MPQ scores in 9 patients and opiate reduction in 8 patients. The variability in responses may be due to differences in pain characteristics or localization. In addition, it again must be emphasized that this is an open-label, nonplacebo controlled study, so that interpretation is limited. Devices were recovered intact from 7 patients, all showing chromaffin cell viability and catecholamine production. No significant adverse effects associated with the xenogeneic implants were noted except for those related to intrathecal drug administration systems such as spinal headache.

Summary

The results of these studies are encouraging and suggest the possibility that cellular implants may provide a source of pain-reducing analgesic substances such as opioids on a local and continually available basis for pain control. Although adrenal medullary allografts and isolated chromaffin cell xenografts have been most utilized for these purposes thus far, it is likely that the future of this approach will depend on the identification of cell lines engineered to produce appropriate and controllable levels of analgesic substances for widespread application of this approach in clinical pain management.

This work was supported in part by NIH grant NS25054.

REFERENCES

Adams, J.U., Andrews, J.S., Hiller, J.M., Simon, E.J., and Holtzman, S.G. (1987). Effects of stress and β-funaltrexamine pretreatment on morphine analgesia and opioid binding in rats. *Life Sci.* **41,** 2835–2844.

Aebischer, P., Buchser, E., Joseph, J.M., Favre, J., de Tribolet, N., Lysaght, M., Rudnick, S., and Goddard, M. (1994). Transplantation in humans of encapsulated xenogeneic cells without immunosuppression. *Transplantation.* **58,** 1275–1277.

Bennett, G.J., and Xie, Y.-K. (1988). A peripheral mononeuropathy in rat that produces disorders of pain sensation like those seen in man. *Pain.* **33,** 87–107.

Burgess, F.W., Goddard, M., Savarese, D., and Wilkonson, H. (1996). Subarachnoid bovine adrenal chromaffin cell implants for cancer pain management. *Amer. Pain Soc. Abstr.* **15,** A-33.

Carmichael, S.W., and Stoddard, S. L. (1993). *The adrenal medulla 1989–1991.* Boca Raton: CRC Press.

Chaminade, M., Foutz, A.S., and Rossier, J. (1984). Co-release of enkephalins and precursors with catecholamines from the perfused cat adrenal gland *in situ. J. Physiol.* **353,** 157–169.

Colpaert, F.C. (1987). Evidence that adjuvant arthritis in the rat is associated with chronic pain. *Pain.* **28,** 201–222.

Comb, M., Liston, D., Martin, M., Rosen, H., and Herbert, E. (1985). Expression of the human proenkephalin gene in mouse pituitary cells: Accurate and efficient mRNA production and proteolytic processing. *EMBO J.* **4,** 3115–3122.

Czech, K.A., and Sagen, J. (1995). Update on cellular transplantation into the CNS as a novel therapy for chronic pain. *Prog. Neurobiol.* **46,** 507–529.

Donnerer, J., Cardinale, G., Coffey, J., Lisek, C.A., Jardine, I., and Spector, S. (1987). Chemical characterization and regulation of endogenous morphine and codeine in the rat. *J. Pharmacol. Exp. Ther.* **242,** 583–587.

Drasner, K., and Fields, H.F. (1988). Synergy between the antinociceptive effects of intrathecal clonidine and systemic morphine in the rat. *Pain.* **32,** 309–312.

Elliott, K., Hynansky, A., and Inturrisi, C.E. (1994). Dextromethorphan attenuates and reverses analgesic tolerance to morphine. *Pain.* **59,** 361–368.

Evans, C., Hammond, D.L., and Frederickson, R.C.A. (1988). The opioid peptides. In *The opiate receptors,* ed. G.W. Pasternak. Totowa, NJ: New Jersey: Humana Press, pp. 23–71.

Evans, C.J., Weber, E., and Barchas, J.D. (1981). Isolation and characterization of α-N-acetyl β-endorphin (1–26) from the rat posterior/intermediate lobe. *Biochem. Biophys. Res. Commun.* **102,** 897–904.

Fournié-Zaluski, M.-C., Chaillet, P., Bouboutou, R., Coulanud, P., Cherot, G., Waksman, G.,

Costentin, J., and Roques, B.P. (1984). Analgesic effects of kelatorphan, a new highly potent inhibitor of multiple enkephalin degrading enzymes. *Eur. J. Pharmacol.* **102,** 524–534.

Ginzburg, R., and Seltzer, Z. (1990). Subarachnoid spinal cord transplantation of adrenal medulla suppresses chronic neuropathic pain behavior in rats. *Brain Res.* **523,** 147–150.

Goldstein, A., Barrett, R.W., James, I.F., Lowney, L.I., Weitz, C.J., Knipmeyer, L. I., and Rapoport, H. (1985). Morphine and other opiates from beef brain and adrenal. *Proc. Natl. Acad. Sci. U.S.A.* **82,** 5203–5207.

Hama, A.T., Pappas, G.D., and Sagen, J. (1996). Adrenal medullary implants reduce transsynaptic degeneration in the spinal cord of rats following chronic constriction nerve injury. *Exp. Neurol.* **137,** 81–93.

Hama, A.T., and Sagen, J. (1993). Reduced pain-related behavior by adrenal medullary transplants in rats with experimental painful peripheral neuropathy. *Pain.* **52,** 223–231.

Hama, A.T., and Sagen, J. (1994a). Alleviation of neuropathic pain symptoms by xenogeneic chromaffin cell grafts in the spinal subarachnoid space. *Brain Res.* **651,** 345–351.

Hama, A., and Sagen, J. (1994b). Induction of a spinal NADPH-diaphorase by nerve injury is attenuated by adrenal medullary transplants. *Brain Res.* **640,** 345–351.

Hathaway, C.B., and Epple, A. (1990). Catecholamines, opioid peptides, and true opiates in the chromaffin cells of the eel: Immunohistochemical evidence. *Gen. Comp. Endocrinol.* **79,** 393–405.

Hexum, T.D., Yang, H.-Y.T., and Costa, E. (1980). Biochemical characterization of enkephalin-like immunoreactive peptides of adrenal glands. *Life Sci.* **27,** 1211–1216.

Höllt, V. (1986). Opioid peptide processing and receptor selectivity. *Ann. Rev. Pharmacol. Toxicol.* **26,** 59–77.

Höllt, V., Haarman, I., Grimm, C., Herz, A., Tulunay, F.C., and Loh, H.H. (1982). Proenkephalin intermediates in bovine brain and adrenal medulla: Characterization of immunoreactive peptides related to BAM-22P and peptide F. *Life Sci.* **31,** 1883–1886.

Höllt, V., Tulunay, F.C., Woo, S.K., Loh, H.H., and Herz, A. (1982). Opioid peptides derived from pro-enkephalin A but not from pro-enkephalin B are substantial analgesics after administration into the brain of mice. *Eur. J. Pharmacol.* **85,** 355–356.

Hook, V.Y. H., Heisler, S., Sabol, S.L., and Axelrod, J. (1982). Corticotropin releasing factor stimulates adrenocorticotropin and β-endorphin release from AtT-20 mouse pituitary tumor cells. *Biochem. Biophys. Res. Comm.* **106,** 1364–1371.

Iadorola, M.J., Tang, J., Costa, E., and Yang, Y.-Y.T. (1986). Analgesic activity and release of [Met^5]enkephalin-Arg^6-Gly^7-Leu^8 from rat spinal cord *in vivo. Eur. J. Pharmacol.* **121,** 39–48.

Ibuki, T., Hama, A., Wang, X.-T., Pappas, G.D., and Sagen, J. (1997). Loss of GABA-immunoreactivity in the spinal dorsal horn of rats with peripheral nerve injury and promotion of recovery by adrenal medullary grafts. *Neuroscience.* **76,** 845–858.

Inturrisi, C.E., Umans, J.G., Wolff, D., Stern, A.S., Lewis, R.V., Stein, S., and Udenfriend, S. (1980). Analgesic activity of the naturally occurring heptapeptide [Met^5]enkephalin-Arg^6-Phe^7. *Proc. Natl. Acad. Sci. U.S.A.* **77,** 5512–5514.

Kilpatrick, D.L., Howells, R.D., Fleminger, G., and Udenfriend, S. (1984). Denervation of rat adrenal glands markedly increases preproenkephalin mRNA. *Proc. Natl. Acad. Sci. USA.* **81,** 7221–7223.

Kilpatrick, D.L., Jones, B.N., Lewis, R.V., Stern, A.S., Kojima, K., Shively, J.E., and Udenfriend, S. (1982). An 18,200-dalton adrenal protein that contains four [Met]enkephalin sequences. *Proc. Natl. Acad. Sci. U.S.A.* **79,** 3057–3061.

Kim, P.H., Seasholtz, A.F., and Sagen, J. (1996). Generation of a met-enkephalin producing PC12 cell line for chronic pain therapy. *Am. Soc. Neural. Transpl. Abstr.* **3,** 34.

Kraicer, J., and Morris, A.R. (1976). In vitro release of ACTH from dispersed rat pars intermedia cells. II. Effect of neurotransmitter substances. *Neuroendocrinology.* **21,** 175–192.

Kuraishi, Y., Hirota, N., Satoh, M., and Takagi, H. (1985). Antinociceptive effects of intrathecal opioids, noradrenaline and serotonin in rats: Mechanical and thermal algesic tests. *Brain Res.* **326,** 168–171.

Larson, A.S., Vaught, J.L., and Takemori, A.E. (1980). The potentiation of spinal analgesia by leucine enkephalin. *Eur. J. Pharmacol.* **61,** 381–383.

Lazorthes, Y., Bès, J.C., Sagen, J., Tafani, M., Tkaczuk, J., Sallerin, B., Nahri, I., Verdié, J.C., Ohayon, E., Caratero, C., and Pappas, G.D. (1995). Transplantation of human chromaffin cells for control of intractable cancer pain. *Acta Neurochir.* **64,** 97–100.

Lemaire, S., Shukla, V.J., Rogers, C., Ibrahim, I.H., Lapierre, C., Parent, P., and Dumont, M. (1993). Isolation and characterization of histogranin, a natural peptide with NMDA receptor antagonist activity. *Eur. J. Pharmacol.* **245,** 247–256.

Lewis, R., Stern, A.S., Kimura, S., Rossier, J., Stein, S., and Udenfriend, S. (1980). An about 50,000-dalton protein in adrenal medulla: A common precursor of [Met]- and [Leu]Enkephalin. *Science.* **208,** 1459–1461.

Liston, D., Datey, G., Rossier, J., Verbanck, J.-J., and Vanderhaeghem, J.-J. (1984). Processing of proenkephalin is tissue specific. *Science.* **225,** 734–737.

Livett, B.G., Dean, D.M., Whelan, L.G., Udenfriend, S., and Rossier, J. (1981). Co-release of enkephalin and catecholamines from cultured adrenal chromaffin cells. *Nature.* **289,** 317–319.

Long, J.B., Rigamonti, D.D., de Costa, B., Rice, K.C., and Martinez-Arizala, A. (1989). Dynorphin A-induced rat hindlimb paralysis and spinal cord injury are not altered by the kappa opioid antagonist nor-binaltorphimine. *Brain Res.* **497,** 155–162.

Mao, J., Proce, D.D., Caruso, F.S., and Mayer, D.J. (1996). Oral administration of dextromethorphan prevents the development of morphine tolerance and dependence in rats. *Pain.* **67,** 361–368.

Mizuno, K., Minamino, N., Kangawa, K., and Matsuo, K. (1980). A new family of endogenous "big" met-enkephalins from bovine adrenal medulla: Purification and structure of docosa- (BAM-22P) and eicosapeptide (BAM-20P) with very potent opiate activity. *Biochem. Biophys. Res. Comm.* **47,** 1283–1290.

Mjanger, E., and Yaksh, T.L. (1991). Characteristics of dose-dependent antagonism by betafunaltrexamine of the antinociceptive effects of intrathecal mu agonists. *J. Pharmacol. Exp. Ther.* **258,** 544–550.

Nguyen, T.T., and De Léan, A. (1987). Nonadrenergic modulation by clonidine of the cosecretion of catecholamines and enkephalins in adrenal chromaffin cells. *Can. J. Physiol. Pharmacol.* **65,** 823–827.

Ortega, J., and Sagen, J. (1993). Pharmacologic characterization of opioid peptide release from chromaffin cell transplants using a brain slice superfusion method. *Exp. Brain Res.* **95,** 381–387.

Ortega-Alvaro, A., Gibert-Rahola, J., Chover, A.J., Tejedor-Real, P., Casas, J., and Mico, J.A. (1994). Effect of amitriptyline on the analgesia induced by adrenal medullary tissue transplanted in the rat spinal subarachnoid space as measured by an experimental model of acute pain. *Exp. Neurol.* **130,** 9–14.

Pacheco-Cano, M.T., Garcia-Hernandez, F., Hiriart, M., Komisaruk, B.R., and Drucker-Colin, R. (1990). Dibutyryl cAMP stimulates analgesia in rats bearing a ventricular adrenal medulla transplant. *Brain Res.* **531,** 290–293.

Palkovits, M., Mezey, D., Chiueh, C.G., Krieger, D.T., Gallatz, K., and Brownstein, M.J. (1986). Serotonin-containing elements of the rat pituitary intermediate lobe. *Neuroendocrinology.* **42,** 522–525.

Pittius, C. W., Kley, N., Loeffler, J.P., and Höllt, V. (1985). Quantitation of proenkephalin A messenger RNA in bovine brain, pituitary, and adrenal medulla: Correlation between mRNA and peptide levels. *EMBO J.* **4,** 1257–1260.

Porreca, F., Jiang, Q., and Tallarida, R.J. (1990). Modulation of morphine antinociception by peripheral [Leu^5]enkephalin: A synergistic interaction. *Eur. J. Pharmacol.* **179,** 463–468.

Randle, J.C.R., Moor, B.C., and Kraicer, J. (1983). Differential control of the release of proopimelanocortin-derived peptides from the pars intermedia of the rat pituitary. *Neuroendocrinology.* **37,** 131–140.

Reggiani, A., Carenzi, A., Frigeni, V., and Della Bella, D. (1984). Effect of bestatin and thiorphan on [Met^5]enkephalin-Arg^6-Phe^7-induced analgesia. *Eur. J. Pharmacol.* **105,** 361–375.

Russell, R.D., and Chang, K.-J. (1989). Altered delta and mu receptor activation: A strategem for limiting opioid tolerance and dependence. *Peptides.* **12,** 151–160.

Russell, R.D., Leslie, J.B., Su, Y.-F., Watkins, W.D., and Chang, K.-J. (1987). Continuous intrathecal opioid analgesia: Tolerance and cross-tolerance of mu and delta spinal opioid receptors. *J. Pharmacol. Exp. Ther.* **240,** 150–158.

Ruz-Franzi, J.I., and Gonzalez-Darder, J.M. (1991). Study of the analgesic effects of the implant of adrenal medullary into the subarachnoid space in rats. *Acta Neurochir.* **52,** 39–41.

Sabol, S.T. (1980). Storage and secretion of β-endorphin and related peptides by mouse pituitary tumor cells: Regulation by glucocorticoids. *Arch. Biochem. Biophys.* **203,** 37–48.

Sagen, J., and Kemmler, J.E. (1989). Increased levels of Met-enkephalin-like immunoreactivity in the spinal cord CSF of rats with adrenal medullary transplants. *Brain Res.* **502,** 1–10.

Sagen, J., Pappas, G.D., and Perlow, M.J. (1996). Adrenal medullary tissue transplants in rat spinal cord reduce pain sensitivity. *Brain Res.* **384,** 189–194.

Sagen, J., Pappas, G.D., and Pollard, H.B. (1996). Analgesia induced by isolated bovine chromaffin cells implanted in the rat spinal cord. *Proc. Nat. Acad. Sci. U.S.A.* **83,** 7522–7526.

Sagen, J., and Wang, H. (1990). Prolonged analgesia by enkephalinase inhibition in rats with spinal cord adrenal medullary transplants. *Eur. J. Pharmacol.* **179,** 427–433.

Sagen, J., Wang, H., and Pappas, G.D. (1990). Adrenal medullary implants in rat spinal cord reduce nociception in a chronic pain model. *Pain.* **42,** 69–79.

Sagen, J., Wang, H., Tresco, P.A., and Aebischer, P. (1993). Transplants of immunologically isolated xenogeneic chromaffin cells provide a long-term source of pain reducing neuroactive substances. *J. Neurosci.* **13,** 2415–2423.

Saitoh, Y., Taki, T., Arita, N., Ohnishi, T., and Hayakawa, T. (1995a). Analgesia induced by transplantation of encapsulated tumor cells secreting β-endorphin. *J. Neurosurg.* **82,** 630–634.

Saitoh, Y., Taki, T., Arita, N., Ohnishi, T., and Hayakawa, T. (1995b). Cell therapy with encapsulated xenogeneic tumor cells secreting β-endorphin for treatment of peripheral pain. *Cell Transpl.* 4 Suppl. **1,** S13–S17.

Sakly, M., Schmitt, G., and Koch, B. (1982). CRF enhances release of both MSH and ACTH from anterior and intermediate pituitary. *Neuroendocrinol. Lett.* **4,** 289–293.

Saland, C., Gutierrez, L., Kraner, J., and Samora, A. (1988). Corticotropin-releasing factor (CRF) and neurotransmitters modulate melanotropic peptide release from rat neurointermediate pituitary in vitro. *Neuropeptides.* **12,** 59–66.

Sherman, S.E., Loomis, C.W., Milne, B., and Cervenko, F.W. (1988). Intrathecal oxymetazoline produces analgesia via spinal α-adrenoceptors and potentiates spinal morphine. *Eur. J. Pharmacol.* **148,** 371–380.

Siegan, J.B., Hama, A.T., and Sagen, J. (1996a). Alterations in spinal cord cGMP by peripheral nerve injury and adrenal medullary transplantation. *Neurosci. Lett.* **215,** 49–52.

Siegan, J.B., Hama, A.T., and Sagen, J. (1996b). Histogranin attenuates chronic pain induced by peripheral neuropathy, formalin-induced nociception, and direct application of NMDA. *Soc. Neurosci. Abstr.* **22,** 1361.

Siegan, J.B., and Sagen, J. (1995). Attenuation of NMDA-induced spinal hypersensitivity by adrenal medullary transplants. *Brain Res.* **680,** 88–98.

Siegan, J.B., and Sagen, J. (1997). Attenuation of formalin pain responses in the rat by adrenal medullary transplants in the spinal subarachnoid space. *Pain.* **70,** 279–285.

Smyth, D.G. (1983). β-endorphin and related peptides in pituitary, brain, pancreas, and antrum. *Br. Med. Bull.* **39,** 25–30.

Song, Z.H., and Takemori, A.E. (1991). Antagonism of morphine antinociception by intrathecally administered corticotropin-releasing factor in mice. *J. Pharmacol. Exp. Ther.* **256,** 909–912.

Stern, A.S., Lewis, R.V., Kimura, S., Rossier, J., Stein, S., and Udenfriend, S. (1980). Opioid hexapeptides and heptapeptides in adrenal medulla and brain: Possible implications on the biosynthesis of enkephalins. *Arch. Biochem. Biophys.* **205,** 606–613.

Stevens, K.E., Leslie, F.M., Evans, C.J., Belluzzi, J.C., and Stein, L. (1988). BAM-18: Analgesia, hyperalgesia, and locomotor effects. *Neuropeptides.* **12,** 21–27.

Takemori, A.E., and Portoghese, P.S. Evidence for the interaction of morphine with kappa and delta opioid receptors to induce analgesia in β-funaltrexamine-treated mice. *Pain.* **243,** 91–94.

Tiseo, P.J., and Yaksh, T.L. (1993). Dose-dependent antagonism of spinal opioid receptor agonists by naloxone and naltrindole: Additional evidence for delta-opioid receptor subtypes in the rat. *Eur. J. Pharmacol.* **236,** 89–96.

Unsicker, K. (1993). The trophic cocktail made by adrenal chromaffin cells. *Exp. Neurol.* **123,** 167–173.

Unsicker, K., Krieglstein, K., Bieger, S., Deimling, F., Huber, K., Schober, A., Cole, T., Monaghan, P., Schmid, W., Schütz, G., Blottner, D., Flanders, K.C., Wolf, N., Kalcheim, C., Schober, A., Minichello, L., and Klein, R. (1996). Molecular cues for development and maintenance of adrenal chromaffin cells and their innervation. *Int. Catecholamine Sympos. Abstr.* **8,** 204.

Vale, W., Vaughn, J., Smith, M., Yamamoto, G., Rivier, J., and Rivier, C. (1983). Effects of synthetic ovine corticotropin-releasing factor, glucocorticoids, catecholamines, neurohypophysial peptides, and other substances on cultured corticotropic cells. *Endocrinology.* **113,** 1121–1131.

Vaquero, J., Arias, A., Oya, S., and Zurita, M. (1991). Chromaffin allografts into arachnoid of spinal cord reduce basal pain responses in rats. *Neuroreport.* **2,** 149–151.

Viveros, O.H., Diliberto, E.J., Jr., Hazum, E., and Chang, K.-J. (1979). Opiate-like materials in the adrenal medulla: Evidence for storage and secretion with catecholamines. *Molec. Pharmacol.* **16,** 1101–1108.

Wang, H., and Sagen, J. (1991). Pain reduction by transplants of pineal and pituitary gland tissues in the spinal cord. *Anat. Rec.* **229,** 91A.

Wang, H., and Sagen, J. (1993). Role of opiate receptor subtypes in mediating antinociception by adrenal medullary transplants in the rat spinal subarachnoid space. *Soc. Neurosci. Abstr.* **19,** 1410.

Wang, H., and Sagen, J. (1994a). Optimization of adrenal medullary allograft conditions for pain alleviation. *J. Neural Transpl. Plastic.* **5,** 49–64.

Wang, H., and Sagen, J. (1994b). Absence of appreciable tolerance and morphine cross-tolerance in rats with adrenal medullary transplants in the spinal cord. *Neuropharmacology.* **33,** 681–692.

Wang, H., and Sagen, J. (1995). Attenuation of pain-related hyperventilation in adjuvant arthritic rats with adrenal medullary transplants in the spinal subarachnoid space. *Pain.* **63,** 313–320.

Wilcox, G.L., Carlsson, K., Jochim, A., and Jurna, I. (1987). Mutual potentiation of antinociceptive effects of morphine and clonidine on motor and sensory responses in rat spinal cord. *Brain Res.* **405,** 84–93.

Wilson, S.P. (1991). Processing of proenkephalin in adrenal chromaffin cells. *J. Neurochem.* **57,** 876–881.

Winnie, A.P., Pappas, G.D., Das Gupta, T.K., Wang, H., Ortega, J.D., Sagen, J. (1993). Alleviation of cancer pain by adrenal medullary transplants in the spinal subarachnoid space: A preliminary report. *Anesthesiology.* **79,** 644–653.

Wu, H.H., McLoon, S.C., and Wilcox, G.L. (1993). Antinociception following implantation of AtT-20 and genetically modified AtT-20/hENK cells in rat spinal cord. *J. Neural Transpl. Plastic.* **4,** 15–26.

Wu, H.H., Wilcox, G.L., and McLoon, S.C. (1994). Implantation of AtT-20 or genetically modified AtT-20-hENK cells in mouse spinal cord induced antinociception and opioid tolerance. *J. Neurosci.* **14,** 4806–4814.

Yaksh, T.L. (1987). Spinal opiates: A review of their effect on spinal function with emphasis on pain processing. *Acta Anaesthesiol. Scand.* 31 Suppl. **1,** 25–37.

Yaksh, T.L., and Harty, G.J. (1982). Effects of thiorphan on the antinociceptive actions of intrathecal [D-Ala^2-Met^5]enkephalin. *Eur. J. Pharmacol.* **79,** 293–300.

Yaksh, T.L., Huang, S.P., and Rudy, T.A. (1977). The direct and specific opiate-like effect of Met^5-enkephalin and analogues on the spinal cord. *Neuroscience.* **2,** 593–596.

Yaksh, T.L., Kohl, R.L., and Rudy, T.A. (1977). Induction of tolerance and withdrawal in rats receiving morphine in the spinal subarachnoid space. *Eur. J. Pharmacol.* **42,** 275–284.

Yaksh, T.L., and Noueihed, R. (1985). The physiology and pharmacology of spinal opiates. *Ann. Rev. Pharmacol. Toxicol.* **25,** 433–462.

Yaksh, T.L., and Reddy, S.V.R. (1981). Studies in the primate on the analgesic effects associated with intrathecal actions of opiates, alpha-adrenergic agonists, and baclofen. *Anesthesiology.* **54,** 451–467.

Yaksh, T.L., and Wilson, R.R. (1979). Spinal serotonin terminal system mediates antinociception. *J. Pharmacol. Exp. Ther.* **208,** 446–453.

Yang, H.-Y.T., Hexum, T., and Costa, E. (1980). Opioid peptides in adrenal gland. *Life Sci.* **27,** 1119–1125.

Yeomans, D.C., Sioussat, T.M., Michalewicz, P., Lu, Y., and Pappas, G.D. (1996). Antinociceptive effects of spinally transplanted synthetic foam scaffolds impregnated with bovine adrenal chromaffin cells in the rat Aδ-C foot withdrawal test. *Soc. Neurosci. Abstr.* **22,** 1021.

Yu, L.C., Hansson, P., and Lundeberg, T. (1995). Opioid antagonists naloxone, beta-funaltrexamine and naltrindole, but not nor-binaltorphimine, reverse the increased hindpaw withdrawal latency in rats induced by intrathecal administration of the calcitonin gene-related peptide antagonist CGRP8–37. *Brain Res.* **698,** 23–29.

Yu, W., Hao, J.-X., Xu, X.-J., Saydoff, J., Haegerstrand, A., and Wiesenfeld-Hallin, Z. (1996). Intrathecal bovine chromaffin cells alleviate chronic allodynia-like response in spinally injured rats. *Int. Assn. Study of Pain Abstr.* **8,** 379.

Zhu, Y.-S., Branch, A.D., Robertson, H.D., Huang, T.H., Franklin, S.O., and Inturrisi, C.E. (1992). Time course of enkephalin mRNA and peptides in cultured rat adrenal medulla. *Molec. Brain Res.* **12,** 173–180.

CHAPTER NINE

Clinical Implications of Physicochemical Properties of Opioids

CHRISTOPHER M. BERNARDS

All opiates in clinical use produce analgesia via the same molecular mechanism, that is, binding to G-protein–coupled opioid receptors with subsequent inhibition of adenylate cyclase, activation of inwardly rectifying K^+ channels, and inhibition of voltage-gated Ca^{2+} channels, all of which decrease neuronal excitability. Given the commonality of the mechanism, one might reasonably ask why there are such clear clinical differences among opioids with respect to pharmacokinetic and pharmacodymanic characteristics such as minimal effective plasma concentration, elimination half-time, and volume of distribution (Table 9.1).

The net analgesic effect of any opiate is the result of numerous processes that must occur prior to G-protein activation. Opiates must first redistribute from their site of administration (IV, IM, epidural, intrathecal) to their site of action (brain, spinal cord, peripheral opioid receptors), they must traverse anatomic and physiologic barriers (blood-brain-barrier, spinal meninges), they must diffuse through tissue (brain, spinal cord) to reach opioid receptors, they must bind to their receptor, and finally they must induce a conformational change in the receptor to activate the G-protein. The rate and extent to which any individual opiate completes these steps is largely dependent on its molecular structure and its physicochemical properties. This chapter discusses what is known about which physicochemical properties (Table 9.1) underlie the clinical pharmacology of opiates.

Intrinsic Efficacy

Intrinsic efficacy refers to the amount of "activity" generated when an agonist binds to a receptor. Alternatively, intrinsic efficacy can be viewed as the percentage of receptors that must be occupied to achieve the maximum possible biologic effect. In the case of opiates, intrinsic efficacy could be quantified as the increase in K^+ flux that occurs when one opiate molecule binds to a single receptor, or as the percentage of available receptors that must be occupied in order to produce maximal inhibition of neurotransmitter release.

Determining intrinsic efficacy has become somewhat easier since the μ opioid receptor was cloned. Emmerson and colleagues (1996) used membranes from C6

Christoph Stein, ed., *Opioids in Pain Control: Basic and Clinical Aspects*. Printed in the United States of America.

Table 9.1. *Physicochemical, Pharmacokinetic, and Pharmacodynamic Properties of Selected Opioid Agonists and Antagonists*

	Mol. Wt.	λοω 7.4	pka	% Nonionized (pH 7.4)	Protein Binding (%)	Vd_{ss} (liters)	Clearance (ml/min/kg)	Slow Redistribution Half-Time ($T_{1/2}$ α, min)	Elimination Half-Time ($T_{1/2}$ β, hr)	Minimal Effective Plasma Concentration (ng/ml)	Equivalent IV Analgesic dose (mg)
Morphine-like agonists											
Morphine	285.33	1	7.9	23	35	224	15–20	1.5–4.4	1.7–3.3	10–15	10
Hydromorphone	285.33	1.28	NA	NA	7–14	84–168	14–23	NA	2.4–3	NA	1.5
Heroin	369.4	4.6	7.6	39	20–39	NA	31	NA	≈0.05	Inactive "pro drug"	0.5
Piperadine-derived agonists											
Meperidine	247.35	39	8.5	7	70	305	8–18	4–16	3 –5	200	75
Alfentanil	416.52	128	6.5	89	92	27	4–9	9.5–17	1.4–1.5	15	1
Fentanyl	336.46	816	8.4	9	84	335	10–20	9.2–19	3.1–6.6	0.6	0.1
Sufentanil	386.55	1757	8	20	93	123	10–15	17.7	2.2–4.6	0.03	0.01
Remifentanil	360.44	NA	7.26	58	66–93	30	40–60	2–3.7	0.17–0.33	NA	0.05
Diphenylpropylamines											
Methadone	345.9	120	9.26	1.36	90	≈350	2	NA	15	NA	10
Propoxyphene	339.48	NA	NA	NA	80	≈175	7–20	NA	8–12	NA	240
Antagonists											
Naloxone	327.37	33.5	7.82	28	40	≈180–210	20–30	NA	0.9–1.9	NA	—
Naltrexone	341.41	13.08	8.13	16	20	≈200	20	NA	3–9	NA	—
Nalorphine	311.39	28.16	7.59	39	NA	NA	NA	NA	NA	NA	—

NA = not available. Note that values for pharmacokinetic variables are averages; kinetic values can vary by severalfold between different studies.
$λοω_{7.4}$ = octanol:buffer (pH 7.4) partition coefficient.
Vd_{ss} = volume of distribution at steady state.

glioma cell lines expressing rat μ opioid receptors to quantify G-protein activation elicited by multiple opioids. They found the intrinsic activity rank order to be etonitazine = sufentanil = DAMGO = PLO17 = fentanyl > morphine > profadol > meperidine > butorphanol = nalbuphine = pentazocine > cyclazocine = nalorphine > levallorphan > naltrexone. Others have reported similar, although not identical results, using comparable techniques in different cell lines (Knapp et al., 1995; Selley et al., 1997).

There are certainly structure-activity relationships that underlie the observed differences in efficacy among these opioid molecules and some of these have been identified (Kutter and Herz, 1970; Hosztafi et al., 1995). For example, substitution of an allyl group for the N-methyl group of morphinelike compounds converts them from agonists to antagonists. However, there is no identifiable relation between any physicochemical property of these agonists and their intrinsic efficacy. As an example of this fact, consider the analgesic effects of the opioid antagonists naloxone and naltrexone, the partial agonist nalorphine, and the full agonists morphine, fentanyl, and methadone. All these compounds bind to the μ opioid receptor, yet they have markedly different intrinsic activities that cannot be predicted from their physicochemical properties (see Table 9.1).

Receptor Binding

Opioid-mediated G-protein activation can occur only after the opioid agonist binds to the opioid receptor, and, not surprisingly, receptor binding affinity has been shown to correlate with intrinsic efficacy (Emmerson et al., 1996). However, there is no correlation between any physicochemical property and receptor binding affinity (Leysen et al., 1983).

Physicochemical Properties and Bioavailability

Because physicochemical properties do not predict an opioid's affinity for its receptor or its intrinsic efficacy, we must look elsewhere to understand how these properties affect opioid pharmacology. As we shall see, physicochemical properties have a pronounced effect on opioid bioavailability – that is, on the ability to get from their site of administration to their site of action. And, importantly, the effect of different physicochemical properties on bioavailability depends markedly on their site of administration, for example, intravenous versus epidural versus intrathecal.

Blood-Brain Barrier

To function properly, the brain must tightly regulate the content of electrolytes, neurotransmitters, hormones, energy substrates, and other biologically active molecules in its extracellular environment. To better regulate its environment, the brain and spinal cord are separated from the chemical milieu of the body by the blood-brain barrier (BBB). Notable exceptions are brain areas with a neuroendocrine function (e.g., circumventricular organs, the hypothalamus), which lack a tight BBB.

The BBB consists of both anatomic and physiologic components. Anatomically, the capillaries of the brain are largely responsible for the permeability characteristics of the BBB (Janzer, 1993). Brain capillaries differ from those in the remainder of the body in that they lack fenestrations, and the endothelial cells are connected to one another by tight junctions with very high electrical resistance (i.e., even small electrolytes have great difficulty passing between them). In addition, brain capillary endothelial cells are surrounded by extensions of astrocytes called foot processes, which appear to be responsible for inducing and maintaining BBB properties in brain endothelial cells (Goldstein, 1988; Abbott et al., 1992; Janzer, 1993).

Lipid Solubility

Because the BBB severely restricts permeability, compounds required by the brain (e.g., glucose, amino acids) are actively transported across the BBB by receptor-mediated endocytosis. Because of endothelial tight junctions, molecules that are not actively transported must pass directly through the endothelial cell to reach the brain. This process requires that drugs (1) partition from the blood into the endothelial cell membrane at the endothelial cell lumenal surface; (2) partition from the lipid bilayer of the endothelial cell membrane into the largely aqueous cytosol; (3) diffuse through the cytosol to reach the portion of the endothelial cell membrane that abuts the brain (and in the process avoid being sequestered in intracellular organelles); (4) again partition into the lipid bilayer of the endothelial cell membrane; and finally (5) partition from the endothelial cell membrane into the brain's aqueous extracellular space.

One can appreciate that passage through the BBB will be most rapid for drugs that most easily negotiate the multiple aqueous/lipid bilayer interfaces separating blood from brain. This explains why hydrophobic character (loosely referred to as lipid solubility) is probably the most important determinant of a drug's ability to cross the BBB (Fig. 9.1). Hydrophobic character is usually quantified as a drug's partition coefficient (P or log P) between an aqueous phase and an organic solvent. Which organic solvent is most representative of the BBB (e.g., hexane, octanol, olive oil) and what is the appropriate pH for the aqueous phase (e.g., pH = 7.4 or the pH at which the molecule is completely unionized) have been the subjects of much discussion; however, there is a reasonably good correlation between a drug's permeability coefficient in any solvent system and its BBB permeability.

Although lipid solubility correlates well with permeability, the relationship may not be as linear as some have suggested. For example, Hansch and colleagues (1987) have suggested that there is an optimal log P for BBB permeability. They suggest that a log P of approximately 2 (octanol:buffer$_{7.4}$ solvent system) results in maximal BBB penetration and that drugs with significantly higher log P values are likely to be less permeable. Figure 9.1 hints at this in that cerebrovascular permeability drops off for drugs with an octanol:buffer partition coefficient greater than 100 (i.e., log P greater than 2).

The reason that extremes of lipid solubility decrease permeability is not precisely known, but the result presumably reflects the interaction between drugs and lipid components of the barrier they are traversing. Increasing lipid solubility improves a

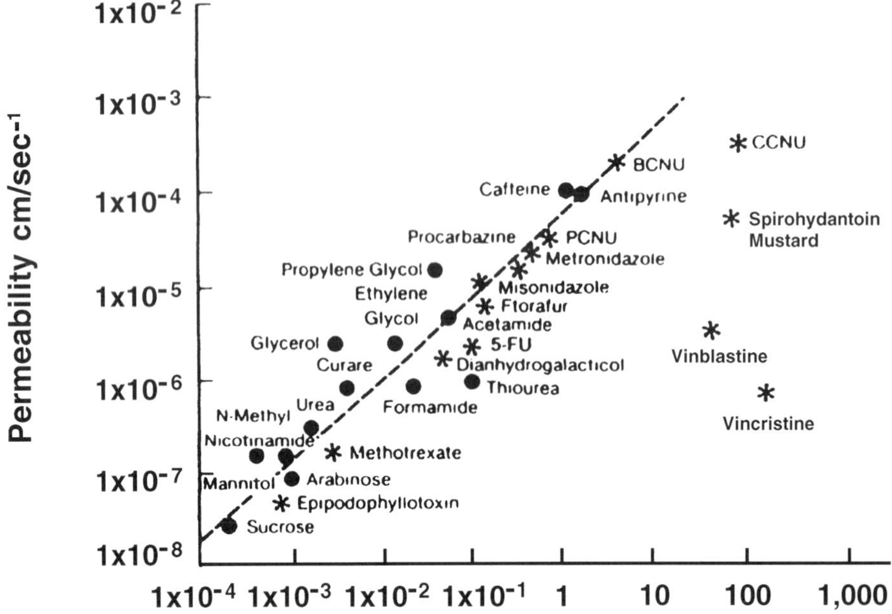

Figure 9.1. Relationship between octanol:buffer (pH 7.4) partition coefficient and blood brain barrier (BBB) permeability. Note that BBB permeability increases as lipid solubility increases, but appears to reach a maximum at a partition coefficient of approximately 100 (log P = 2). Thereafter, further increases in lipid solubility result in decreased BBB permeability. (Reprinted with permission from Rapoport, S.I. Drug delivery to the brain: Barrier modification and drug modification methodologies, In Frankenheim, J.F., and Brown, R.M., eds., *Bioavailability of drugs to the brain and blood-brain barrier,* NIDA research Monograph 120. Washington, DC: Government Printing Office, 1992.)

drug's ability to enter the lipid bilayer of the brain endothelial cells because lipid-soluble drugs are thermodynamically more stable in lipid environments. However, as lipid solubility increases further, drugs will essentially become sequestered in lipid environments because the "activation energy" necessary to leave the lipid environment and re-enter an aqueous environment is too high. Thus, extremely lipid-soluble drugs will have essentially the same problem encountered by hydrophilic drugs – that is, they will have difficulty negotiating the multiple aqueous:lipid bilayer interfaces necessary to pass from the blood to the brain.

In addition, increasing lipid solubility may result in greater nonspecific binding to brain lipid. Evidence of this comes from work by Scott and co-workers (1985), who used EEG to quantitate the narcotic effect of fentanyl and alfentanil in surgical patients. They reported that there was a significantly longer time lag between plasma concentration and brain effect with fentanyl than alfentanil. One interpretation of this clinical phenomenon is that, owing to its greater lipid solubility, fentanyl must "fill" nonspecific lipid-binding sites before sufficient free drug is available to bind at opioid receptors.

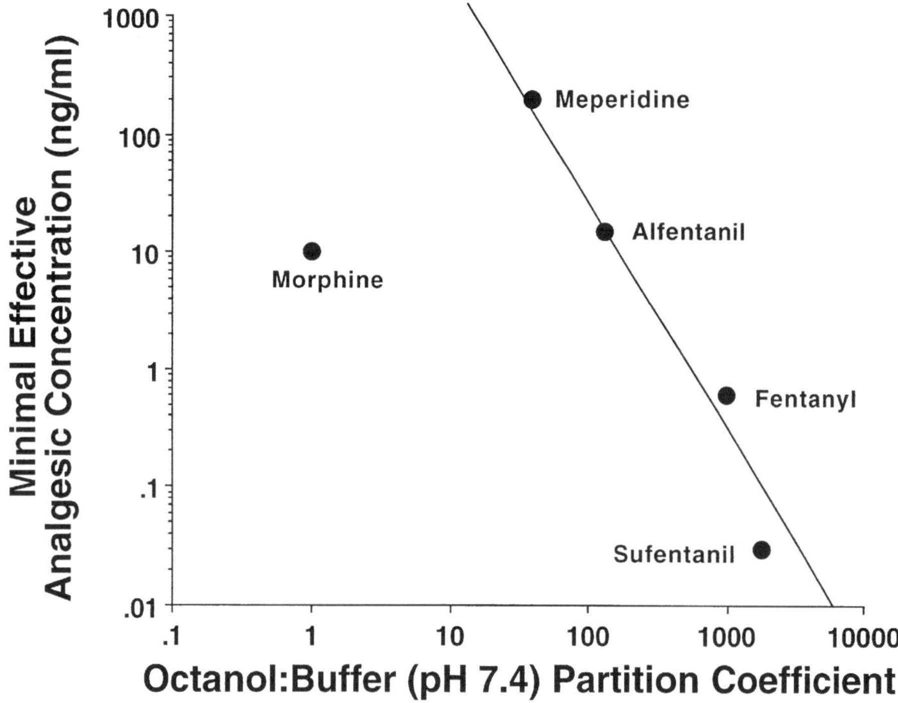

Figure 9.2. Log:log plot demonstrating the relationship between octanol:buffer$_{7.4}$ distribution coefficient and minimal effective analgesic concentration (MEAC) of five commonly used opioids. There is a strong correlation between lipid solubility and minimal effective plasma concentration for the four phenylpiperidine opioids, suggesting that lipid solubility accurately predicts opioid receptor bioavailability for these drugs. Of note, the potency of morphine is significantly greater than would be predicted based on its lipid solubility alone. (MEAC data from Coda, B.A. Opioids. In Barash, P.G., Cullen, B.F., and Stoelting, R.K., *Clinical anesthesia,* 3rd ed. Philadelphia: Lippincott-Raven, 1997.)

Consistent with this interpretation, Hug and Murphy (1981) have shown that the brain:serum concentration ratio for fentanyl in rats is 5:1, whereas it is the opposite for alfentanil (i.e., 0.2:1) (Scott et al., 1985). These data suggest that fentanyl's greater lipid solubility results in greater entry into the brain, but also correspondingly greater nonspecific binding to brain lipid and consequently less drug available at the receptor. The take-home message is that we must be careful about worshipping at the altar of lipid solubility as we look to design or employ more effective opiates; at some point increasing a drug's lipid solubility is likely to decrease its ability to reach opioid receptors.

Despite the caveat about extremes of lipid solubility, there is reasonably good correlation between the octanol:buffer partition coefficients of clinically used opioids and their potency as determined by their minimal effective plasma concentration (Fig. 9.2). These potency differences largely reflect differences in ability to cross the BBB and access brain opioid receptors.

Although the anatomic barrier presented by the BBB has been known for nearly

100 years, the physiologic barrier presented by brain endothelial cells is a more recent discovery. Several investigators have identified multiple enzyme systems (e.g., cytochrome P450, UDP-glucuronosyltransferase) capable of metabolizing opioids and other xenobiotics (Minn et al., 1991; Ghersi-Egea et al., 1995). Whether drug metabolism occurs to an appreciable extent has not yet been determined for brain endothelial cells; however, the possibility exists.

Another physiologic component of the BBB is the membrane-bound transporters that can transport various drugs. One of the most interesting of these transporters with respect to opioid pharmacology is p-glycoprotein (*MDR1* gene product). P-glycoprotein is a nonspecific transporter for a variety of dissimilar xenobiotics (Ford and Hait, 1990), including morphine-6-glucuronide (Huwyler et al., 1996). Morphine-6-glucuronide is a morphine metabolite that is many times more potent than morphine as an analgesic (47–360 times) when administered intracerebroventricularly but not when administered intravenously (Frances et al., 1992). Active exclusion of morphine-6-glucuronide by P-glycoprotein, and not simply its hydrophilic character, may be responsible for morphine-6-glucuronide's low BBB permeability (Wu et al., 1997) and consequently its low intravenous potency.

More direct evidence that P-glycoprotein may be responsible for excluding opioids from the central nervous system comes from the work of Schinkel et al. (1996). These investigators administered loperamide, a peripherally acting antidiarrheal opiate that does not cross the BBB to wild-type mice and knock-out mice, which lack the gene coding for P-glycoprotein. Oral loperamide induced typical opiatelike behavior in the knock-out mice but no such behavior in the wild-type animals. The obvious implication is that loperamide is normally prevented from crossing the BBB by active P-glycoprotein–mediated exclusion.

Which physicochemical properties, if any, make opioids potential targets for metabolism by brain endothelial cells or for active exclusion by P-glycoprotein remains to be determined. However, both mechanisms need to be considered as potentially important determinants of opioid bioavailability and thus analgesic efficacy.

pk_a

A drug's dissociation constant is another physicochemical property that plays an important role in opioid bioavailability. For drugs that are either weak acids or bases, the pk_a (i.e., negative logarithm of the dissociation constant) is the pH at which a molecule exists in equal concentrations as the acid and its corresponding conjugate base – that is, half the molecules are ionized and half are not ionized. The importance of this with respect to BBB penetration is that unionized molecules have an octanol:buffer partition coefficient that is as much as 1,000-fold greater than their ionized conjugates (Rapaport, 1976).

For drugs with a pk_a near the physiologic pH range, even relatively small changes in pH can have dramatic effects on the proportion of ionized and unionized molecules. Since only the unionized form of the molecule can penetrate the BBB, pH changes can have marked effects on a drug's BBB penetration and consequently its clinical effect. For example, Schulman and colleagues (1984) have shown that morphine penetration into the brain was two- to threefold higher in alkalotic rats (pH 7.62; morphine 15% ionized) compared to acidotic rats (pH 7.16; morphine 33% ionized) (Schulman et al., 1984). Similarly, moderate hypocarbia has been shown to increase the brain concentration of fentanyl in dogs (Ainslie et al., 1979) and the clinical effects of sufentanil in humans (Matteo et al., 1992). As predicted by the Henderson-Hasselbach equation, respiratory alkalosis increases the proportion of unionized morphine, fentanyl, and sufentanil in plasma, thereby increasing their apparent octanol:water partition coefficients and presumably their ability to cross the BBB. Thus, one of the most important clinical consequences of a drug's pk_a is that it makes lipid solubility a dynamic property instead of a static one.

Protein Binding

In plasma, a percentage of all opioids is bound to proteins (principally albumin and α_1 acid glycoprotein [AAG]), whereas the remainder is free in solution. Importantly, it is only the "free fraction" that is available to move from plasma into brain or other tissues. Thus, protein binding is another property of opioids that may affect their ability to penetrate the BBB and thus their clinical pharmacology.

Whether protein binding alters BBB penetration depends on the rate at which the opioid is able to dissociate from the protein. As blood passes through a brain capillary, unbound drug leaves the plasma to enter the brain, depleting the concentration of unbound drug in plasma and disturbing the equilibrium between the free and the protein-bound drug. If bound opioid dissociates from the protein rapidly enough, the free fraction in plasma can be "replenished" in less time than it takes the blood to transit the capillary, and protein binding will not limit BBB penetration. However, if the drug is so strongly protein bound that the dissociation is relatively slow, then protein binding may be rate limiting. Unfortunately, the kinetics of opioid dissociation from plasma proteins during transit through brain capillaries is not known.

However, there is conflicting evidence that protein binding may alter opioid pharmacokinetics. Macfie and colleagues (1992) compared alfentanil kinetics in burn patients with a control group. The burned patients had significantly higher AAG concentrations and consequently a 38% decrease in free alfentanil concentration and a significantly reduced volume of distribution. Though not determined, one might expect that alfentanil penetration of the BBB was likewise reduced. In contrast, studies in Crohn's disease patients with increased AAG concentrations have failed to find any correlation between AAG and alfentanil pharmacodynamics or pharmacokinetics, suggesting that changes in protein binding were not limiting in this patient group (Gesink-van der Veer et al., 1989, 1993). Additional work is necessary to clarify if other conditions that alter plasma protein concentrations (e.g., malignancy, age extremes, renal and hepatic failure) also alter opioid pharmacokinetics or pharmacodynamics.

Plasma Pharmacokinetics

Systemically administered opioids are distributed to and removed from the brain by blood flow. Although the blood concentration of an opioid is certainly not the same as the receptor concentration, there is a defined relation between the two, so that plasma concentration plays an important role in determining the rate, magnitude, and duration of opioid effects. In turn, the physicochemical properties of an opioid play an important role in determining plasma pharmacokinetics.

After an intravenous bolus, opioids reach peak concentrations in the plasma almost immediately. Thereafter, plasma concentration falls non-linearly as the drug is removed from the plasma by multiple mechanisms. Initially, the bulk of any drug dose is delivered to organs that are highly perfused (often termed the vessel-rich group), including the brain, heart, lung, and kidney. As blood passes through these organs, the drug is taken up in proportion to its capillary permeability and its relative "solubility" in tissue and blood. In fact, a drug may be concentrated in tissues if tissue solubility exceeds blood solubility.

One measure of the extent to which a drug is concentrated in tissues is the apparent volume of distribution (Vd), which is calculated as Vd = total amount of drug administered/resultant plasma concentration (i.e., the volume a dose of drug would have to be dissolved in to yield the measured plasma concentration). Importantly, the Vd is simply a mathematical construct; it does not give any information regarding the tissues into which the drug has distributed, nor does it tell the actual drug concentration in those tissues.

Drugs that leave the plasma readily and are concentrated in tissues may have volumes of distribution that greatly exceed total body volume. This is most likely to be the case for drugs that are relatively lipid soluble and not very highly protein bound. For example, because fentanyl is highly lipid soluble and not avidly protein bound, it can readily leave the plasma and be concentrated in tissues, resulting in a Vd of 335 L. In contrast, alfentanil is a highly protein-bound, moderately lipid-soluble drug and consequently has a Vd of only 27 L.

The volume of distribution can also give useful insights into the mechanism by which an opioid's clinical effects are terminated. For example, following a single intravenous bolus, fentanyl is rapidly delivered to and concentrated in the brain and other highly perfused organs. As its large Vd suggests, fentanyl's initially high plasma concentration falls relatively rapidly as the drug is distributed to and concentrated in the large mass of peripheral tissues such as muscle and, finally, fat. As fentanyl's plasma concentration falls, the drug moves out of the brain to re-enter plasma for redistribution to peripheral tissues. Therefore, following a single bolus, the termination of fentanyl's clinical effects is largely the result of redistribution to peripheral

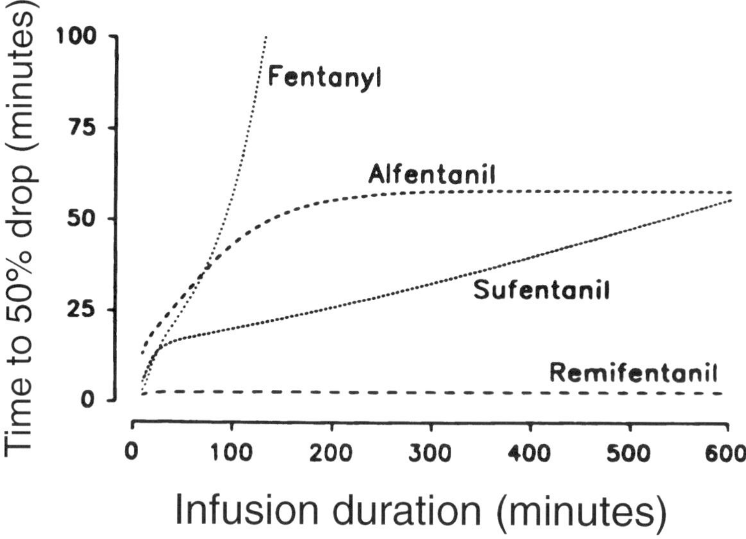

Figure 9.3. Computer simulation of the time required for a 50% decrease in plasma concentration of fentanyl, sufentanil, alfentanil, and remifentanil as a function of infusion duration – that is, context-sensitive half-time. Fentanyl's context-sensitive half-time increases dramatically because its high lipid solubility and relatively low protein binding result in large drug concentrations in peripheral tissues. Remifentanil's context-sensitive half-time does not change over time because it is rapidly metabolized in tissue and plasma and, therefore, elimination is not dependent on redistribution. (Reprinted with permission from Egan, T.D., Lemmens, H.J.M., Fiset, P., et al. [1993]. The pharmacokinetics of the new short acting opioid remifentanil (G187084B) in healthy adult male volunteers. *Anesthesiology.* **79,** 881.)

tissues and not hepatic metabolism. In contrast, alfentanil has a relatively small volume of distribution, indicating that it is not extensively taken up by peripheral tissues, and the termination of its clinical effect is largely the result of hepatic metabolism and not redistribution.

Importantly, the role of redistribution in terminating a drug's effect depends on whether the drug is administered as a single bolus or as a continuous infusion. As a drug is administered for longer and longer periods of time, the tissue sites to which it redistributes become increasingly "full," and redistribution decreases correspondingly. Drugs heavily dependent on redistribution to decrease their plasma concentration will have increasingly longer plasma half-times as redistribution diminishes and metabolism becomes the sole mechanism for removal from plasma. This fact was nicely demonstrated by Hughes and colleagues (1992), who proposed the term "context-sensitive half-time" to describe the change in central compartment (i.e., plasma) kinetics that occurs during opioid infusions. Figure 9.3 shows the context-sensitive half-times of fentanyl, alfentanil, sufentanil, and remifentanil. The plasma half-time of fentanyl increases markedly as the duration of infusion increases because the peripheral tissues are increasingly full, resulting in little capacity for redistribution to peripheral sites. In addition, fentanyl stored in peripheral tissues readily re-enters the central compartment to slow the fall in plasma concentration resulting from hepatic metabolism.

In contrast, the half-times of alfentanil and sufentanil increase only modestly during continuous infusion. Their greater protein binding (and in the case of alfentanil its lower lipid solubility) renders them less dependent on redistribution to decrease plasma concentration, and neither is present at very high concentrations in peripheral tissues. The context-sensitive half-time for remifentanil does not change over time because it is rapidly metabolized by tissue and plasma esterases and is not dependent on redistribution.

Spinal Opioid Administration

The discussion so far makes clear that an opioid's physicochemical properties have important effects on its BBB permeability and plasma pharmacokinetics and consequently on its clinical pharmacology following intravenous administration. Physicochemical properties also have important consequences for opioid pharmacology following epidural or intrathecal administration. However, as we shall see, properties that enhance brain bioavailability actually impair spinal bioavailability.

Spinal opioid administration seeks to deliver drugs to opioid receptors in the spinal cord dorsal horn at concentrations that are not generally attainable following IV administration. An equally important goal is to restrict opioids to their spinal site of action so as to avoid dose-limiting side effects mediated through brain opioid receptors (e.g., respiratory depression, sedation, nausea). Unfortunately, all epidurally and intrathecally administered opioids redistribute to extraspinal sites, where they can produce the same untoward and potentially fatal side effects that are associated with systemic opioid administration. Redistribution occurs both by uptake into the systemic circulation and by rostral spread in the cerebral spinal fluid (CSF). Understanding the factors that govern this redistribution is essential if one is to choose drugs whose physicochemical properties maximize redistribution to spinal opioid receptors while simultaneously limiting redistribution to extraspinal sites.

Unlike opioids administered into the plasma, epidurally and intrathecally administered opioids must diffuse relatively long distances to reach their site of action in the spinal cord dorsal horn. In so doing, they are subject to the same laws of thermodynamics that govern the movement of molecules in any other chemical environment. Specifically, they diffuse in random directions from their site of administration, and they partition into the chemical micro-environments in which they are thermodynamically most stable. The epidural space, intrathecal space, and spinal cord contain many different micro-environments, including epidural fat, collagen, arachnoid cell membranes, intracellular organelles, CSF, axons, myelin, neuronal cell bodies, extracellular fluid, and glycocalyx (Fig. 9.4). Which of these microenvironments a given

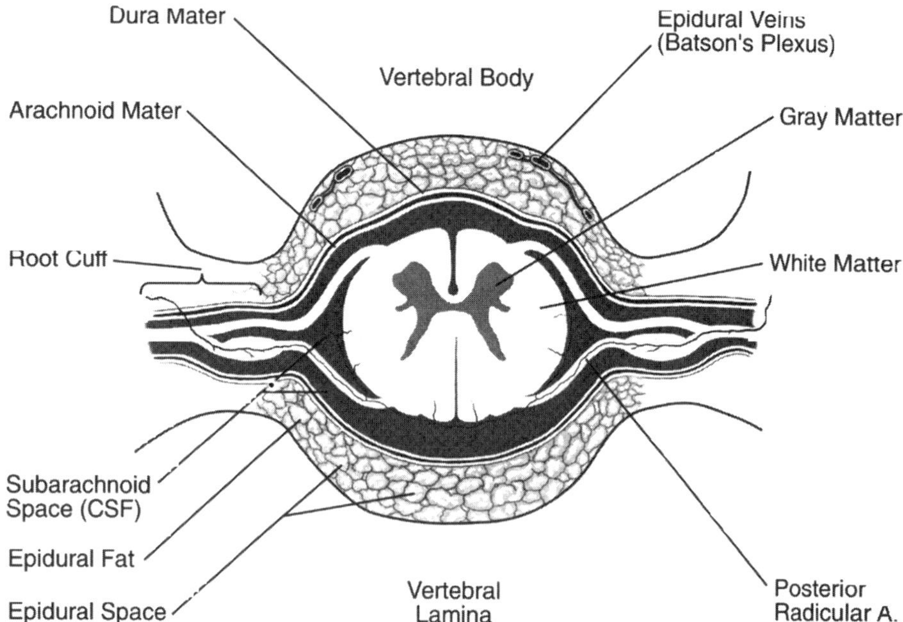

Figure 9.4. Cross section of the spinal cord depicting the multiple barriers and environments that must be negotiated by spinally administered opioids before they reach opioid receptors "buried" in the gray matter of the spinal cord dorsal horn.

molecule preferentially partitions into will depend on that molecule's particular physicochemical properties, and the pattern of partitioning will play a crucial role in determining the bioavailability of a given drug molecule at its spinal cord effect site.

Epidural Administration

To understand how physicochemical properties govern the rate and extent to which epidurally administered opioids redistribute to the spinal cord, it is necessary to understand how opioids reach the spinal cord from the epidural space. Over the years, several mechanisms have been proposed: (1) diffusion through the spinal meninges; (2) preferential diffusion through the spinal nerve root cuff (Cousins et al., 1971); and (3) diffusion through the walls of spinal radicular arteries with subsequent carriage to the spinal cord via radicular blood flow (Cousins et al., 1984). However, experimental animal studies have shown that epidurally administered drugs do not preferentially diffuse through the spinal nerve root cuff (Bernards and Hill, 1991), nor are they carried to the spinal cord by radicular blood flow (Bernards et al., 1994). Thus, to date the only mechanism shown to be responsible for drug movement between the epidural space and the spinal cord is diffusion thorough the spinal meninges (Bernards and Hill, 1990, 1992) with subsequent diffusion through the CSF and the spinal cord white matter to reach the spinal cord dorsal horn.

Contrary to the conventional wisdom, the arachnoid mater, not the dura mater, is the principal meningeal permeability barrier accounting for nearly 95% of the resistance to drug diffusion through the spinal meninges (Bernards and Hill, 1990). Histologically, the arachnoid barrier is composed of multiple tiers of overlapping cells connected to one another by frequent tight junctions. As with the endothelial cells of the BBB, the intercellular tight junctions are largely responsible for the low permeability of the arachnoid mater (Nabeshima et al., 1975; Vandenabeele et al., 1996). Another similarity between the BBB and the spinal meninges is the presence of enzyme systems potentially capable of metabolizing exogenously administered drugs (Zajac et al., 1987; Mitro and Lojda, 1988; Haninec and Grim, 1990; Volk et al., 1991; Ghersi-Egea et al., 1995; Kern et al., 1996; Kern and Bernards, 1997; Ummenhofer and Bernards, in press), including opioids.

Bernards and Hill (1992) investigated the role of physicochemical properties in governing drug permeability through the spinal meninges and found that no measure of physical size (i.e., molecular weight, molecular volume, molecular surface area, length of the major molecular axis) had an effect on a drug's meningeal permeability. However, hydrophobicity was shown to be an important determinant, although the relation between permeability and lipid solubility was not linear (Fig. 9.5). Just as Hansch et al. (1987) suggested for BBB permeability, meningeal permeability was optimal at an octanol:buffer$_{7.4}$ partition coefficient of about 100 (i.e., log P = 2). Thus, drugs of intermediate lipid solubility, for example, alfentanil, were significantly more permeable than were drugs that were less hydrophobic, for example, morphine, or more hydrophobic, for example, fentanyl and sufentanil.

The reason for this effect of hydrophobicity is not precisely known, but presumably it reflects differences in how hydrophobic and hydrophilic drugs negotiate the arachnoid cell membrane. One would expect that hydrophobic drugs would readily partition into the lipid bilayer of the arachnoid cell membrane because their hydrophobic character would render them thermodynamically more stable there. For the same reason, however, hydrophobic drugs would have difficulty partitioning out of the cell membrane to re-enter the aqueous intra- or intercellular space. Consequently, hydrophobic drugs may be temporarily sequestered in the lipid bilayer and their rate of penetration slowed proportionately. Yet, hydrophilic drugs would be expected to have difficulty entering the lipid bilayer of the arachnoid cell membrane, and their permeability would be slowed accordingly. In contrast, drugs of intermediate hydrophobicity presumably move through the arachnoid mater most rapidly because they are able to negotiate the aqueous:lipid interface of the arachnoid cell membranes more readily than drugs on either end of the "lipid-solubility" spectrum.

Importantly, meningeal permeability is not the only determinant of an opioid's spinal cord bioavailability following epidural administration. Drugs may partition into multiple different environments in the epidural space and thus be unavailable for transfer across the spinal meninges. In particular, the epidural fat may serve as a sequestration site for lipid-soluble drugs. In fact, following simultaneous epidural

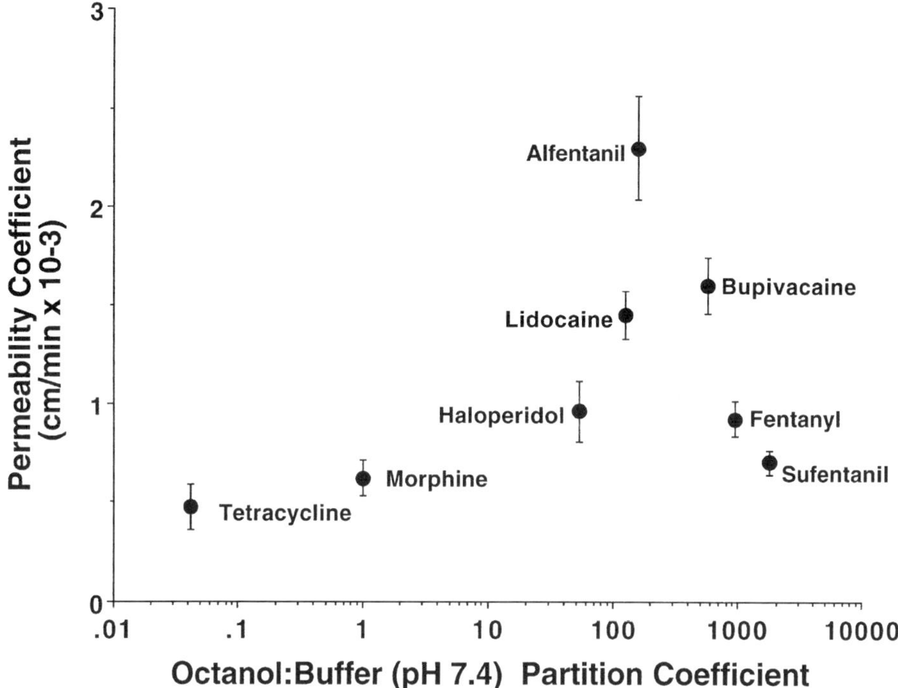

Figure 9.5. Relationship between octanol:buffer$_{7.4}$ partition coefficient and meningeal permeability. Note that permeability is maximal at a partition coefficient of approximately 100 (log P = 2). This is similar to what has been described for blood-brain–barrier permeability. (Data from Bernards, C.M., and Hill, H.F. (1992). Physical and chemical properties of drug molecules governing their diffusion through the spinal meninges. *Anesthesiology.* **77,** 750–756.)

administration of equal doses of morphine and sufentanil to pigs, Bernards (in preparation) has found that the concentration of sufentanil in the epidural fat is as much as 60 times greater than the concentration of morphine. Consequently, much less sufentanil is bioavailable to cross the spinal meninges than is the more hydrophilic drug morphine. It has also been suggested that epidurally administered drugs can be cleared from the epidural space by direct uptake through the wall of epidural veins (Batson's plexus). Despite claims to the contrary, however, this mechanism for drug clearance has never been demonstrated.

Intrathecal Drug Administration

Opioids injected directly into the CSF are cleared by two competing mechanisms – diffusion into the spinal cord or diffusion into the epidural space. Of note, epidurally administered drugs that reach the CSF can also diffuse back across the meninges into the epidural space, but unless and until the drug's concentration in the epidural space falls below that in the CSF, net drug transfer will be from the epidural space and into the CSF.

It is important to understand what fraction of an intrathecally administered opioid dose is cleared into the epidural space because this amount of drug is essentially unavailable to the spinal cord. Unfortunately, the necessary studies have not been performed in humans because it is not possible to measure drug concentration in spinal cord or epidural space. However, Bernards and colleagues (in preparation) have recently employed microdialysis techniques to measure the time course of morphine, fentanyl, and alfentanil in the CSF and epidural space following intrathecal delivery in pigs. The rate at which the opioids were cleared from the CSF was sufentanil > > alfentanil > morphine, which, not surprisingly, is the reverse order of their aqueous solubility. As one would predict based on their longer CSF residence times, morphine and alfentanil underwent significantly greater rostral spread than did sufentanil. Very surprising, however, was the finding that nearly 88% of the administered sufentanil dose was cleared into the epidural space, whereas only 40% and 42% of the administered morphine and alfentanil doses, respectively, were lost to the epidural space. Sufentanil's greater lipid solubility presumably results in its being sequestered in epidural fat, which acts as an "infinite sink" to maintain a high concentration gradient for movement of sufentanil into the epidural space.

There are also important differences among drugs with respect to their ability to penetrate the spinal cord to reach opioid receptors "buried" in laminae I, II, and V. Anatomically, the spinal cord is arranged into an outer mantle of white matter surrounding the gray matter core. The white matter consists of myelinated axons coursing between the spinal cord and brain. Importantly, myelin is 70% lipid, so that the white matter is a relatively hydrophobic environment. In contrast, the gray matter, which consists of neuronal cell bodies and short stretches of unmyelinated axons, is a relatively hydrophilic environment.

To determine how hydrophobicity affects a drug's ability to penetrate the spinal cord, Bernards (in preparation) used microdialysis to measure the penetration of equal doses of morphine and fentanyl following simultaneous application to the surface of the spinal cord of anesthetized pigs. Morphine penetrated the spinal cord much faster and much deeper than did fentanyl (Fig. 9.6). However, when the relative concentration of both drugs was measured in the superficial layer of the cord, the concentration of fentanyl was found to be three times greater than that of morphine. The presumed explanation is that fentanyl's greater lipid solubility results in its being sequestered in the hydrophobic domain of the myelin surrounding axons in the white matter and is thus unavailable to move extensively through the aqueous extracellular space. This finding is consistent with work by Herz and Teschemacher (1971), who reported that fentanyl preferentially accumulated in brain white matter following intraventricular CSF administration in rabbits, whereas morphine preferentially accumulated in gray matter.

These pharmacokinetic data suggest that extremes of lipid solubility limit the bioavailability of opioids at their target receptors in the spinal cord dorsal horn because they are sequestered either in epidural fat or in the hydrophobic environment

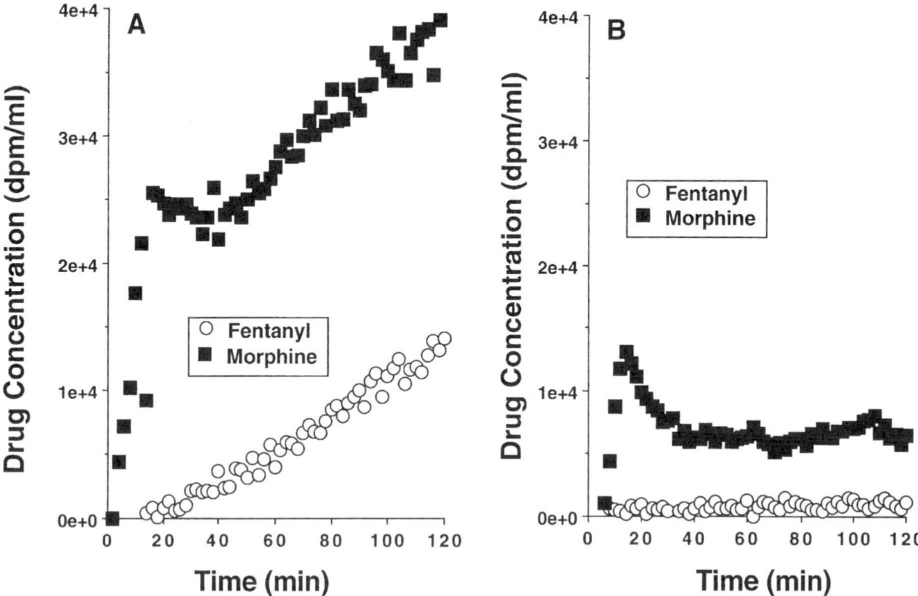

Figure 9.6. Concentration versus time profile of morphine and fentanyl within the spinal cord following simultaneous application of equal doses of both drugs to the surface of the spinal cord. Drug samples were obtained using microdialysis probes inserted into the white matter at a depth of 1.5 mm (A) and in the gray matter at a depth of 2.5 mm (B). Radiotracer methods were used to measure drug concentration, which is presented in units of dpm/ml. Note that morphine penetrates the cord much more rapidly and to a greater depth than does fentanyl, which is virtually undetectable in the gray matter. (Data from Bernards, C.M., manuscript in preparation.)

of spinal cord white matter. Consistent with these pharmacokinetic data, McQuay and colleagues (1989) have shown that the analgesic potency of intrathecally administered opioids in rats is inversely proportional to the drug's lipid solubility.

Clinical Correlations

The animal data presented here suggest that "extremes" of lipid solubility will limit the analgesic effectiveness of spinally administered opioids. As it turns out, much of the available human clinical data are consistent with this view.

Chrubasik and colleagues (1993) used historical data to calculate the epidural/IV potency ratio for several epidurally administered opioids. Their data are plotted against the drug's octanol buffer distribution coefficient in Figure 9.7, which shows that the most hydrophilic drug, morphine, is nine times more potent when delivered epidurally than when delivered systemically. However, as lipid solubility increases, the relative epidural potency of these opioids decreases; in fact, nearly 70% of the variability in potency can be explained by differences in lipid solubility.

In clinical studies aimed at determining the efficacy of epidural fentanyl, both

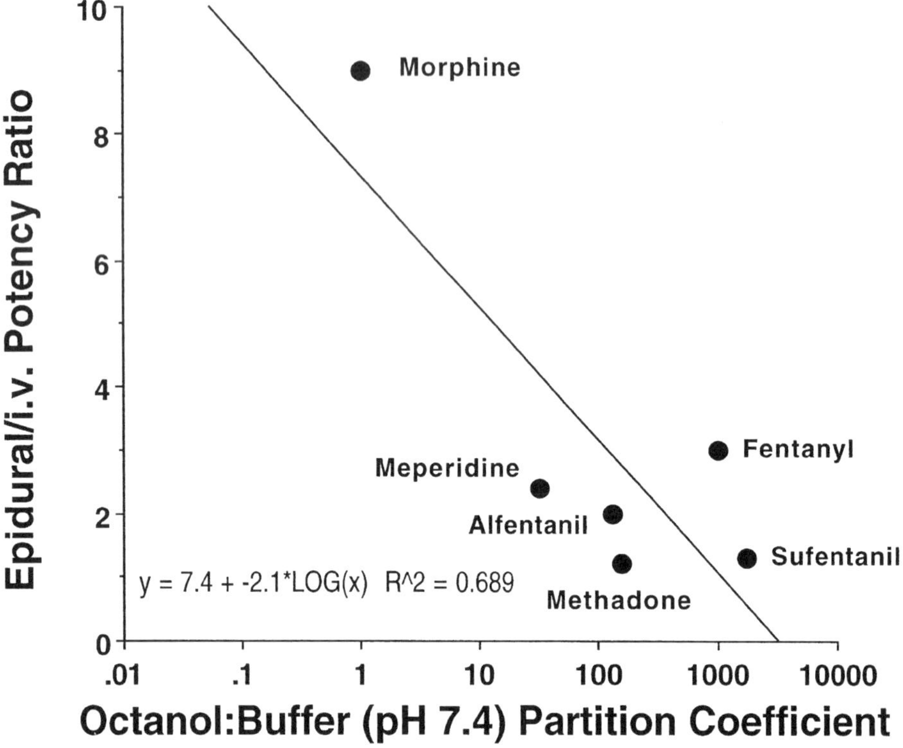

Figure 9.7. Relationship between epidural/IV potency ratio and octanol:buffer$_{7.4}$ partition coefficient for several epidurally administered opioids. Note that the analgesic potency of the hydrophilic opioid morphine is markedly greater when administered epidurally than when administered intravenously. In contrast, the more lipid-soluble opioids are relatively less potent epidurally; in fact, sufentanil and methadone are essentially equipotent whether administered epidurally or intravenously. (Data for epidural/IV potency ratios from Chrubasik, J., Chrubasik, S., and Martin, E. [1993]. The ideal epidural opioid – fact or fantasy? *Eur. J. Anaesthesiol.* **10,** 79–100.)

Loper et al. (1990) and Ellis et al. (1990) found that the fentanyl plasma concentration required to produce a similar degree of postoperative analgesia was the same whether the drug was administered epidurally or intravenously. Likewise, Guinard and colleagues (1992) found that the dose of fentanyl required to produce comparable analgesia following thoracotomy was the same whether the drug was administered into the lumbar epidural space, the thoracic epidural space, or intravenously. The same investigators demonstrated that patients randomized to receive fentanyl either intravenously or epidurally required equivalent doses, which resulted in equivalent plasma concentrations and pharmacodynamic effects during intraoperative administration (Guinard et al., 1992; Miguel et al., 1994). In a well-designed prospective double blind cross-over PCA study, Glass et al. (1992) demonstrated that analgesic effect and fentanyl plasma concentrations were the same within one hour of patients initiating either intravenous or epidural fentanyl administration. These studies strongly suggest that the mode of action for epidurally administered fentanyl is uptake into the systemic circulation with subsequent distribution to brain opioid receptors. There is no evidence of a selective spinal site of action. This fact is disturbing given the large number of patients whose epidural spaces are currently being instrumented for delivery of fentanyl; this mode simply represents an expensive and invasive way to give an intravenous injection.

Similarly, Miguel and colleagues (1994) demonstrated that the sufentanil dose, quality of analgesia, frequency of side effects, and, importantly, sufentanil plasma concentrations were the same whether sufentanil was administered into the thoracic epidural space or intravenously following intra-abdominal surgery. As with fentanyl, these data suggest that epidural sufentanil produces analgesia by uptake into the systemic circulation with subsequent distribution to brain opioid receptors. Therefore, it is difficult to justify administering sufentanil epidurally.

Finally, Coda et al. (1995) have shown that most, though not all, of the analgesic effect derived from epidurally administered alfentanil is also the result of systemic redistribution to brain. In contrast, multiple studies clearly demonstrate that epidural morphine produces analgesia by a predominately spinal site of action (Nordberg et al., 1983; Murakawa et al., 1989; Killbride et al., 1992; Erikkson-Mjoberg et al., 1997).

These clinical studies suggest that bioavailability of lipid-soluble opioids at spinal cord opioid receptors is limited following epidural administration and that analgesia produced by these drugs is largely the result of uptake into the systemic circulation with subsequent redistribution to brain opioid receptors. In contrast, the potent analgesia produced by modest doses of the hydrophilic drug morphine is largely the result of redistribution from the epidural space to spinal cord opioid receptors.

Fewer studies have examined the efficacy of intrathecally administered fentanyl or sufentanil, but the available information is again consistent with limited spinal cord bioavailability of these highly lipid-soluble opioids. Sundershan and colleagues (1995) demonstrated that intrathecal fentanyl improved the quality of analgesia and decreased morphine use in patients receiving IV PCA morphine for post-thoracotomy pain. However, the fentanyl dose administered (50 μg) is equivalent to 5 mg of morphine based on their relative intravenous potencies. Since most patients obtain excellent analgesia with as little as 0.25 mg of intrathecal morphine (and often with much smaller doses), this dose of fentanyl is roughly equivalent to 20 times the dose of intrathecal morphine necessary to provide complete spinal analgesia.

Similarly, Herman and colleagues (1997) determined the ED_{95} for intrathecal sufentanil in laboring women to be 8.9 μg. Given their relative intravenous potencies, this dose of sufentanil represents roughly 71 times the intrathecal dose of morphine that can be expected to provide good-quality spinal analgesia.

Thus, both epidural and intrathecal studies in humans suggest that the relative analgesic potency of lipid-soluble opioids is significantly less than that of the hydrophilic opioid morphine. Based on the available animal studies, we can reasonably surmise that lipid-soluble drugs are sequestered in lipid environments in and around the cord and are thus much less bioavailable at spinal opioid receptors.

Whether opioids are administered intravenously or spinally, their physicochemical properties have marked effects on their bioavailability and therefore their clinical pharmacology. Importantly, the effect of physicochemical properties, particularly lipid solubility, on bioavailability is entirely dependent on the site of administration. Clinicians must keep this in mind as they seek to employ opioids in the most effective way, and pharmaceutical developers should consider designing drugs for site-specific use.

REFERENCES

Abbott, J.J., Revest, P.A., and Romero, I.A. (1992). Astrocyte-endothelial interaction: Physiology and pathology. *Neuropathol. Appl. Neurobiol.* **18,** 424–433.

Ainslie, S., Eisele, J., and Corkill, G. (1979). Fentanyl concentrations in brain and serum during respiratory acid-base changes in the dog. *Anesthesiology.* **51,** 293–297.

Bernards, C.M., and Hill, H.F. (1992). Physical and chemical properties of drug molecules governing their diffusion through the spinal meninges. *Anesthesiology.* **77,** 750–756.

Bernards, C.M., and Hill, H.F. (1990). Morphine and alfentanil permeability through the spinal dura, arachnoid, and pia mater of dogs and monkeys. *Anesthesiology.* **73,** 1214–1219.

Bernards, C.M., and Hill, H.F. (1991). The spinal nerve root sleeve is not a preferred route for redistribution of drugs from the epidural space to the spinal cord. *Anesthesiology.* **75,** 827–832.

Bernards, C.M., and Sorkin, L.S. (1994). Radicular artery blood flow does not redistribute fentanyl from the epidural space to the spinal cord. *Anesthesiology.* **80,** 872–878.

Chrubasik, J., Chrubasik, S., and Martin, E. (1993). The ideal epidural opioid – fact or fantasy? *Eur. J. Anaesthesiol.* **10,** 79–100.

Coda, B., Brown, M., Schaffer, R., Donaldson, G., and Shen, D. (1995). A pharmacokinetic approach to resolving spinal and systemic contributions to epidural alfentanil analgesia and side effects. *Pain.* **62,** 329–337.

Cousins, M., and Bromage, P. (1987). Epidural neural blockade. In Cousins, M., Bridenbaugh, P., eds., *Neural blockade in clinical anesthesia and management of pain.* Philadelphia: J.B. Lippincott, pp. 253–360.

Cousins, M., and Mather, L. (1984). Intrathecal and epidural administration of opioids. *Anesthesiology.* **61,** 276–310.

Ellis, D.J., Millar, W.L., and Reisner, L. (1990). A randomized double-blind comparison of epidural versus intravenous fentanyl infusion for analgesia after Cesarean section. *Anesthesiology.* **72,** 981–986.

Emmerson, P.J., Clark, M.J., Mansour, A., Akil, H., Woods, J.H., and Medzihradsky, F. (1996). Characterization of opioid agonist efficacy in a C_6 glioma cell line expressing the μ opioid receptor. *JPET.* **278,** 1121–1127.

Erikkson-Mjoberg, M., Svensson, J., Almkvist, O., Olund, A., and Gustafsson, L. (1997). Extradural morphine gives better pain relief than patient-controlled i.v. morphine after hysterectomy. *Br. J. Anaesth.* **78,** 10–16.

Ford, J.M., and Hait, W.N. (1990). Pharmacology of drugs that alter multidrug resistance in cancer. *Pharmacol. Rev.* **42,** 155–199.

Frances, B., Gout, R., Monsarrat, B., Cros, J., and Zajac, J.M. (1992). Further evidence that morphine-6-beta-glucuronide is a more potent opioid agonist than morphine. *J. Pharmacol. Exp. Ther.* **262,** 25–31.

Gesink-van der Veer, B., Burm, A., Hennis, P., and Bovill, J. (1989). Alfentanil requirement in Crohn's disease: Increased alfentanil dose requirement in patients with Crohn's disease. *Anaesthesia.* **44,** 209–211.

Gesink-van der Veer, B., Burm, A., Vletter, A., and Bovill, J. (1993). Influence of Crohn's disease on the pharmacokinetics and pharmacodynamics of alfentanil. *Br. J. Anaesth.* **71,** 827–834.

Ghersi-Egea, J.F., Leininger-Muller, B., Cecchelli, R., and Fenstermacher, J.D. (1995). Blood-brain interfaces: Relevance to cerebral drug metabolism. *Toxicol. Lett.* **December,** 645–653.

Ghersi-Egea, J.F., Leininger-Muller, B., Cecchelli, R., and Fenstermacher, J.D. (1995). Blood-brain interfaces: Relevance to cerebral drug metabolism. *Toxicol. Lett.* **82/83,** 645–653.

Glass, P., Estok, P., Ginsberg, B., Goldberg, J., and Sladen, R. (1992). Use of patient-controlled analgesia to compare the efficacy of epidural to intravenous fentanyl administration. *Anesth. Analg.* **74,** 345–351.

Goldstein, G.W. (1988). Endothelial cell-astrocyte interactions. A cellular model of the blood-brain barrier. *Ann. N.Y. Acad. Sci.* **529,** 31–39.

Guinard, J.P., Mavrocordatos, P., Chiolero, R., and Carpenter, R.L. (1992). A randomized comparison of intravenous versus lumbar and thoracic epidural fentanyl for analgesia after thoracotomy. *Anesthesiology.* **77,** 1108–1115.

Haninec, P., and Grim, M. (1990). Localization of dipeptidylpeptidase IV and alkaline phosphatase in developing spinal cord meninges and peripheral nerve coverings of the rat. *Int. J. Develop. Neurosci.* **8,** 175–185.

Hansch, C., Björkroth, J.P., and Leo, A. (1987). Hydrophobicity and central nervous system agents: On the principle of minimal hydrophobicity in drug design. *J. Pharm. Sci.* **76,** 663–686.

Herman, N.L.C.R., Van Decar, T.K., Conlin, G., and Tilton, J. (1997). Determination of the dose-response relationship for intrathecal sufentanil in laboring patients. *Anesth. Analg.* **84,** 1256–1261.

Herz, A., and Teschemacher, H. (1971). Activities and sites of antinociceptive action of morphine-like analgesics and kinetics of distribution following intravenous, intracerebral and intraventricular application. In N. Harper and A. Simmonds, eds., *Advances in drug research.* London: Academic Press, pp. 79–119.

Hosztafi, S., Friedmann, T., and Furst, Z. (1993). Structure-activity relationship of synthetic and semisynthetic opioid agonists and antagonists. *Acta Pharm. Hung.* **63,** 335–349.

Hug, Jr., C., and Murphy, M. (1981). Tissue redistribution of fentanyl and termination of its effect in rats. *Anesthesiology.* **55,** 369–375.

Hughes, M.A., Glass, P.S., and Jacobs, J.R. (1992). Context-sensitive half-time in multicompartment pharmacokinetic models for intravenous anesthetic drugs. *Anesthesiology.* **76**(3), 334–341.

Huwyler, J., Drewe, J., Klusemann, C., and Fricker, G. (1996). Evidence for P-glycoprotein-modulated penetration of morphine-6-glucuronide into brain capillary endothelium. *Br. J. Pharmacol.* **118,** 1879–1885.

Janzer, R.C. (1993). The blood-brain barrier: Cellular basis. *J. Inherit. Metab. Dis.* **16,** 639–647.

Kern, C., and Bernards, C.M. (1997). Ascorbic acid inhibits spinal meningeal catechol-o-methyl transferase *in vitro* resulting in a marked increase in epinephrine bioavailability. *Anesthesiology.* **86,** 405–409.

Kern, C., Mautz, D., and Bernards, C.M. (1996). Epinephrine is metabolized by the spinal meninges of monkeys and pigs. *Anesthesiology.* **83,** 1078–1081.

Kilbride, M., Senagore, A., Mazier, W., Ferguson, C., and Ufkes, T. (1992). Epidural analgesia. *Surg. Gynecol. Obstet.* **174,** 137–140.

Knapp, R.J., Waite, S., Landsman, R., et al. (1995). Efficacy of peptide and nonpeptide agonists at the cloned human δ opioid receptor. *Proc. West. Pharmacol. Soc.* **38,** 141–143.

Kutter, E., Herz, A., Teschemacher, H., and Hess, R. (1970). Structure-activity correlates, using regression analysis in the series of morphine-like analgesics. *Naunyn Schmiedebergs, Arch. Pharmacol.* **266,** 386–387.

Leysen, J.E., Gommeren, W., and Niemegeers, C.J.E. (1983). [^{3}H]Sufentanil, a superior ligand for μ-opiate receptors: Binding properties and regional distribution in rat brain and spinal cord. *Eur. J. Pharmacol.* **87,** 209–225.

Loper, K., Ready, L.B., Downey, M., et al. (1990). Epidural and intravenous fentanyl infusions are clinically equivalent after knee surgery. *Anesth. Analg.* **70,** 72–75.

Macfie, A., Magides, A., and Reilly, C. (1992). Disposition of alfentanil in burns patients. *Br. J. Anaesth.* **69,** 447–450.

Matteo, R., Ornstein, E., Schwartz, A., Young, W., Weinstein, J., and Cain, C. (1992). Effects of hypocarbia on the pharmacodynamics of sufentanil in humans. *Anesth. Analg.* **75,** 186–192.

McQuay, H.J., Sullivan, A.F., Smallman, K., and Dickenson, A.H. (1989). Intrathecal opioids, potency and lipophilicity. *Pain.* **36,** 111–115.

Miguel, R., Barlow, I., Morrell, M., Scharf, J., Sanusi, D., and Fu, E. (1994). A prospective, randomized, double-blind comparison of epidural and intravenous sufentanil infusions. *Anesthesiology.* **81,** 346–352.

Minn, A., Ghersi-Egea, J., Leininger, B., and Siest, G. (1991). Drug metabolizing enzymes in the brain and cerebral microvessels. *Brain Res.* **16,** 65–82.

Mitro, A., and Lojda, Z. (1988). Histochemistry of proteases in ependyma, choroid plexus and leptomeninges. *Histochemistry.* **88,** 645–646.

Murakawa, T., Baba, S., Isozaki, K., Kudo, M., Matsuki, A., and Oyama, T. (1989). Plasma morphine levels during its continuous epidural infusion. *Masui.* **38,** 1166–1170.

Nabeshima, S., Reese, T.S., Landis, D.M.D., and Brightman, M.W. (1975). Junctions in the meninges and marginal glia. *J. Comp. Neur.* **164,** 127–170.

Nordberg, G., Hedner, T., Mellstrand, T., and Dahlstrom, B. (1983). Pharmacokinetic aspects of epidural morphine analgesia. *Anesthesiology.* **58,** 545–551.

Rapaport, S. (1976). *Blood-brain barrier in physiology and medicine.* New York: Raven Press, pp. 1–316.

Schinkel, A.H., Wagenaar, E., Mol, C.A.A.M., and van Deemter, L. (1996). P-Glycoprotein in the blood-brain barrier of mice influences the brain penetration and pharmacological activity of many drugs. *J. Clin. Invest.* **97,** 2517–2524.

Schulman, D., Kaufman, J., Eisenstein, M., and Rapoport, S. (1984). Blood pH and brain uptake of 14C-morphine. *Anesthesiology.* **61,** 540–543.

Scott, J., Ponganis, K., and Stanski, D. (1985). EEG quantitation of narcotic effect: The comparative pharmacodynamics of fentanyl and alfentanil. *Anesthesiology.* **62,** 234–241.

Selley, D.E., Sim, L.J., Xiao, R., Liu, Q., and Childers, S.R. (1997). μ-Opioid receptor-stimulated guanosine-5′-O-(γ-thio)-triphosphate binding in rat thalamus and cultured cell lines: Signal transduction mechanisms underlying agonist efficacy. *Mol. Pharmacol.* **51,** 87–96.

Sudarshan, G., Browne, B.L., Matthews, J.N., and Conacher, I.D. (1995). Intrathecal fentanyl for post-thoracotomy pain. *Br. J. Anaesth.* **75,** 19–22.

Ummenhofer, W., and Bernards, C.M. (in press). The spinal meninges of monkeys and pigs possess significant cholinesterase activity. *Anesthesiology.*

Vandenabeele, F., Creemers, J., and Lambrichts, I. (1996). Ultrastructure of the human spinal arachnoid mater and dura mater. *J. Anat.* **189,** 417–430.

Volk, B., Hettmannsperger, U., Papp, T., Amelizad, Z., Oesch, F., and Knoth, R. (1991). Mapping of phenytoin-inducible cytochrome P450 immunoreactivity in the mouse central nervous system. *Neuroscience.* **42,** 215–235.

Wu, D., Kang, Y.S., Bickel, U., and Pardridge, W.M. (1997). Blood-brain barrier permeability to morphine-6-glucuronide is markedly reduced compared with morphine. *Drug Metab. Dispos.* **25,** 768–771.

Zajac, J.-M., Charnay, Y., Soleilhac, J.-M., Sales, N., and Roques, B.P. (1987). Enkephalin-degrading enzymes and angiotensin-converting enzyme in human and rat meninges. *F.E.B.S. Lett.* **216,** 118–122.

CHAPTER TEN

Clinical Pharmacology and Adverse Effects

LAURENCE E. MATHER AND MAREE T. SMITH

This chapter is not intended to be a comprehensive pharmacopoeial treatment of opioid pharmacology; rather, its purpose is to emphasize principles using the main opioid analgesics in current clinical practice as examples.

Overview of the Use of Opioid Analgesics

Opioid analgesics are first-line medication for moderate to severe nociceptive pain. Their clinical effectiveness in this role is traditional and unquestioned. They are highly effective, inexpensive, and relatively simple to use. In addition, they may produce a sense of well-being, and, by control over pain, they promote restful sleep. Nevertheless, the results of most surveys indicate that pain management is suboptimal (Bruster et al., 1994; Zhukowsky et al., 1995). When current analgesic medications can be so effective, why is pain management not always excellent? There are many reasons. Although attitudes, teaching, and unfavorable logistics among medical and nursing staff may contribute, perhaps compounded by vagaries associated with inappropriate dosage regimens, fickle routes of administration, and unfavorable individual pharmacokinetics, the drugs themselves are not blameless. Opioid analgesics have a spectrum of side effects that can limit their usefulness, so that some patients may even prefer to endure pain than to withstand the side effects of the therapy.

Development of new agents over the past decades has never significantly dissociated the adverse from the salutary actions of opioid analgesics. The deficiencies of opioid analgesics include their potential for initiating drug dependence; life-threatening ventilatory depression; untoward central nervous system (CNS) responses such as somnolence, excitation, and dysphoria; and gastrointestinal disturbances, particularly nausea, emesis, gastroparesis, and constipation; and for generating a miscellany of lesser studied effects such as pruritus, altered immunocompetence, and impaired micturition. In addition, the complex legal issues associated with their use contributes to their frugal use in patients and, sometimes, by patients. There is still not a single agent with a clear therapeutic advantage for general use. Hence "multimodal" analgesia has evolved as a way of using lower doses of analgesic agents acting by different mechanisms (e.g., opioids with local anesthetics or nonsteroidal anti-inflammatory drugs) in concert to maximize therapeutic effects and minimize side effects associated with any one component (Kehlet, 1997).

On the positive side, opioids are now available with ultrahigh (e.g., remifentanil) to very low (e.g., methadone) clearances, with many agents in between. Moreover, the options for administration now allow for several direct, albeit highly invasive (e.g., intracerebroventricular and intrathecal), methods and many indirect but non-invasive routes (e.g., transdermal and transmucosal) with pharmaceutic improvements still being made to conventional methods (e.g., oral controlled release).

Dosage regimens, particularly for postoperative pain management, have evolved to allow a large measure of patient participation as a demonstrated means of improving the clinical outcome. Opioid analgesic agents are used, broadly, in two discrete dosage ranges: analgesic doses for conscious patients and antinociceptive ("anesthetic") doses for unconscious patients (usually surgical and intensive care patients). They are used, for the most part, for two discrete time ranges, acutely over days (such as in postsurgical pain), and chronically over weeks to months (such as in cancer pain). This difference has implications for routes of administration and dosage regimens as well as for the choice of agent, the activity of metabolites, and the costs. However, despite the range of agents listed in pharmacopoeias and research literature, the choices of agents in local formularies still tend to be driven more by traditional issues such as local prejudice, price, and availability than by theoretical or demonstrated pharmacology. It is also now recognized that an effective replacement and/or a reliable supplement for postoperative opioid analgesia is highly desirable, especially because the shortcomings of existing agents are accentuated by the advance of day-case surgery, making demands for speedy discharge of patients and for availability of reliable pain management in patients' home environments.

Pharmacologic Significance of the Metabolism of Opioid Analgesics

When considering the pharmacology of opioid analgesics it also necessary to consider that of their metabolites. Although it has been generally taught that the hydrophilic products of xenobiotic metabolism are pharmacologically inactive excretion products, many experiments have amply demonstrated that this is not the case for many of the metabolites of opioids.

Opioid analgesics undergo one or more major metabolic biotransformations relevant to their chemical structures (Fig. 10.1): glucuronidation and dealkylation products have decreased lipophilicity, and hydrolysis products may or may not retain activity as their parents. Lesser biotransformations also occur, but these are unlikely to have much pharmacologic significance.

Opioids structurally related to morphine (benzomorphans) with intact 3- and/or 6-OH groups are conjugated with the hydrophilic sugar moiety glucuronic acid (Milne et al., 1996). The resultant metabolites of morphine, morphine 3-O-glucuronide (M3G), and morphine 6-O-glucuronide (M6G) have become well known since reliable assay methods for their quantification were first described in the mid-1980s.

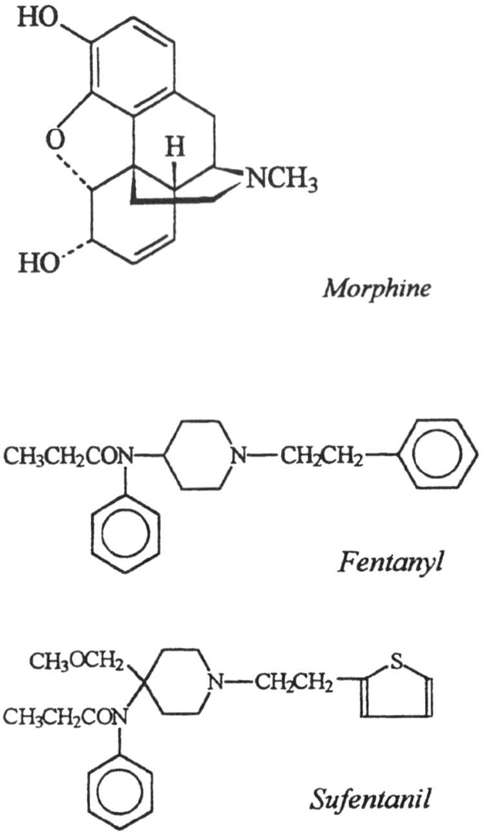

Morphine

Fentanyl

Sufentanil

Figure 10.1. Chemical formulas showing the benzomorphan structure of morphine (top) and the nonbenzomorphan structures of fentanyl and sufentanil (center and bottom) to explain the functional group features that pertain to their major routes of metabolism. Morphine undergoes glucuronide conjugation on the 3-OH (phenolic, upper) and 6-OH (alcoholic, lower) sites, as well as N-dealkylation of the N-methyl substituent. Fentanyl and sufentanil undergo hydrolysis of the amide group; as well, fentanyl undergoes N-dealkylation of the N-phenylethyl substituent, and sufentanil undergoes N-dealkylation of the N-thienylethyl substituent.

Indeed, the literature now abounds with studies of the pharmacokinetics and/or effects of morphine and its glucuronide metabolites as well as of some related opioids.

Whereas once M6G and M3G were commonly thought to be too hydrophilic to enter the CNS, it is now clear that these glucuronides can have CNS activity when administered peripherally or produced by metabolism. Single-dose studies in rodents have shown that when injected directly into the CNS, M6G is 10- to more than 100-fold more potent an antinociceptive agent than morphine, and it is longer acting when given in equieffective doses (Abbott and Palmour, 1988; Paul et al., 1989; Gong et al., 1991; Frances et al., 1992; Stain et al., 1995). When injected peripherally, M6G is more potent than morphine, but the margin is smaller (less than 10-fold). Such findings are consistent with M6G's slower rate of penetration into the CNS relative to morphine (Barjavel et al., 1994; Aasmundstad et al., 1995; Kalman et al., 1997; Vancrugten et al., 1997; Hasselström and Säwe, 1993; Mignat et al., 1995; Wu et al., 1997). The same argument has been used in rationalizing the activities of more potent/more lipophilic drugs, such as fentanyl, with morphine (Mather, 1983).

M3G has no intrinsic analgesic actions, consistent with its poor affinity for classical inhibitory opioid receptors in vitro (Chen et al., 1991; Bartlett, Dodd, and Smith,

1994; Loser et al., 1996). However, a variety of studies in experimental animals have now shown that M3G does have pharmacologic activity. Following intracerebroventricular (ICV) and intrathecal administration, M3G evokes dose-dependent excitatory behavioral effects in rats (Labella et al., 1979; Yaksh et al., 1986; Bartlett, Cramond, and Smith, 1994). It has also been shown to attenuate morphine activity by nonopioid or nonconventional opioid receptor–mediated mechanisms. ICV M3G can attenuate morphine- or M6G-induced antinociception (Faura et al., 1996; Gong et al., 1992; Smith et al., 1990), and ventilatory depression (Pelligrino et al., 1989; Gong et al., 1992), as well as counter the inhibitory effects of morphine and M6G on the micturition response (Igawa et al., 1993). In other studies it has been indicated that there is a significant inverse correlation between the mean degree of antinociception achieved and the mean plasma and ECF molar concentration ratio, M3G/morphine, following administration of various dosage regimens of morphine to rats (Smith and Smith, 1995; Barjavel et al., 1995).

Clinically, the plasma and CSF concentrations of M3G exceed those of morphine by several-fold after single doses of morphine (Hasselström and Säwe, 1993) and by as much as 10–20-fold in patients receiving morphine chronically (Cramond et al., 1993). Hence, it is essential to give serious consideration to the pharmacology of M3G and to whether it has significant antimorphine action in clinical practice, and if so, whether its antimorphine actions show cross-over to nonbenzomorphan opioids such as fentanyl.

In patients dosed with morphine, M6G is thought to augment morphine's effects (Portenoy et al., 1992). There is evidence that M6G may augment respiratory depression and mental confusion in some patients, especially if it is associated with poor renal function, but there is no convincing evidence that it is involved in myoclonus (Tiseo et al., 1995). M6G has recently been used in trials in humans as an analgesic agent, and the results differ as to its effectiveness. After single doses, M6G has been found to be analgetically superior to morphine (Osborne et al., 1992), of similar activity (Thompson et al., 1995), and devoid of analgesic activity (Geisslinger et al., 1997). As noted earlier, M6G enters the CNS, but its efficacy is more reliable when it is given directly into the CNS. When injected intrathecally, M6G has been found to be more potent than morphine, but not devoid of opioid side effects (Hanna et al., 1990; Grace and Fee, 1996).

Many opioid analgesics have an N-methyl group that is traditionally considered to be important for pharmacologic activity. N-demethylation of morphine to normorphine is a minor metabolic pathway compared with glucuronidation, and normorphine is a weaker analgesic than morphine, due probably to its slower CNS penetration. Normorphine also undergoes glucuronidation, particularly in rodents (Evans and Shanahan, 1995). N-demethylation is a significant feature of pethidine, methadone, and propoxyphene metabolism because the metabolites have a longer residence time in the body and appear to be more toxic than their respective parent drugs. Norpethidine, in particular, is a sufficiently potent CNS excitant to be classified as neurotoxic (Plummer et al., 1995). If the excitatory side effects of norpethidine are observed, pethidine should be discontinued immediately and another opioid substituted in the pain management plan. Fentanyl, alfentanil, and sufentanil are also N-dealkylated (Labroo et al., 1995; Tateishi et al., 1996).

The enzyme (CYP2D6) catalyzing the O-dealkylation of codeine (3-O methyl morphine) to morphine shows genetic polymorphism such that it is bimodally distributed among humans (Sindrup et al., 1993; Mikus et al., 1994). Many studies suggest that individuals who have this enzyme ("extensive metabolizers," approximately 90% Caucasians) also obtain analgesia from codeine, whereas individuals genetically deficient in this enzyme ("poor metabolizers," approximately 10% Caucasians) do not. However, given the recent evidence showing that codeine and its glucuronide conjugate codeine-6-glucuronide have intrinsic antinociceptive effects in rodents (Srinivasan et al., 1996), it may be premature to conclude that "poor metabolizers" do not obtain analgesia from codeine.

Ester groups such as occur in diamorphine (heroin), meperidine (pethidine), and remifentanil are hydrolyzed by one or more plasma and/or liver esterases. Diamorphine undergoes two, essentially sequential, hydrolytic reactions (Skopp et al., 1997). Rapid hydrolysis of the 3-acetyl group gives 6-monoacetyl morphine, which undoubtedly contributes potent morphinoid effects. The second and slower hydrolysis step gives morphine. Remifentanil has two ester groups, one of which is hydrolyzed extremely rapidly, thereby terminating the opioid effects (Dershwitz et al., 1996). The metabolic products of meperidine and remifentanil hydrolysis do not contribute significantly to opioid actions. Fentanyl (also remifentanil) contains an amide group in place of the ester group found in meperidine, but the hydrolysis product does not have significant opioid actions.

Using a traditional mass balance approach, human studies show that approximately 10% of an intravenous dose of morphine appears in the urine as unmetabolized morphine, 55% as M3G, and 10% as M6G; other routes of metabolism and further metabolites probably make up the remainder of the dose (Milne et al., 1996). The respective role of the kidneys versus the liver in morphine disposition has been debated (Mather, 1995). Some insight has come from recent direct measurements in sheep, which have shown that the magnitude of morphine extraction by the kidneys is almost as great as that by the liver and that the contribution of the kidneys to the overall clearance of morphine is diminished by renal pathology (e.g., Milne et al., 1993, 1995; Dhonneur et al., 1994). However, it is not known whether the same is true for humans. Hepatic dysfunction does alter morphine dose-effect relationships, but the body has a larger reserve for metabolism of morphine (Shelly et al., 1989; Hasselström et al., 1990) than for excretion of the glucuronide metabolites (Davies et al., 1996).

Relevant Clinical Pharmacokinetics of Opioid Analgesics

The most important outcome of the plethora of pharmacokinetic studies of opioid analgesics has been to document the variability between patients in dose-plasma drug concentration relationships and in plasma drug concentration-clinical effect

Table 10.1. *Comparison of Intravenous Pharmacokinetics of Selected Opioid Analgesics (typical mean values)*

Drug	Subjects	V_D (L/kg)	CL_T (ml/kg/minute)	$T_{1/2}$ (hour)	$t_{1/2}K_{eo}$ (minute)
Morphine	Normal	2.8	15.5	2.5	NA
Hydromorphone	Normal	4.1	22.7	3.0	NA
Levorphanol	Chronic pain	10	10.5	11	NA
Pethidine	Preoperative	2.6	12	3.5	NA
Methadone	Chronic pain	3.4	1.6	23	NA
Fentanyl	Normal	4.6	21	3	6
Alfentanil	Normal	0.9	7.6	1.5	0.6
Sufentanil	Surgical	2.5	11.3	2.5	6
Remifentanil	Surgical	0.2	34	0.2	1.3
Buprenorphine	Postoperative	2.8	17.2	3	NA
Oxycodone	Cancer pain	3.3	12.5	3	NA

V_D = apparent volume of distribution; CL_T = mean total body clearance; $T_{1/2}$ = elimination half-life; $t_{1/2}K_{eo}$ = half-life of equilibration between blood and brain as derived from quantitative EEG analysis; NA = not available.
Sources: Adapted from Scott, et al., 1991; Leow, et al., 1992; Hill and Mather, 1993; Egan, 1995; Rosow, 1995; Minto et al., 1997.

relationships. A brief synopsis of the pharmacokinetic characteristics of some important opioid analgesics is given in Table 10.1. Several general points are relevant (Mather and Woodhouse, 1997). (1) As judged by V_D, there are differences in the tissue:blood distribution of opioids; the larger the value, the more likely the opioid effects are terminated by redistribution than by clearance, and the more likely cumulation will take place on repeated (continuous) administration. (2) As judged by CL_T, there is a wide range of rates of metabolism; the larger the value, the more likely effects will dissipate rapidly after cessation of administration. (3) $T_{1/2}$ is not a reliable guide to the duration of opioid effects because it is a derivative of both distribution and clearance; the actual range of drug concentrations being influenced needs to be considered at the same time. (4) Studies are often performed under different paradigms – some in healthy subjects, others in patients with pathology, and others in anesthetized subjects before, during, and after surgery: because of physiologic vagaries, comparison of data between such paradigms and populations is hazardous.

A noninvasive approach to studying the rate of opioid uptake into the brain comes from a combined pharmacokinetic-quantitative EEG model. The model, originally developed to study drugs used for the induction of anesthesia (Youngs and Shafer, 1994; Lemmens et al., 1994; Kapila et al., 1995), links the arterial blood–drug concentration time relationship with the time course of changes in a parameter of the

EEG, typically the 95% spectral edge. The parameters derived for the drug are the half-life of equilibration of drug between blood and biophase in the brain ($t_{1/2}K_{eo}$) and the concentration of half maximal drug effect. Using this approach, values of $t_{1/2}K_{eo}$ have been tabulated for a variety of opioids, giving a comparative index for the speed of onset of drug effect (Table 10.1). This approach, although useful empirically, does not have a known basis pertinent to pain management.

Principles of Pharmacotherapy with Opioid Analgesics

Factors including the indications, duration, frequency, and route of administration have implications for the choice and dose of opioid analgesics as well as for the side effects encountered.

The extent to which there is a reliable relationship between plasma concentrations and analgesic response is often not clear for opioid analgesics because alleviation of pain in conscious patients is influenced by individual differences in factors such as local tissue damage and coexisting pathology, the turnover of local hormones and endogenous opioids and by psychosocial factors relating to previous experiences, the significance of the injury, the surroundings, and the extent of caring offered by hospital staff and others. When considered in conjunction with individual differences in opioid pharmacokinetics, it is not surprising that there are large differences in responses between, and even within, individual patients to opioid analgesics (Hill and Mather, 1993). Traditional tables of dosage equivalents that are often found in the literature or in pharmaceutical companies' promotional materials provide only starting estimates. Indeed, the need for individualization of dosage, sometimes combined with creative dosage regimens, is a hallmark of opioid pharmacotherapy (Hunt and Bruera, 1995).

As noted elsewhere, opioid analgesics are the first-line treatment for nociceptive pain. For acute nociceptive pain opioid doses can be adjusted under close supervision until the desired therapeutic effect is achieved or unacceptable side effects supervene. Cancer pain is usually regarded as a combination of repeated acute nociceptive and neurogenic stimuli, biased by emotional responses, and may have superimposed the consequences of surgical and other painful treatments. Whereas the nociceptive pain can be treated successfully with opioids, combination or multimodal drug therapy is usually required, along with other nonpharmacologic support mechanisms (Hanks and Forbes, 1997). Nevertheless, opioid-related side effects can be problematic. Opioid treatment of chronic nonmalignant and neuropathic pain is still controversial (Hanks and Forbes, 1997; Stein, 1997) and without widespread medical support. Iatrogenic drug dependence is just one side effect of concern.

Side Effects of Opioid Analgesics

It is clear that all opioid analgesics can cause side effects, but not all opioid side effects are equally important to patients or their clinicians. Whereas many side effects are extensions of the therapeutic effects, others appear more related to the duration of administration. The side effect of tolerance is considered at the outset because it impinges on the issue of acute versus chronic opioid administration.

Tolerance

Analgesic tolerance and cross tolerance to opioids can be regarded as a side effect (Moulin et al., 1988). There are countless reports of tolerance in laboratory animals, but this effect is particularly poorly characterized in humans receiving opioids for pain control. It is arguable from laboratory studies that tolerance is produced rapidly – from even the first perioperative exposure (Ling et al., 1989; Kissin et al., 1991), and this is supported by circumstantial evidence in patients after surgery (Cooper et al., 1997). There is little disagreement that tolerance occurs in patients treated for acute pain for more than 5 to 7 days or for chronic pain or that tolerance also develops to other side effects of opioids, such as ventilatory depression. Anecdotal clinical reports that the benzomorphan opioids, morphine and hydromorphone, show incomplete or no cross tolerance to the structurally dissimilar opioids sufentanil, ketobemidone, and methadone in cancer patients (Sjogren et al., 1994; Vigano et al., 1996) are supported by recent pharmacologic studies in mice (Bilsky et al., 1996). These studies showed that although NMDA antagonists attenuated the development of antinociceptive tolerance to morphine, the same NMDA antagonists were ineffective in preventing tolerance to the structurally dissimilar μ opioids fentanyl, DAMGO and PL017, deltorphin II (δ opioid peptide), or endogenous opioids released following a swim-stress stimulus. Clearly, these findings imply that different mechanisms underlie the development of tolerance to benzomorphan and nonbenzomorphan opioids, which may relate to the fact that benzomorphan opioids, such as morphine or hydromorphone, are metabolized to 3-O-glucuronides, which have been proposed to play a causal role in the development of tolerance to these opioids (Smith et al., 1990; Smith and Smith, 1995; Barjavel et al., 1995). Implications for the clinical setting are that co-administration of NMDA antagonists (e.g., ketamine, dextromethorphan, and dextrorphan) with opioids may be beneficial only in attenuating tolerance development when the opioid administered is morphine or a close structural analog such as hydromorphone.

Ventilatory Depression

Ventilatory depression is the side effect most feared in clinical practice because it may be life threatening. Depression of the medullary respiratory center neurones is a universal property of traditional opioid analgesics thought to involve μ_2, δ, and κ receptor responses, although the involvement of μ_1 opioid receptors has again been suggested recently (Shook et al., 1990; Chen et al., 1996). Ventilatory depression is characterized by several physiologically and clinically detectible signs – notably, decreased tidal volume and minute ventilation, right-shifted CO_2 response, bradypnea, hypercapnia, hypoxia, and decreased oxygen saturation (Borison, 1977). The various agonist-type opioid analgesics do not appear to differ in their potential for ventilatory depression in humans, so there is probably no advantage of one pure agonist over another.

It is likely that blood opioid concentration is a reasonable guide to the probability of ventilatory depression, so that the route of introducing the drug into the blood – intravenous, intramuscular, and so on – is less important than the dose or the dosage rate. Pain is often said to stimulate respiration, and experimental pain has been shown to do so in healthy volunteers (Borgbjerg et al., 1996). However, there is a marked difference between this and poor ventilatory parameters due to splinting and inability to cough in a subject with pain. Sometimes there is a fine line in ventilatory parameters between patients who are underdosed and those who are overdosed with opioid analgesic, particularly if the latter is combined with sleep, although the physiology and pharmacology differ dramatically. Moreover, the extremes of age are thought to provide particularly sensitive subjects (Vaughn et al., 1996). In high doses the fentanyl opioids may additionally produce a chest wall rigidity syndrome that further compromises ventilation. In clinical practice, hourly observation of respiratory rate has been shown to be next to useless to ascertain this side effect; continuous monitoring is the only reliable method (Catley et al., 1985; Bulow et al., 1995).

Tramadol, a relatively recent synthetic opioid analgesic, is a racemic 4-phenylpiperidine analog of codeine. Both enantiomers of tramadol bind only very weakly to opioid receptors (μM affinity), but (+)-tramadol preferentially inhibits serotonin reuptake, whereas (–)-tramadol mainly inhibits noradrenaline reuptake (Reimann and Hennies, 1994). The actions of the two enantiomers, along with those of its metabolites, are complementary in producing the analgesic effect. Tramadol, regarded as a "weak" opioid for management of postoperative pain, is essentially devoid of significant ventilatory depressant effects (Lehmann, 1997).

Recent experience with spinal opioids indicates that ventilatory depression is not a special problem with this route in adults for acute (Chung et al., 1997) or chronic (Rawal et al., 1996) pain management. Nevertheless, the literature continues to record case reports of ventilatory depression from spinal opioids in children (Bozkurt et al., 1997), perhaps indicating that the technique is not yet optimized. Intracerebroventricular injections are more likely to produce ventilatory depression than the spinal routes, but the incidence is acceptably small given the problem being treated (Ballantyne et al., 1996). Perhaps some of the cases of ventilatory depression from epidural administration correspond to inadvertent dural punctures (Swenson et al., 1996).

Emesis, Gastroparesis, Constipation

Regardless of the many causes of postoperative nausea and vomiting, it is well recognized that emetogenic effects of opioids used in the perioperative period are especially troublesome to patients (Haigh et al., 1993; Toner et al., 1996; Woodhouse and Mather, 1997a). Moreover, emesis in day-surgery patients is probably the most frequent reason for their delayed discharge. Although tramadol has not been found to produce opioid side effects, it is not free from causing nausea and vomiting (Lehmann, 1997).

All μ-opioid agonists can cause naloxone-reversible spasm of the sphincter of Oddi and subsequent biliary tract hypertension (Thune et al., 1990). Such effects of the agonist/antagonists are less than those of the agonists and are unlikely to be clinically significant (Vieria et al., 1993).

All μ-opioid agonists delay gastric emptying and decrease intestinal motility (Bennett et al., 1994). Indeed, the antidiarrheal side effect of opioids is an ancient indication for opium and a current indication for codeine. Constipation is brought about through direct interaction with opioid receptors in the gut wall and through central opioidergic mechanisms in the CNS (Massi et al., 1994; Thorn et al., 1996). Following morphine dosing, it is clear from ICV studies in rodents (Paul et al., 1989) and humans (Cramond et al., 1993) that M6G contributes significantly to this side effect. Thus, patients receiving chronic opioids may require regular use of an appropriate apperient. Opioids of the agonist/antagonist type cause less inhibition of gastrointestinal activity in animal tests than do pure agonists (Bhounsule et al., 1996), but at present data are insufficient to determine whether this effect also applies to humans.

Nonanalgetic CNS Effects – Sedation, Lightheadedness, Pupillary Constriction, Excitatory Effects

Opioids are sometimes given for their sedating effects, for example, in premedication, but this effect can be troublesome. It is not clear whether sedation/somnolence from opioids is more dose or drug related. The sometimes beneficial euphoric effects of opioids in most patients may become dysphoric effects in others. Furthermore, volunteer subjects receiving opioids are more likely to become dysphoric than patients being treated for pain. Dysphoria may be a protective perceptual response during rapidly changing blood opioid concentrations because it is exacerbated by movement in the supine position, as well as by vertical posture, and seems much less frequent when blood opioid concentrations are relatively stable. Lightheadedness is commonly reported by patients and volunteers alike receiving most, if not all, opioid analgesics.

Pupillary constriction, a hallmark of morphinoid drug action, is due to opioid stimulation of the Edinger-Westphal nuclei in the brainstem. Apart from its commonly used role in diagnosis of opioid intoxication, the pupillary response is a useful research tool to evaluate drug effect. As examples, the onset of pupillary constriction is at least as fast with morphine as with the more lipophilic opioid alfentanil (Miller et al., 1990); the central effects of systemically absorbed alfentanil make a significant contribution after epidural injection (Coda et al., 1994).

Excitatory side effects such as allodynia, hyperalgesia, myoclonus, and seizures may occur in patients receiving chronic high-dose opioids. A clear temporal relationship between increasing doses of morphine and exacerbation of excitatory behaviors has been observed in many cases (Reutens and Stewart-Wynne, 1989; Sjogren et al., 1993, 1994; Vigano et al., 1996), with the excitatory side effects gradually disappearing following the discontinuation of morphine treatment (Sjogren et al., 1994). For example, following chronic pethidine, particularly in patients with impaired renal function, norpethidine has been reported to accumulate in plasma and CSF and to have a temporal association with the occurrence of myoclonus and seizures in a range of patients (Reutens and Stewart-Wynne, 1989). Similarly, a number of reports have described the occurrence of hyperalgesia, myoclonus, and seizures in patients following chronic high doses of oral, SC (Potter et al., 1989), intravenous (Sjogren et al., 1993) or spinal (Parkinson et al., 1990; De Conno et al., 1991; Rozan et al., 1995) morphine, and/or hydromorphone for the management of cancer pain. It is clear from studies in rodents (Labella et al., 1979; Yaksh et al., 1986; Bartlett, Cramond, and Smith, 1994) that M3G has a 10-fold higher excitatory potency than its parent, morphine (Bartlett, Cramond, and Smith, 1994). Given the high concentrations of M3G likely to be in CSF following chronic systemic dosing of patients with high-dose morphine, M3G is probably the primary causative agent of these excitatory side effects. The mechanism(s) responsible for the excitatory side effects of opioids are not currently known, although it is clear from rodent studies that these effects are not reversed by subsequent administration of naloxone (Labella et al., 1979; Frenk et al., 1984; Yaksh et al., 1986). If anything, the excitatory side effects may be exacerbated by naloxone, consistent with the view that they are not mediated by classical inhibitory opioid receptors.

Many authors have suggested that the excitatory side effects of high-dose morphine in patients may be due to disinhibition of inhibitory glycinergic neurotransmission in the spinal cord or to activation of NMDA receptors in the CNS (Werz and MacDonald, 1982; Yaksh et al., 1986; Yaksh, 1989; Sjogren et al., 1993). Although these mechanisms cannot be ruled out entirely, Bartlett, Cramond, and Smith (1994) showed that neither M3G nor morphine bound with high affinity to strychnine-sensitive glycine receptors in calf spinal cord or bound significantly to any of the known binding sites on NMDA receptors in rat brain. Additionally, they showed that neither M3G nor morphine prevented the reuptake or enhanced the release of the excitatory amino acid glutamate from presynaptic nerve terminals in the CNS (Bartlett and Smith, 1996). Thus, based on the in vitro evidence, it is unlikely that either of these mechanisms is responsible for the excitatory side effects of high-dose morphine in humans, unless M3G and/or morphine interact with novel binding sites on these receptors, which have yet to be characterized.

Although studies in rodents have shown that ICV administration of the competitive NMDA antagonist LY274614 or midazolam (agonist at $GABA_A$-benzodiazepine receptor complex) significantly attenuated the excitatory behavioral effects of ICV

M3G (Bartlett, Cramond, and Smith, 1994), subsequent in vitro studies in a range of brain tissue preparations (Bartlett, Dodd, and Smith, 1994; Bartlett and Smith, 1996) indicate that this attenuation occurs by raising the excitatory threshold in the rat brain at a functional level rather than by competitive antagonism at NMDA receptors or at the $GABA_A$-benzodiazepine receptor complex.

In cancer patients, these excitatory side effects secondary to high-dose morphine have proved difficult to manage (De Conno et al., 1991; Sjogren et al., 1993). A variety of approaches with varying degrees of success have been reported, including a reduction in opioid dosage (De Conno et al., 1991; De Armendi et al., 1993; Mercandante, 1995), changing to a different opioid ("opioid rotation") (Sjogren et al., 1994; Vigano et al., 1996), and co-administration of the anticonvulsants diazepam (De Conno et al., 1991; Sjogren et al., 1993), clonazepam (Eisele et al., 1992), and midazolam (Holdsworth et al., 1995) or the antispasmodic dantrolene (Mercadante, 1995).

The observations (Sjogren et al., 1994; Vigano et al., 1996) that the excitatory side effects of high-dose opioids in cancer patients gradually resolve after rotation to structurally dissimilar opioids are intriguing. Specifically, Sjogren et al., (1994) reported four cases in which changing the administered opioid from morphine to a structurally dissimilar (nonbenzomorphan) opioid – for example, methadone, ketobemidone, or sufentanil – resulted in resolution of the hyperalgesia, allodynia and myoclonus over a relatively short period of time (hours to days). Vigano et al., (1996) reported a similar case in which changing the administered opioid from hydromorphone (another benzomorphan) to methadone (open-chain opioid) resulted in resolution of myoclonus and a marked improvement in pain control for 3 months. Marked escalation (12-fold) of the patient's methadone dose in the fourth month resulted in myoclonus, sedation, delirium, and poor pain control, which again resolved after rotation of the patient's opioid from methadone back to parenteral hydromorphone (600–990 mg/day). After another month of hydromorphone, the patient developed intractable nausea and drowsiness, which again resolved when the patient's opioid was rotated back to methadone (60 mg/day).

Such clinical observations clearly imply that the excitatory side effects evoked by the benzomorphan opioids (morphine and hydromorphone) and the nonbenzomorphan opioids methadone (open-chain opioid) and sufentanil (anilinopiperidine) are mediated by distinctly different CNS mechanisms and that cross tolerance does not appear to occur. One possible factor contributing to the apparently higher excitatory potency of the benzomorphan opioid agonists is that many of these drugs are metabolized avidly to 3-O-glucuronides, several of which (noroxymorphone-3-glucuronide (Yaksh and Harty, 1987), M3G (Labella et al., 1979; Woolf, 1981; Yaksh and Harty, 1987; Smith et al., 1990; Bartlett, Cramond, and Smith, 1994), normorphine-3-glucuronide (Smith et al., 1997), and hydromorphone-3-glucuronide (Smith, unpublished results) have been shown to be potent CNS excitants in rodents.

Many studies (Cramond et al., 1993; Goucke et al., 1994, for example) have now shown that CSF concentrations of M3G can be manyfold higher than those of morphine following chronic oral or SC administration of morphine. It is probable that the 3-O-glucuronide metabolites of hydromorphone and oxymorphone would also be present in high CSF concentration relative to their parent opioids with chronically high doses, thereby having the potential to produce a similar spectrum of excitatory side effects (Rozan et al., 1995).

Pruritus

Pruritus was first thought to be related to the spinal route of opioid administration, but it is now clear that it also occurs, but probably less frequently, after systemic routes of administration (Woodhouse et al., 1996). Various empirical treatments and preventative measures have been suggested, but its mechanism is not clearly understood (Kam and Tan, 1996).

Other – Effects on the Heart and Circulation, Urinary Retention

Many opioids cause release of histamine from mast cells (Barke and Hough, 1993). This can lead to a multitude of histamine-related effects. Many opioids may cause arterial and venous dilatation due to either direct activity or histamine release (Doenicke et al., 1995; Grossman et al., 1996). The propensity for each action depends on the particular drug. For example, both morphine and meperidine may have both actions, but fentanyl has neither.

Although all opioids appear capable of causing some direct myocardial depression at high dosage used for opioid "anesthesia," the magnitude may differ between the different agents. Meperidine also has atropine-like effects, which may result in appreciable vagal stimulation at normal doses or appreciable vagal blockade at high doses. The newer μ agonists alfentanil, sufentanil, and remifentanil exert minimal cardiovascular effects while maintaining analgesic effects (Egan, 1995). Myocardial depression is minimal or absent in the normal analgesic dose range of most opioids, but meperidine may cause a direct, brief, myocardial depressant effect when injected rapidly intravenously (Huang et al., 1994). Mixed agonist/antagonists such as nalbuphine are without appreciable myocardial depressant effects (Elmauer et al., 1994).

Urinary retention, characterized by an increased urgency and an increased tone of the vesical sphincter, is not uncommon in patients who are naive to opioids. It was noticed consistently during studies of epidural opioids and often attributed to the route of administration (Cousins and Mather, 1983; Chaney, 1995). However, its incidence was not dose related and was higher in volunteers than in patients (Cousins and Mather, 1983). It also occurs after intravenous and intramuscular injections of opioids. Tolerance to this effect appears to develop rapidly, so that it is rarely a problem of long-term administration. It is reversible by naloxone. Recent studies have suggested that the incidence is less after epidural agonist/partial agonist/antagonist than pure agonists (Parker et al., 1997).

Principles of Administration of Opioid Analgesics

It is clear that selective targeting of opioid receptors in the CNS or in inflamed tissues with directed low doses of opioid analgesics has the potential to provide analgesia with minimal side effects. However, this approach, by its nature, is much more invasive than the more common indirect approach of supplying blood-borne drug to the receptors. Direct administration using intrathecal, epidural, and ICV injections, and even intra-articular injections, with or without apparatus for repeated or prolonged administration, falls into the classification of specialist techniques that are not universally applicable. Many analyses of the effectiveness of such direct techniques have been made (Cousins and Mather, 1983; Chrubasik et al., 1993).

Most patients are best dosed with the simplest, least invasive, most passive method available. If the patient has a functioning gastrointestinal tract and can swallow, then the oral route of administration is preferred. Accordingly, many opioid analgesic preparations have been developed for oral administration, each seeking a commercial advantage through an improved pharmacokinetic profile (Maccarone et al., 1994). It should be remembered that pharmacokinetic manipulations by way of controlled-release formulations do not alter the intrinsic bioavailability, but regulate the peak and trough plasma concentrations with respect to dose. Thus, the average oral bioavailability of morphine is approximately 25%, but the range is large. Again, the message is clear that individualized dosage needs to be based upon observation of the patient.

Rectal administration also provides a useful method for the administration of many opioid analgesics. Correctly placed suppositories will have higher bioavailability than oral preparations because a large portion of the drug dose avoids portal-hepatic extraction en route to the systemic circulation. Because rectal opioids usually have a slower rate of absorption, this route can provide basal analgesia in a patient unable to take the medication orally (Bruera et al., 1995; Olkolla et al., 1995). However, the potential for incorrect placement in the rectum, leading to either substantial portal-hepatic extraction if placed too high or expulsion if placed too low, along with some patients' dislike of the method, makes this a secondary technique.

If intravenous access is available, then intravenous infusion is an appropriate way to administer most opioid analgesics, particularly in the acute setting. Infusion rather than bolus injection is preferred because the latter is generally more disorienting and distressing to the patient. Furthermore, infusion allows control over the time course of effects and allows the dose to be stopped if necessary.

Intramuscular (Kirkpatrick et al., 1988) or subcutaneous (Semple et al., 1997) injections have been the standard methods for parenteral administration of opioid analgesics without the need for intravenous access. Both routes are capable of adequate drug delivery provided it is remembered that both are subject to inter- and intrapatient variability in rate of drug absorption due to differences in perfusion of the injected site. Hence, neither a predictable dose-effect relationship nor a predictable time course of effect is assured. The injections may hurt, and many patients, particularly children, have a significant fear of injections.

A number of noninvasive methods are now in clinical use, and others are receiving research attention. Several methods have been designed around fentanyl because it is sufficiently potent that only submilligram doses need to be delivered for effect. A marked improvement in the delivery of transdermal fentanyl (Grond et al., 1997; Jeal and Benfield, 1997) across the skin comes in the form of a fentanyl iontophoresis device that appears to be rapidly enough responding to be suitable for patient-controlled analgesia (Nimmo, 1992; Ashburn et al., 1995). Oral transmucosal delivery of fentanyl from a dosage form popularly known as the "fentanyl lollipop" but properly known as the Oralet has been useful for induction of sleep in children (Epstein et al., 1996) or anxiolysis in adults (Macaluso et al., 1996). This method involves the subject absorbing the fentanyl across the buccal mucosa, but variability in dose effect can occur, and predictability can be problematic because different subjects swallow different portions of the dose, and fentanyl that is swallowed has very low bioavailability.

Pulmonary delivery of opioids has been tried with different degrees of success. Various studies reporting nebulized delivery of morphine and fentanyl have usually had a low bioavailability, and pain relief has not been reliable. Recent developments to improve the pulmonary bioavailability of opioids administered by oral inhalation have been based upon control over particle size along with the incorporation of a pneumotachography circuit to sense the air flow so that the dose is delivered into the inspired air when predetermined conditions of flow rate and inspired volume coincide. Prototype devices based on these principles have been tried for delivery of morphine from an aqueous solution (AERx) and for delivery of fentanyl from a chlorofluorocarbon solution of fentanyl base (SmartMist). Both have been found to give time courses of plasma concentrations of the respective opioid analgesics that are similar to those after intravenous injection (Mather et al., 1997; Ward et al., 1997).

Despite improvements in drug delivery, the marked variability in opioid dosing requirements among patients makes it very difficult to provide reliable pain management from predetermined prescriptions. For postoperative pain management in particular, a major shift in philosophy evolved during the 1980s that allowed patients to determine their timing and frequency of dosage with opioid analgesics. Concurrently, devices evolved with various levels of control that allowed orders to be written for patient-controlled analgesia (PCA), which permitted variability in the choice of opioid, the incremental dose (i.e., dose per demand), a lock-out interval (i.e., a minimum time between incremental doses), the maximum dose per unit of time, and a background infusion. During the 1980s, the dosing route was almost exclusively intravenous, but today the philosophy is also applied to the epidural route of administration. Continued research has found that virtually every opioid analgesic has been successfully used in PCA, that adjusting the incremental dose is critical to success or failure, that a lock-out interval should be kept as short as possible to promote patient confidence in the system, that a maximum dose per unit of time denies the premise of patient control, and that a background infusion usually should not be used (Woodhouse and Mather, 1997a). However, PCA is not equal to a "set it and forget it" philosophy because patients still require a regular assessment for optimal efficacy and safety. Moreover, it has been found that PCA does not necessarily provide superior pain relief to nurse-controlled analgesia. Most patients, however, prefer the control over their own management (Woodhouse and Mather, 1997b).

REFERENCES

Aasmundstad, T.A., Morland, J., and Paulsen, R.E. (1995). Distribution of morphine-6-glucuronide and morphine across the blood-brain barrier in awake, freely moving rats investigated by in vivo microdialysis sampling. *J. Pharmacol. Exp. Therap.* **275,** 435–441.

Abbott, F.V., and Palmour, R.M. (1988). Morphine-6-glucuronide: Analgesic effects and receptor binding profile in rats. *Life Sci.* **43,** 1685–1695.

Ashburn, M.A., Streisand, J., Zhang, J., Love, G., Rowin, M., Niu, S., Kievit, J.K., Kroep, J.R., and Mertens, M.J. (1995). The iontophoresis of fentanyl citrate in humans. *Anesthesiology.* **82,** 1146–1153.

Ballantyne, J.C., Carr, D.B., Berkey, C.S., Chalmers, T.C., and Mosteller, F. (1996). Comparative efficacy of epidural, subarachnoid, and intracerebroventricular opioids in patients with pain due to cancer. *Reg. Anesth.* **21,** 542–556.

Barjavel, M., Sandouk, P., Plotkine, M., and Scherrmann, J.M. (1994). Morphine and morphine metabolite kinetics in the rat brain as assessed by transcortical microdialysis. *Life Sci.* **55,** 1301–1308.

Barjavel, M.J., Scherrmann, J.M., and Bhargava, H.N. (1995). Relationship between morphine analgesia and cortical extracellular fluid levels of morphine and its metabolites in the rat: A microdialysis study. *Br. J. Pharmacol.* **116,** 3205–3210.

Barke, K.E., and Hough, L.B. (1993). Opiates, mast cells and histamine release. *Life Sci.* **53,** 1391–1399.

Bartlett, S.E., Cramond, T., and Smith, M.T. (1994). The excitatory effects of morphine-3-glucuronide are attenuated by LY274614, a competitive NMDA receptor antagonist, and by midazolam, an agonist at the benzodiazepine site on the $GABA_A$ receptor complex. *Life Sci.* **54,** 687–694.

Bartlett, S.E., Dodd, P.R., and Smith, M.T. (1994). Pharmacology of morphine and morphine-3-glucuronide at opioid, excitatory amino acid, GABA and glycine binding sites. *Pharmacol. Toxicol.* **75,** 73–81.

Bartlett, S.E., and Smith, M.T. (1996). Effects of morphine-3-glucuronide and morphine on the K^+-evoked release of $[^3H]$glutamic acid and $[^{14}C]$gamma-aminobutyric acid from rat brain synaptosomes. *Life Sci.* **58,** 447–454.

Bennett, M.W., Shah, M.V., and Bembridge, J.L. (1994). A comparison of the effect on gastric emptying of alfentanil or morphine given during anaesthesia for minor surgery. *Anaesthesia.* **49,** 155–156.

Bhounsule, S.A., D'Sa, S., Fernandes, N., D'Souza, R.D., and Dhume, V.G. (1996). Gastrointestinal actions of buprenorphine: Are different receptors involved?. *Eur. J. Pharmacol.* **316,** 253–256.

Bilsky, E.J., Inturrisi, C.E., Sadee, W., Hruby, V.J., and Porreca, F. (1996). Competitive and non-competitive NMDA antagonists block the development of antinociceptive tolerance to morphine, but not to selective mu or delta opioid agonists in mice. *Pain.* **68,** 229–237.

Borgbjerg, F.M., Nielsen, K., and Franks, J. (1996). Experimental pain stimulates respiration and attenuates morphine-induced respiratory depression – a controlled study in human volunteers. *Pain.* **64,** 123–128.

Borison, H.L. (1977). Central nervous respiratory depressants – narcotic analgesics. *Pharmacol. Ther.* (Part B). **3,** 227–237.

Bozkurt, P., Kaya, G., and Yeker, Y. (1997). Single-injection lumbar epidural morphine for postoperative analgesia in children – a report of 175 cases. *Reg Anesth.* **22,** 212–217.

Bruera, E., Watanabe, S., Fainsinger, R.L., Spachynski, K., Suarez-Almazor, M., and Inturrisi, C. (1995). Custom-made capsules and suppositories of methadone for patients on high-dose opioids for cancer pain. *Pain.* **62,** 141–146.

Bruster, S., Jarman, B., Bosanquet, N., Weston, D., Erens, R., and Delbanco, T.L. (1994). National survey of hospital patients. *Br. Med. J.* **309,** 1542–1546.

Bulow, H.H., Linnemann, M., Berg, H., Langjensen, T., Lacour, S., and Jonsson, T. (1995). Respiratory changes during treatment of postoperative pain with high dose transdermal fentanyl. *Acta Anaesth. Scand.* **39,** 835–839.

Catley, D.M., Thornton, C., Jordan, C., Lehane, J.R., Royston, D., and Jones, J.G. (1985). Pronounced, episodic oxygen desaturation in the postoperative period: Its association with ventilatory pattern and analgesic regimen. *Anesthesiology.* **63,** 20–28.

Chaney, M.A. (1995). Side effects of intrathecal and epidural opioids. *Can. J. Anaesth.* **42,** 891–903.

Chen, S.W., Maguire, P.A., Davies, M.F., Beatty, M.F., and Loew, G.H. (1996). Evidence for mu(1)-opioid receptor involvement in fentanyl-mediated respiratory depression. *Eur. J. Pharmacol.* **312,** 241–244.

Chen, Z.R., Irvine, R.J., Somogyi, A.A., and Bochner, F. (1991). Mu receptor binding of some commonly used opioids and their metabolites. *Life Sci.* **48,** 2165–2171.

Chrubasik, J., Chrubasik, S., and Mather, L.E. (1993). *Postoperative epidural opioids.* Berlin, Heidelberg, and New York: Springer-Verlag.

Chung, J.H., Sinatra, R.S., Sevarino, F.B., and Fermo, L. (1997). Subarachnoid meperidine-morphine combination – an effective perioperative analgesic adjunct for cesarean delivery. *Reg. Anesth.* **22,** 119–124.

Coda, B.A., Brown, M.C., Schaffer, R., Donaldson, G., Jacobson, R., Hautman, B., and Shen, D.D. (1994). Pharmacology of epidural fentanyl, alfentanil, and sufentanil in volunteers. *Anesthesiology.* **81,** 1149–1161.

Cooper, D.W., Lindsay, S.L., Ryall, D.M., Kokri, M.S., Eldabe, S.S., and Lear, G.A. (1997). Does intrathecal fentanyl produce acute cross-tolerance to i.v. morphine? *Br. J. Anaesth.* **78,** 311–313.

Cousins, M.J., and Mather, L.E. (1983). Intrathecal and epidural administration of opioids. *Anesthesiology.* **61,** 276–310.

Cramond, T., Wright, A.W.E., Stuart, G.S., and Smith, M.T. (1993). Plasma and CSF concentrations of morphine (M), morphine-3-glucuronide (M3G) and morphine-6-glucuronide (M6G) in cancer patients receiving morphine by the intracerebroventricular (icv) route. *Proc. Seventh World Congress on Pain.* Paris: IASP Press, 531–532.

Davies, G,. Kingswood, C., and Street, M. (1996). Pharmacokinetics of opioids in renal dysfunction. *Clin. Pharmacokin.* **31,** 410–422.
De Armendi, A.J., Fahey, M., and Ryan, J.F. (1993). Morphine-induced myoclonic movements in a pediatric pain patient. *Anesth. Analg.* **77,** 191–192.
De Conno, F., Caraceni, A., Martini, C., Spoldi, E., Salvetti, M., and Ventafridda, V. (1991). Hyperalgesia and myoclonus with intrathecal infusion of high-dose morphine. *Pain.* **47,** 337–339.
Dershwitz, M., Hoke, J.F., Rosow, C.E., Michalowski, P., Connors, P.M., Muir, K.T., and Dienstag, J.L. (1996). Pharmacokinetics and pharmacodynamics of remifentanil in volunteer subjects with severe liver disease. *Anesthesiology.* **84,** 812–820.
Dhonneur, G., Gilton, A., Sandouk, P., Scherrmann, J.M., and Duvaldestin, P. (1994). Plasma and cerebrospinal fluid concentrations of morphine and morphine glucuronides after oral morphine – the influence of renal failure. *Anesthesiology.* **81,** 87–93.
Doenicke, A., Moss, J., Lorenz, W., and Hoernecke, R. (1995). Intravenous morphine and nalbuphine increase histamine and catecholamine release without accompanying hemodynamic changes. *Clin. Pharmacol. Ther.* **58,** 81–89.
Egan, T.D. (1995). Remifentanil pharmacokinetics and pharmacodynamics. A preliminary appraisal. *Clin Pharmacokin.* **29,** 80–94.
Eisele, J.H., Grisby, E.J., and Den, G. (1992). Clonazepam treatment of myoclonic contractions associated with high-dose opioids: Case report. *Pain.* **49,** 213–232.
Elmauer, S., Dick, W., Otto, S., and Muller, H. (1994). Perioperative analgesia in the cardiovascular risk patient: A comparison on haemodynamic side effects following eight different opioids. *Anaesthesist.* **43,** 743–749.
Epstein, R.H., Mendel, H.G., Witkowski, T.A., Waters, R., Guarniari, K.M., Marr, A.T., and Lessin, J.B. (1996). The safety and efficacy of oral transmucosal fentanyl citrate for preoperative sedation in young children. *Anesth. Analg.* **83,** 1200–1205.
Evans, A.M., and Shanahan, K. (1995). The disposition of morphine and its metabolites in the in-situ rat isolated perfused liver. *J. Pharm. Pharmacol.* **47,** 333–339.
Faura, C.C., Olaso, M.J., Garcia Cabanes, C., and Horga, J.F. (1996). Lack of morphine-6-glucuronide antinociception after morphine treatment. Is morphine-3-glucuronide involved?. *Pain.* **65,** 25–30.
Frances, B., Gout, R., Monsarrat, B., Cros, J., and Zajac, J.M. (1992). Further evidence that morphine-6β-glucuronide is a more potent opioid agonist than morphine. *J. Pharmacol. Exp. Ther.* **262,** 25–29.
Frenk, H., Watkins, L.R., and Mayer, D.J. (1984). Differential behavioural effects induced by intrathecal microinjection of opiates: Comparison of convulsive and cataleptic effects produced by morphine, methadone and D-Ala2-methionine-enkephalinamide. *Brain Res.* **299,** 31–42.
Geisslinger, G., Brune, K., Kobal, G., and Lotsch, J. (1997). Intravenous morphine-6-glucuronide (m6g) is devoid of analgesic activity in man. *Pain.* **70,** 289–290.
Gong, Q.L., Hedner, J., Bjorkman, R., and Hedner, T. (1992). Morphine-3-glucuronide may functionally antagonise morphine-6-glucuronide induced antinociception and ventilatory depression in the rat. *Pain.* **48,** 249–255.
Gong, Q.L., Hedner, T., Hedner, J., Bjorkman, R., and Nordberg G. (1991). Antinociceptive and ventilatory effects of the morphine metabolites: Morphine-6-glucuronide and morphine-3-glucuronide. *Eur. J. Pharmacol.* **193,** 47–56.
Goucke, C.R., Hackett, L.P., and Ilett, K.F. (1994). Concentrations of morphine, morphine-6-glucuronide and morphine-3-glucuronide in serum and cerebrospinal fluid following morphine administration to patients with morphine-resistant pain. *Pain.* **56,** 145–149.

Grace, D., and Fee, J.P.H. (1996). A comparison of intrathecal morphine-6-glucuronide and intrathecal morphine sulfate as analgesics for total hip replacement. *Anesth. Analg.* **83,** 1055–1059.

Grond, S., Zech, D., Lehmann, K.A., Radbruch, L., Breitenbach, H., and Hertel, D. (1997). Transdermal fentanyl in the long-term treatment of cancer pain: A prospective study of 50 patients with advanced cancer of the gastrointestinal tract or the head and neck region. *Pain.* **69,** 191–198.

Grossmann, M., Abiose, A., Tangphao, O., Blaschke, T.F., and Hoffman, B.B. (1996). Morphine-induced venodilation in humans. *Clin. Pharmacol. Ther.* **60,** 554–560.

Haigh, C.G., Kaplan, L.A., Durham, J.M., Dupeyron, J.P., Harmer, M., and Kenny, G.N. (1993). Nausea and vomiting after gynaecological surgery: A meta-analysis of factors affecting their incidence. *Br. J. Anaesth.* **71,** 517–522.

Hanks, G.W., and Forbes, K. Opioid responsiveness. (1997). *Acta Anaesth. Scand.* **41** (1 Part 2), 154–158.

Hanna, M.H., Peat, S.J., Woodham, M., Knibb, A., and Fung, C. (1990). Analgesic efficacy and CSF pharmacokinetics of intrathecal morphine-6-glucuronide: Comparison with morphine. *Br. J. Anaesth.* **64,** 547–550.

Hasselström, J., and Säwe, J. (1993). Morphine pharmacokinetics and metabolism in humans. Enterohepatic cycling and relative contribution of metabolites to active opioid concentrations. *Clin. Pharmacokin.* **24,** 344–354.

Hasselström, J., Eriksson, S., Persson, A., Rane, A., Svensson, J.O., and Säwe, J. (1990). The metabolism and bioavailability of morphine in patients with severe liver cirrhosis. *Br. J. Clin. Pharmacol.* **29,** 289–297.

Hill, H.F., and Mather, L.E. (1993). Patient-controlled analgesia. Pharmacokinetic and therapeutic considerations. *Clin. Pharmacokin.* **24,** 124–140.

Holdsworth, M.T., Adams, V.R., Chavez, C.M., Vaughan, L.J., and Duncan, M.H. (1995). Continuous midazolam infusion for the management of morphine-induced myoclonus. *Ann. Pharmacother.* **29,** 25–29.

Huang, Y.F., Upton, R.N., Rutten. A.J., and Mather, L.E. (1994). The hemodynamic effects of intravenous bolus doses of meperidine in conscious sheep. *Anesth. Analg.* **78,** 442–449.

Hunt, G., and Bruera, E. (1995). Respiratory depression in a patient receiving oral methadone for cancer pain. *J. Pain Symptom Management.* **10,** 401–404.

Igawa, Y., Westerling, D., Mattiasson, A., and Andersson, K.E. (1993). Effects of morphine metabolites on micturition in normal, unanaesthetized rats. *Br. J. Pharmacol.* **110,** 257–262.

Jeal, W., and Benfield, P. (1997). Transdermal fentanyl. A review of its pharmacological properties and therapeutic efficacy in pain control. *Drugs.* **53,** 109–138.

Kalman, S., Metcalf, K., and Eintrei, C. (1997). Morphine, morphine-6-glucuronide, and morphine-3-glucuronide in cerebrospinal fluid and plasma after epidural administration of morphine. *Reg. Anesth.* **22,** 131–136.

Kam, P.C., and Tan, K.H. (1996). Pruritus – itching for a cause and relief? *Anaesthesia.* **51,** 1133–1138.

Kapila, A., Glass, P.S., Jacobs, J.R., Muir, K.T., Hermann, D.J., Shiraishi, M., Howell, S., and Smith, R.L. (1995). Measured context-sensitive half-times of remifentanil and alfentanil. *Anesthesiology.* **83,** 968–975.

Kehlet, H. (1997). Multimodal approach to control postoperative pathophysiology and rehabilitation. *Br. J. Anaesth.* **78,** 606–617.

Kirkpatrick, T., Henderson, P.D., and Nimmo, W.S. (1988). Plasma morphine concentrations after intramuscular injection into the deltoid or gluteal muscles. *Anaesthesia.* **43,** 293–295.

Kissin, I., Brown, P.T., Robinson, C.A., and Bradley, E.L., Jr. (1991). Acute tolerance in morphine analgesia: Continuous infusion and single injection in rats. *Anesthesiology.* **74,** 166–171.

Labella, F.S., Pinsky, C., and Havlicek, V. (1979). Morphine derivatives with diminished opiate receptor potency show enhanced central excitatory activity. *Brain Res.* **174,** 263–271.

Labroo, R.B., Thummel, K.E., Kunze, K.L., Podoll. T., Trager, W.F., and Kharasch, E.D. (1995). Catalytic role of cytochrome P4503A4 in multiple pathways of alfentanil metabolism. *Drug Metab. Dispos.* **23,** 490–496.

Lehmann, K.A. (1997). Tramadol in acute pain. *Drugs.* **53** (Suppl 2), 25–33.

Lemmens, H.J., Dyck, J.B., Shafer, S.L., and Stanski, D.R. (1994). Pharmacokinetic-pharmacodynamic modeling in drug development: Application to the investigational opioid trefentanil. *Clin. Pharmacol. Ther.* **56,** 261–271.

Leow, K.P., Smith, M.T., Williams, B., and Cramond, T. (1992). Single-dose and steady-state pharmacokinetics and pharmacodynamics of oxycodone in patients with cancer. *Clin. Pharmacol. Ther.* **52,** 487–495.

Ling, G.S.F., Paul, D., Simantov, R., and Pasternak, G.W. (1989). Differential development of acute tolerance to analgesia, respiratory depression, gastrointestinal transit and hormone release in a morphine infusion model. *Life Sci.* **45,** 1627–1636.

Loser, S.V., Meyer, J., Freudenthaler, S., Sattler, M., Desel, C., Meineke, I., and Gundert-Remy, U. (1996). Morphine-6-O-beta-D-glucuronide but not morphine-3-O-beta-D-glucuronide binds to mu-, delta- and kappa-specific opioid binding sites in cerebral membranes. *Arch. Pharmacol.* **354,** 192–197.

Macaluso, A,D., Connelly, A.M., Hayes, W.B., Holub, M.C., Ramsay, M.A., Suit, C.T., Hein, H.A., and Swygert, T.H. (1996). Oral transmucosal fentanyl citrate for premedication in adults. *Anesth. Analg.* **82,** 158–161.

Maccarrone, C., West, R.J., Broomhead, A.F., and Hodsman, G.P. (1994). Single-dose pharmacokinetics of Kapanol, a new oral sustained-release morphine formulation. *Drug Investigation.* **7,** 262–274.

Massi, P., Giognoni, G., Basilico, L., Gori, E., Rubino, T., and Parolaro, D. (1994). Intestinal effect of morphine 6-glucuronide – in vivo and in vitro characterization. *Eur. J. Pharmacol.* **253,** 269–274.

Mather, L.E. (1983). Clinical pharmacokinetics of fentanyl and its newer derivatives. *Clin. Pharmacokinet.* **8,** 422–446.

Mather, L.E. (1995). "The clinical effects of morphine pharmacology" – the JJ Bonica Distinguished Lecture for 1994. *Reg. Anaesth.* **20,** 263–282.

Mather, L.E., and Woodhouse, A. (1997). Pharmacokinetics of opioids in the context of patient controlled analgesia. *Pain Reviews* **4,** 20–32.

Mather, L.E., Woodhouse, A., Ward, M.E., Farr, S.J., Rubsamen, R., and Elthrington, L.G. (submitted). Pulmonary administration of aerosolised fentanyl: Pharmacokinetic evaluation of systemic delivery.

Mercadante, S. (1995). Dantrolene treatment of opioid-induced myoclonus. *Anesth. Analg.* **81,** 1307–1308.

Mignat, C., Jansen, R., and Ziegler, A. (1995). Plasma and cerebrospinal fluid concentrations of morphine and morphine glucuronides in rabbits receiving single and repeated doses of morphine. *J. Pharm. Pharmacol.* **47,** 171–175.

Mikus, G., Bochner, F., Eichelbaum, M., Horak, P., Somogyi, A.A., and Spector, S. (1994). Endogenous codeine and morphine in poor and extensive metabolisers of the CYP2D6 (debrisoquine/sparteine) polymorphism. *J. Pharmacol. Exp. Ther.* **268,** 546–551.

Miller, C.D., Asbury, A.J., and Brown, J.H. (1990). Pupillary effects of alfentanil and morphine. *Br. J. Anaesth.* **65,** 415–417.

Milne, R.W., McLean, C.F., Mather, L.E., Nation, R.L., Runciman, W.B., Rutten, A.J., and Somogyi, A.A. (1995). Comparative disposition of morphine-3-glucuronide during separate intravenous infusions of morphine and morphine-3-glucuronide in sheep – importance of the kidney. *Drug Metab. Dispos.* **23,** 334–342.

Milne, R.W., Nation, R.L., and Somogyi, A.A. (1996). The disposition of morphine and its 3- and 6-glucuronide metabolites in humans and animals, and the importance of the metabolites to the pharmacological effects of morphine. *Drug Metab. Rev.* **28,** 345–472.

Milne, R.W., Sloan, P.A., McLean, C.F., Mather, L.E., Nation, R.L., Runciman, W.B., Rutten, A.J., and Somogyi, A.A. (1993). Disposition of morphine and its 3-glucuronide and 6-glucuronide metabolites during morphine infusion in the sheep. *Drug Metab. Dispos.* **21,** 1151–1156.

Minto, C.F., Schnider, T.W., Egan, T.D., Youngs, E., Lemmens, H.J., Gambus, P.L., Billard, V., Hoke, J.F., Moore, K.H., Hermann, D.J., Muir, K.T., Mandema, J.W., and Shafer, S.L. (1997). Influence of age and gender on the pharmacokinetics and pharmacodynamics of remifentanil. I. Model development. *Anesthesiology.* **86,** 10–23.

Moulin, D.E., Ling, G.S.F., and Pasternak, G.W. (1988). Unidirectional analgesic cross-tolerance between morphine and levorphanol in the rat. *Pain.* **33,** 233–239.

Nimmo, W.S. (1992). Novel delivery systems: Electrotransport. *J. Pain Symptom Management.* **7,** 160–162.

Olkkola, K.T., Hamunen, K., and Maunuksela, E.L. (1995). Clinical pharmacokinetics and pharmacodynamics of opioid analgesics in infants and children. *Clin. Pharmacokin.* **28,** 385–404.

Osborne, R., Thompson, P., Joel, S., Trew, D., Patel, N., and Slevin, M. (1992). The analgesic activity of morphine-6-glucuronide. *Br. J. Clin. Pharmac.* **34,** 130–138.

Osborne, R., Joel, S., Grebenik, K., Trew, D., and Slevin, M. (1993). The pharmacokinetics of morphine and morphine glucuronides in kidney failure. *Clin. Pharmacol. Ther.* **54,** 158–167.

Parker, R.K., Holtmann, B., and White, P.F. (1997). Patient-controlled epidural analgesia: Interactions between nalbuphine and hydromorphone. *Anesth. Analg.* **84,** 757–763.

Parkinson, S.K., Baily, S.L., Little, W.L., and Mueller, J.B. (1990). Myoclonic seizure activity with high-dose spinal opioid administration. *Anesthesiology.* **72,** 743–745.

Paul, D., Standifer, K.M., Inturrisi, C.E., and Pasternak, G.W. (1989). Pharmacological characterization of morphine-6β-glucuronide, a very potent morphine metabolite. *J. Pharmacol. Exp. Ther.* **251,** 477–483.

Pelligrino, D.A., Riegler, F.X., and Albrecht, R.F. (1989). Ventilatory effects of fourth cerebroventricular infusions of morphine-6- or morphine-3-glucuronide in the awake dog. *Anesthesiology.* **71,** 936–940.

Plummer, J.L., Gourlay, G.K., Cmielewski, P.L., Odontiadis, J., and Harvey, I. (1995). Behavioural effects of norpethidine, a metabolite of pethidine, in rats. *Toxicology.* **95,** 37–44.

Portenoy, R.K., Thaler, H.T., Inturrisi, C.E., Friedlander-Klar, H., and Foley, K.M. (1992). The metabolite morphine-6-glucuronide contributes to the analgesia produced by morphine infusion in patients with pain and normal renal function. *Clin. Pharmacol. Ther.* **51,** 422–431.

Potter, J.M., Reid, D.B., Shaw, R.J., Hackett, P., and Hickmann, P.E. (1989). Myoclonus associated with treatment with high doses of morphine: The role of supplemental drugs. *Br. Med. J.* **299,** 150–153.

Rawal, N., Allvin, R., Neumark, J., Sosnowski, M., Kroner, K., Nuutinen, L., Bonnet, F., Hempel, V., Vadaloukas, A., Hirlekar, G., Assaf, R., Capogna, G., Hasenbos, M., Bjorgo S., Campos, R., Banos, J.E., and Canellas, M. (1996). Epidural and intrathecal opioids for postoperative pain management in Europe – a 17-nation questionnaire study of selected hospitals. *Acta Anaesth. Scand.* **40,** 1119–1126.

Reutens, D.C., and Stewart-Wynne, E.G. (1989). Norpethidine induced myolclonus in a patient with renal failure (letter). *J. Neurol. Neurosurg. Psychiatry.* **52,** 1450–1451.

Reimann, W., and Hennies, H.H. (1994). Inhibition of spinal noradrenaline uptake in rats by the centrally acting analgesic tramadol. *Biochem. Pharmacol.* **47,** 2289–2293.

Rosow, C.E. (1995). Newer opioid agonists. *Baillières Clin. Anaesthesiol.* **9,** 67–82.

Rozan, J.P., Kahn, C.H., and Warfield, C.A. (1995). Epidural and intravenous opioid-induced neuroexcitation. *Anesthesiology.* **83,** 860–863.

Scott, J.C., Cooke, J.E., and Stanski, D.R. (1991). Electroencephalographic quantitation of opioid effect: Comparative pharmacodynamics of fentanyl and sufentanil. *Anesthesiology.* **74,** 34–42.

Semple, T.J., Upton, R.N., Macintyre, P.E., Runciman, W.B., and Mather, L.E. (1997). Morphine blood concentrations in elderly postoperative patients following administration via an indwelling subcutaneous cannula. *Anaesthesia.* **52,** 318–323.

Shelly, M.P., Quinn, K.G., and Park, G.R. (1989). Pharmacokinetics of morphine in patients following orthotopic liver transplantation. *Br. J. Anaesth.* **63,** 375–379.

Shook, J.E., Watkins, W.D., and Camporesi, E.M. (1990). Differential roles of opioid receptors in respiration, respiratory disease, and opiate-induced respiratory depression. *Am. Rev. Resp. Dis.* **142,** 895–909.

Sindrup, S.H., Poulsen, L., Brosen, K., Arendt-Nielsen, L., and Gram, L.F. (1993). Are poor metabolisers of sparteine/debrisoquine less pain tolerant than extensive metabolisers? *Pain.* **53,** 335–339.

Sjogren, P., Jensen, N.H., and Jensen, T.S. (1994). Disappearance of morphine-induced hyperalgesia after discontinuing or substitution morphine with other opioid agonists. *Pain.* **59,** 313–316.

Sjogren, P., Jonsson, T., Jensen, N.H., Drenck, N.E., and Jensen, T.S. (1993). Hyperalgesia and myoclonus in terminal cancer patients treated with continuous intravenous morphine. *Pain.* **55,** 93–97.

Skopp, G., Ganssmann, B., Cone, E.J., and Aderjan, R. (1997). Plasma concentrations of heroin and morphine-related metabolites after intranasal and intramuscular administration. *J. Anal. Toxicol.* **21,** 105–111.

Smith, G.D., and Smith, M.T. (1995). Morphine-3-glucuronide: Evidence to support its putative role in the development of tolerance to the antinociceptive effects of morphine in the rat. *Pain.* **62,** 51–60.

Smith, G.D., Prankerd, R.J., and Smith, M.T. (1997). Biochemical synthesis, purification and preliminary pharmacological evaluation of normorphine-3-glucuronide. *Life Sci.* **61,** 95–104.

Smith, M.T., Watt, J.A., and Cramond, T. (1990). Morphine-3-glucuronide: A potent antagonist of morphine analgesia. *Life Sci.* **47,** 579–585.

Srinivasan, V., Wielbo, D., Simpkins J., Karlix J., Sloan K., and Tebbett, I. (1996). Analgesic and immunomodulatory effects of codeine and codeine 6-glucuronide. *Pharm. Res.* **13,** 296–300.

Stain, F., Barjavel, M.J., Sandouk, P., Plotkine, M., Scherrmann, J.M., and Bhargava, H.N. (1995). Analgesic response and plasma and brain extracellular fluid pharmacokinetics of morphine and morphine-6-beta-d-glucuronide in the rat. *J. Pharmacol. Exp. Ther.* **274,** 852–857.

Stein, C. (1997). Opioid treatment of chronic nonmalignant pain. *Anesth. Analg.* **84,** 912–914.

Swenson, J.D., Wisniewski, M., Mcjames, S., Ashburn, M.A., and Pace, N.L. (1996). The effect of prior dural puncture on cisternal cerebrospinal fluid morphine concentrations in sheep after administration of lumbar epidural morphine. *Anesth. Analg.* **83,** 523–525.

Tateishi, T., Krivoruk, Y., Ueng, Y.F., Wood, A.J., Guengerich, F.P., and Wood, M. (1996). Identification of human liver cytochrome P-450 3A4 as the enzyme responsible for fentanyl and sufentanil N-dealkylation. *Anesth. Analg.* **82,** 167–172.

Thompson, P.I., Joel, S.P., John, L., Wedzicha, J.A., Maclean, M., and Slevin, M.L. (1995). Respiratory depression following morphine and morphine 6-glucuronide in normal subjects. *Br. J. Clin. Pharmacol.* **40,** 145–152.

Thorn, S.E., Wattwil, M., Lindberg, G., and Säwe, J. (1996). Systemic and central effects of morphine on gastroduodenal motility. *Acta Anaesth. Scand.* **40,** 177–186.

Thune, A., Baker, R.A., Saccone, G.T., Owen, H., and Toouli, J. (1990). Differing effects of pethidine and morphine on human sphincter of Oddi motility. *Br. J. Surg.* **77,** 992–995.

Tiseo, P.J., Thaler, H.T., Lapin, J., Inturrisi, C.E., Portenoy, R.K., and Foley, K.M. (1995). Morphine-6-glucuronide concentrations and opioid-related side effects – a survey in cancer patients. *Pain.* **61,** 47–54.

Toner, C.C., Broomhead, C.J., Littlejohn, I.H., Samra, G.S., Powney, J.G., Palazzo, M.G., Evans, S.J., and Strunin, L. (1996). Prediction of postoperative nausea and vomiting using a logistic regression model. *Br. J. Anaesth.* **76,** 347–351.

Vancrugten, J.T., Somogyi, A.A., Nation, R.L., and Reynolds, G. (1997). The effect of old age on the disposition and antinociceptive response of morphine and morphine-6-beta-glucuronide in the rat. *Pain.* **71,** 199–205.

Vaughn, P.R., Townsend, S.F., Thilo, E.H., Mckenzie, S., Moreland, S., and Kawato, K. (1996). Comparison of continuous infusion of fentanyl to bolus dosing in neonates after surgery. *J. Pediat. Surg.* **31,** 1616–1623.

Vieria, Z.E., Zsigmond, E.K., Duarte, B., Renigers, S.A., and Hirota, K. (1993). Double-blind comparison of butorphanol and nalbuphine on the common bile duct by ultrasonography in man. *Int. J. Clin. Pharmacol. Ther.* **31,** 564–567.

Vigano, A., Fan, D., and Bruera, E. (1996). Individualized use of methadone and opioid rotation in the comprehensive management of cancer pain associated with poor prognostic indicators. *Pain.* **67,** 115–119.

Ward, M.E., Woodhouse, A., Mather, L.E., Farr, S.J., Schuster, J., and Rubsamen, R. (1997). Pharmacokinetics of morphine following pulmonary administration from a novel inhalation delivery system. *Clin. Pharmacol. Ther.* **62,** 596–609.

Werz, M.A., and MacDonald, R.L. (1982). Opiate alkaloids antagonize postsynaptic glycine and GABA responses: Correlation with convulsant action. *Brain Res.* **236,** 107–119.

Woodhouse, A., Hobbes, A.F., Mather, L.E., Gibson, M. (1996). A comparison of morphine, pethidine and fentanyl in the postsurgical patient-controlled analgesia environment. *Pain.* **64,** 115–121.

Woodhouse, A., and Mather, L.E. (1997a). Nausea and vomiting in the postoperative patient-controlled analgesia (PCA) environment. *Anaesthesia.* **52,** 949–955.

Woodhouse, A., and Mather, L.E. (1997b). Patient-controlled analgesia (PCA) for postoperative pain relief: What have we learned and where do we go from here? *Analgesia.* **3,** 1–14.

Woolf, C.J. (1981). Intrathecal high dose morphine produces hyperalgesia in the rat. *Brain Res.* **209,** 491–495.

Wu, D.F., Kang, Y.S., Bickel, U., and Pardridge, W.M. (1997). Blood-brain barrier permeability to morphine-6-glucuronide is markedly reduced compared with morphine. *Drug Metab. Dispos.* **25,** 768–771.

Yaksh, T.L. (1989). Behavioural and anatomic correlates of tactile evoked allodynia produced by spinal glycine inhibition: Effects of modulatory receptor systems and excitatory amino acid antagonists. *Pain.* **37,** 111–123.

Yaksh, T.L., and Harty, G.J. (1987). Pharmacology of the allodynia in rats evoked by high dose intrathecal morphine. *J. Pharmacol. Exp. Ther.* **244,** 501–507.

Yaksh, T.L., Harty, G.J., and Onofrio, B.M. (1986). High doses of spinal morphine produce a non-opiate receptor-mediated hyperesthesia: Clinical and theoretic implications. *Anesthesiology.* **64,** 590–597.

Youngs, E.J., and Shafer, S.L. (1994). Pharmacokinetic parameters relevant to recovery from opioids. *Anesthesiology.* **81,** 833–842.

Zhukovsky, D.S., Gorowski, E., Hausdorff, J., Napolitano, B., and Lesser M. (1995). Unmet analgesic needs in cancer patients. *J. Pain Symptom Management.* **10,** 113–119.

CHAPTER ELEVEN

Pre-emptive Analgesia by Opioids

CLIFFORD WOOLF AND LESLEY BROMLEY

Introduction

Pre-emptive analgesia is a therapeutic strategy designed to relieve pain by administration of treatment in advance of pain (Woolf et al., 1993). The rationale for this approach comes from the discovery that the sensory barrage initiated by tissue damage and carried by C-fibers sets in train changes in the excitability or sensitivity of neurons within the central nervous system that outlast the initiating stimulus; the phenomenon of central sensitization (Woolf, 1983; Coderre et al., 1993; Dubner and Ruda, 1992; McMahon et al., 1993; Woolf, 1994). Central sensitization manifests as a reduction in the pain threshold, an amplification of the intensity and duration of the pain response to noxious stimuli, the spread of abnormal sensitivity to uninjured tissue, and the generation of pain by normally innocuous inputs (Torebjork et al., 1992; Koltzenburg et al., 1992, 1994; Woolf, 1995).

If tissue damage can be anticipated, as in the case of elective surgery, there may be a clinical advantage in minimizing the establishment or maintenance of central sensitization in the intraoperative and postoperative period. Three potential approaches can be adopted to do this. The first is to block sensory inflow during surgery using regional anesthesia with sodium channel blockers to block conduction in C-nociceptor sensory fibers. The second is to target specifically those transmitters and receptors in the dorsal horn of the spinal cord responsible for initiating central sensitization with, for example, N-methyl-D-aspartic acid receptor antagonists like ketamine or neurokinin receptor antagonists to block the action of glutamate and substance P. The third approach is to both reduce release of transmitters from nociceptor C-fibers presynaptically in the dorsal horn and clamp the dorsal horn neuron at resting membrane potential, preventing voltage-dependent changes. This is precisely the effect that μ opioid receptor agonists can achieve, acting on presynaptic calcium and postsynaptic potassium channels.

This chapter reviews the pathophysiology of pain in the context of functional plasticity and describes the scientific evidence supporting the idea that opioids can interfere with central sensitization. Clinical evidence in favor of a pre-emptive action of opioids is then surveyed, and suggestions are made for the optimization of the

Christoph Stein, ed., *Opioids in Pain Control: Basic and Clinical Aspects*. Printed in the United States of America.

pre-emptive approach to relieve the distress, discomfort, and suffering associated with surgical intervention.

The Pathophysiology of Acute Postoperative Pain

Surgical intervention can activate primary sensory nociceptors in three ways; (1) by direct activation of high-threshold sensory terminals by intense mechanical or thermal tissue-damaging stimuli; (2) by indirect activation of chemosensitive nociceptors following the release of inflammatory mediators; and (3) by reducing the threshold of nociceptors, secondary to the release of inflammatory cytokines, growth factors, and other sensitizing mediators (peripheral sensitization), so that less intense stimuli can activate the nociceptors. The first two kinds of activation will induce a sensory barrage during and immediately after the tissue-damaging stimulus. The last kind will manifest some time after, as the inflammatory response develops. Surgical incision will then, for example, generate three phases of sensory input: an immediate high-frequency short-term discharge of mechanosensitive afferents, low and high threshold, as the scalpel blade cuts through skin and deeper tissue; a later lower level of input from chemosensitive nociceptors activated by the release of potassium ions; a reduction in pH; activation of kininogens; release of histamine, ATP, and serotonin; and, finally, a phase in which innocuous inputs will begin to activate nociceptors sensitized by the inflammatory reaction triggered by the incision (Fig. 11.1) (LaMotte et al., 1992; Treede et al., 1992; Davis et al., 1993; Levine and Taiwo, 1994; Reeh, 1994). There is then a combination of provoked and spontaneous C-fiber input.

Input from nociceptors has the capacity to produce what has been called nociceptive pain. This sensory inflow is not, however, simply passively transferred through sensory pathways to those parts of the brain that interpret the input as pain; it also has the capacity to generate alterations or plasticity in sensory processing in the central nervous system, which is a key factor in the generation of pain sensitivity.

Use-Dependent Plasticity in the Spinal Cord

Apart from the differences in their peripheral transduction sensitivity, caliber, conduction velocity, Schwann-cell-myelin arrangement, and central termination sites in the spinal cord, there is another key difference between Aβ and C-sensory fibers, which is essential in explaining the different central effects they generate: Aβ fibers elicit fast excitatory postsynaptic potentials (EPSPs) only in dorsal horn neurons. These are fast-rising, fast-decaying synaptic potentials that last only for several milliseconds and are largely mediated by the release of glutamate acting on AMPA receptors located on dorsal horn neuron membranes. C-fibers, in contrast, release glutamate and neuropeptides, including substance P and calcitonin gene-related peptide (CGRP). The glutamate acts on AMPA and N-methyl-D-aspartic (NMDA) ionotropic receptors and metabotropic receptors (mGluR), whereas the neuropeptides act on G-protein–coupled metabotropic receptors (Fig. 11.2). This combination

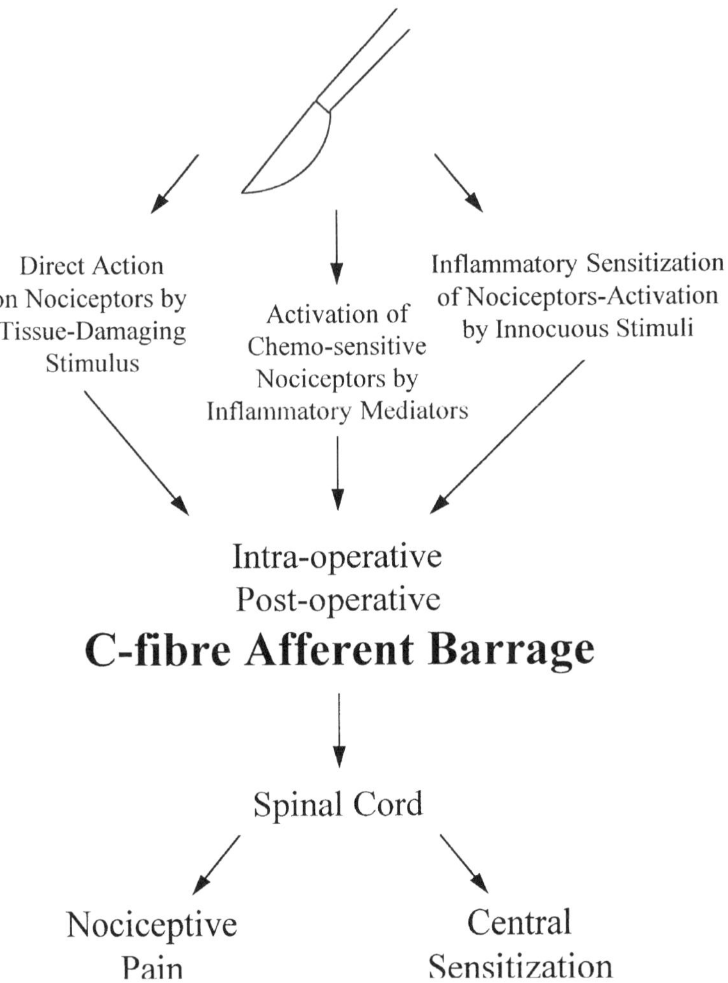

Figure 11.1. A diagrammatic representation of the way in which surgical damage can activate nociceptor C-fibers and the consequences of such an input into the central nervous system.

of multiple transmitters and receptors leads to a postsynaptic response quite different from that of Aβ fibers, a slow synaptic potential that reaches its peak slowly, over several hundred milliseconds, and then declines very slowly, over tens of seconds (Urban and Randic, 1984; Yoshimura and Jessell, 1989; Thompson et al., 1990; Yoshimura and Nishi, 1992; Nagy et al., 1993, 1994; Miller and Woolf, 1996).

Fast synaptic potentials enable high-frequency input in A-fibers to generate responses that encode rapidly changing stimuli faithfully, as in signaling vibration. Slow synaptic potentials offer, in contrast, the possibility of substantial spatial and temporal summation, integrating input. Because the slow potential lasts for so long,

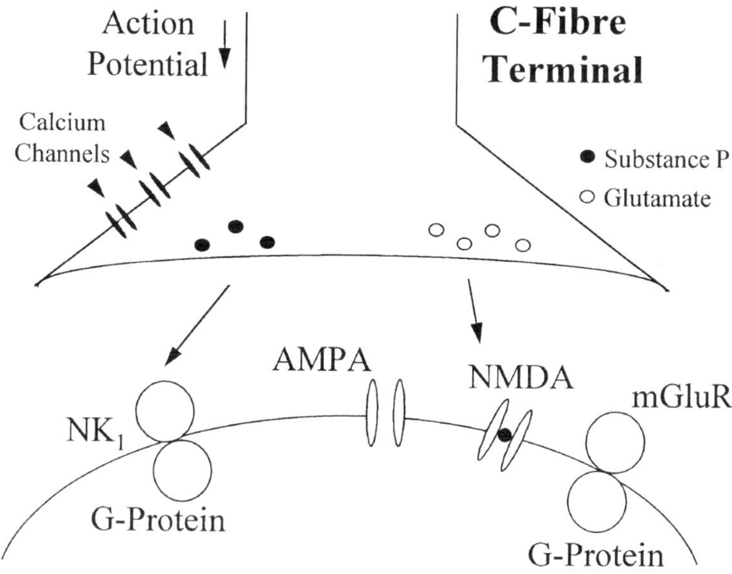

Figure 11.2. A model of the transmitters and receptors involved in synaptic transmission of C-fiber input to the spinal cord. The C-fiber terminal contains excitatory amino acids (e.g., glutamate) and neuropeptides (e.g., substance P) whose release is under the control of presynaptic calcium entry. The post-synaptic membrane contains neuropeptide G-protein–coupled receptors (e.g., the neurokinin NK_1 receptor for substance P) and excitatory amino acid receptors, including ligand-gated ion channels (AMPA receptor and the voltage-gated NMDA channel), and metabotropic G-protein–coupled receptors (mGluR). These transmitters and receptors are responsible for the generation of fast and slow synaptic potentials.

a second input some time afterward (1–2 seconds) can summate with the first input and generate a greater response (Thompson et al., 1990; Sivilotti et al., 1993). Experimentally, this effect is best exemplified by synchronous electrical stimulation of sensory fibers in which a cumulative depolarization due to summation of slow potentials occurs in response to stimulation at 0.5–2Hz (Sivilotti et al., 1993) and that manifests as a progressive increase in action potential activity, known as windup (Mendell and Wall, 1965) (Fig. 11.3). Much more important than this interesting example of use- or activity-dependent plasticity during a set of repeated stimuli are the long-lasting events triggered by the summation of slow synaptic potentials and that manifest after the conditioning input is over (Thompson et al., 1993).

Central Sensitization

A brief barrage of C-fiber activity (20 stimuli at 1 stimulus/second) is capable of greatly increasing the excitability of spinal neurons for a period of tens of minutes

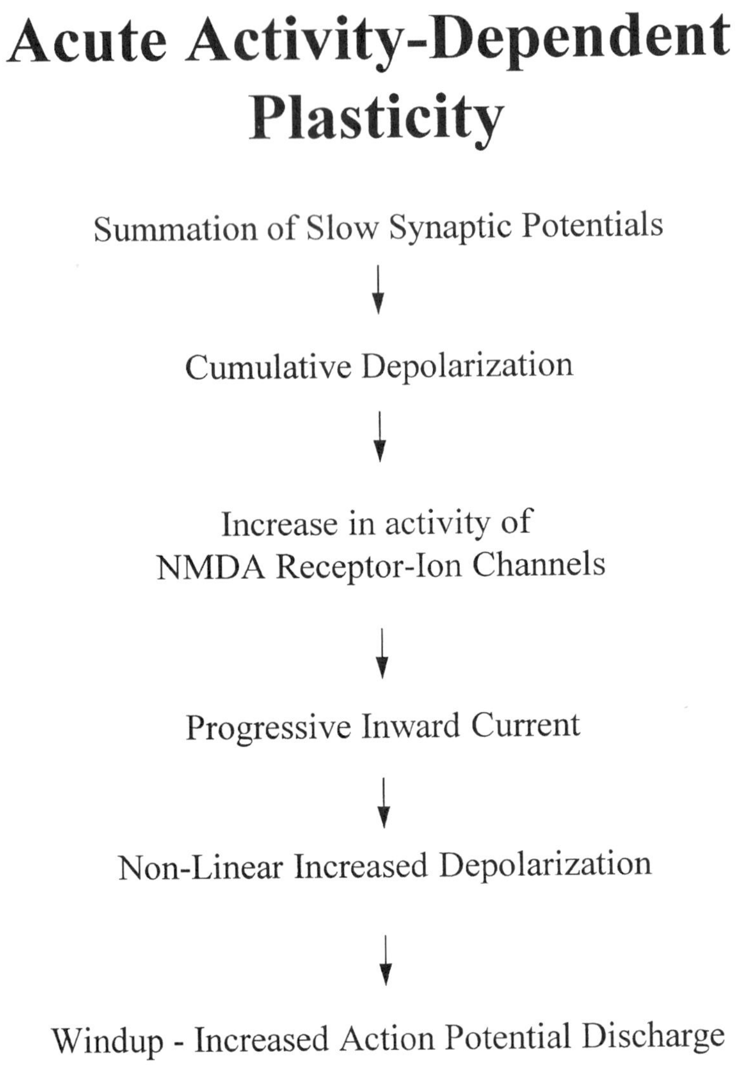

Acute Activity-Dependent Plasticity

Summation of Slow Synaptic Potentials

↓

Cumulative Depolarization

↓

Increase in activity of
NMDA Receptor-Ion Channels

↓

Progressive Inward Current

↓

Non-Linear Increased Depolarization

↓

Windup - Increased Action Potential Discharge

Figure 11.3. By virtue of the slow synaptic potentials generated by C-fibers, there is an opportunity for temporal summation such that low levels of activity in C-fibers will cause an integration of slow postsynaptic events. This causes a cumulative depolarization, which leads to an activity-dependent increase in the output of the cell, which is known as windup.

(Wall and Woolf, 1984; Coderre et al., 1985; Woolf and Wall, 1986a). This increased excitability can be detected by an expansion in the size of the receptive field of dorsal horn neurons, an increase in the response to standard suprathreshold stimuli, and a reduction in threshold (Cook et al., 1987; Simone et al., 1991; Woolf et al., 1994). These changes, which can be detected at the cellular level in laboratory animals, also manifest in human subjects as the development of secondary hyperalgesia and allodynia (Koltzenburg et al., 1992, 1994; Torebjork et al., 1992; Woolf, 1995). The alteration in the response properties of spinal neurons is a reflection of an increase in membrane excitability, such that inputs that normally evoke subthreshold responses now elicit an action potential output (Woolf and King, 1989, 1990). The vast majority of synaptic inputs to any dorsal horn neuron are too small to directly depolarize the cell to the point at which an action potential is elicited. Increasing the excitability of the membrane by recruiting normally subthreshold inputs transforms the functional repertoire of cells manifesting as central sensitization.

Induction of Central Sensitization

How do brief C-fiber inputs produce prolonged changes in neuronal excitability? The answer lies not in the direct postsynaptic actions of transmitters but rather in the intracellular signal-transduction pathways they initiate. The key here is intracellular calcium levels (Fig. 11.4). The calcium level in the cell is highly buffered, and excess calcium is stored in the microsomal compartment. Intracellular calcium levels can, however, be increased in three different ways: first, by passage of calcium down its chemical gradient from the extracellular to the intracellular compartment through ligand-gated ion channels. The best example of this is the NMDA receptor-ion channel complex. This receptor, activated by glutamate, allows sodium and calcium ions to enter the cell, but only when the membrane is depolarized (MacDermott et al., 1986). At normal resting membrane potentials the ion channel is blocked by a magnesium ion. This means that glutamate released presynaptically and binding to the receptor will not generate a postsynaptic response (Mayer et al., 1984). The magnesium block is, however, removed at membrane potentials of about –40mV; this is an example of a voltage-dependent ion channel that operates only when the cell is depolarized. The importance of this voltage dependency is that it provides the means for short-lived activity-dependent plasticity. Stimuli that depolarize a cell sufficiently to remove the magnesium block of the NMDA receptors will then greatly augment the subsequent response of the cell to glutamate. NMDA receptor antagonists have been shown repeatedly to reduce such short-lived plasticity, including windup (Dickenson and Sullivan, 1987).

The second way in which intracellular calcium levels can rise is via voltage-gated calcium channels (Dolphin et al., 1994). These ion channels are not activated by ligands but instead sense the voltage across the membrane and on depolarization allow a calcium inflow. For both NMDA and voltage-gated calcium channels, the only way in which calcium can enter the cell is if the membrane is depolarized. Such depolarization can occur either via nonvoltage-dependent receptor-ion channels such as the AMPA glutamate receptor, which allows sodium influx, or via a blockade of potassium channels.

The third way in which transmitters can increase intracellular calcium is via G-protein–coupled receptors (Heath et al., 1994). These seven transmembrane recep-

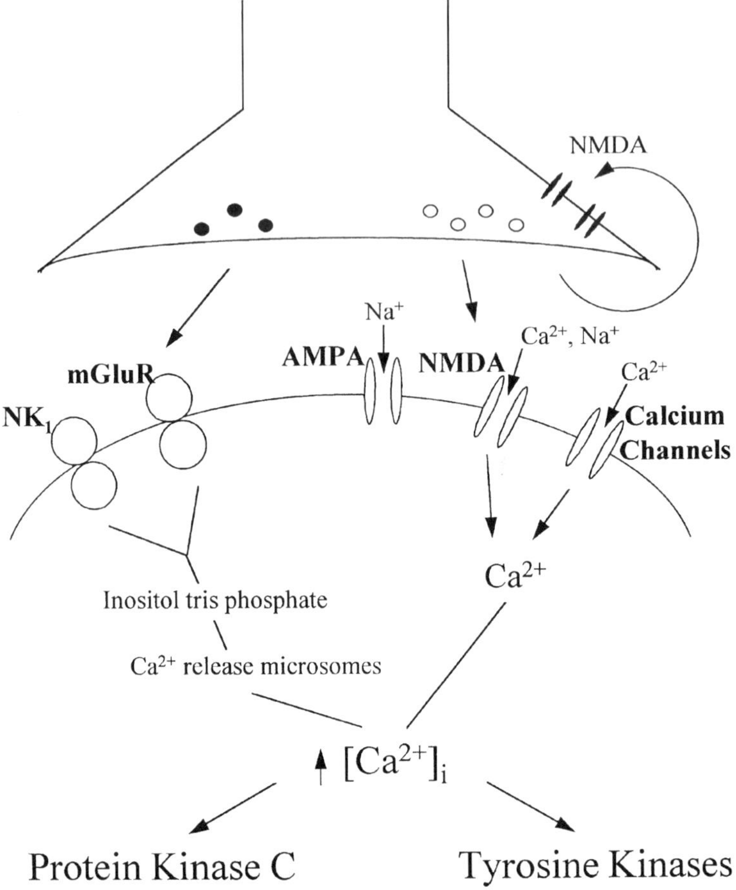

Figure 11.4. Central sensitization is an increase in the excitability of spinal neurons triggered by C-fiber inputs. This diagram summarizes how C-fiber inputs initiate central sensitization by increasing intracellular calcium levels in the postsynaptic cell via G-protein–coupled receptors releasing calcium from intracellular stores or via calcium entry through ion channels. The elevated calcium will bind to calcium-binding proteins, including protein kinase C, which can, by phosphorylating membrane proteins, including the NMDA receptor, alter excitability.

tors do not directly influence calcium flow through the membrane, but, via second messenger pathway activation, particularly inositol trisphosphate production, can induce a release of calcium from intracellular stores in microsomes. These are the metabotropic receptors as opposed to the ionotropic receptors.

Once calcium levels increase, it acts as a second messenger, activating calcium-dependent enzymes and binding to calcium-binding proteins like calmodulin. One key calcium-dependent kinase is protein kinase C (Fig. 11.4). This enzyme, once activated, can phosphorylate a number of cytosolic and membrane-bound proteins.

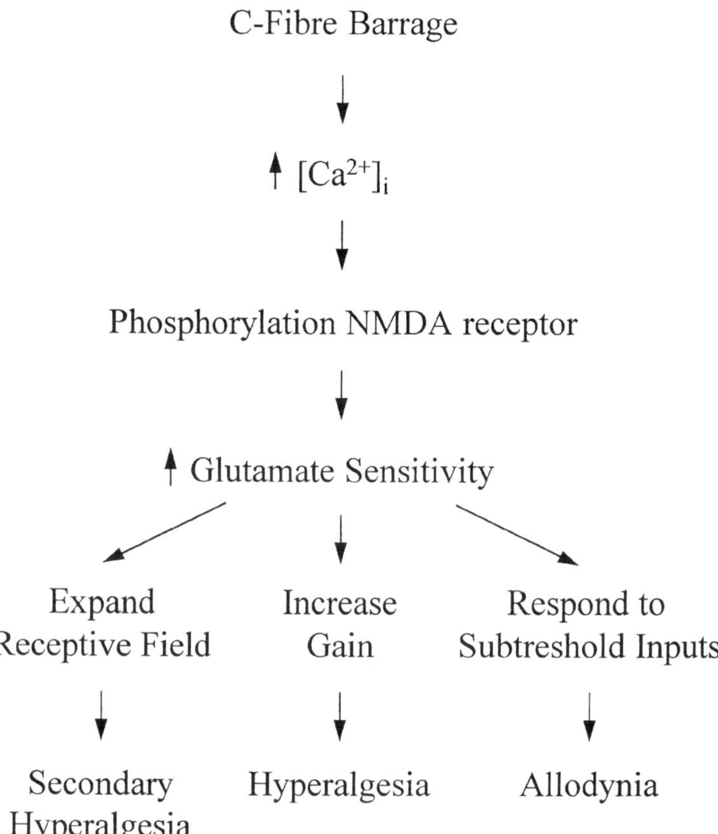

Figure 11.5. Once intracellular calcium levels are increased in spinal neurons as a consequence of a C-fiber barrage (see Fig. 11.3), the resulting increase in excitability produced by phosphorylation of the NMDA receptor changes the receptive field of the neuron, altering its spatial extent, sensitivity, and responsiveness. These changes produce pain hypersensitivity.

This post-translational modification alters the function of the proteins. One protein that is a substrate for post-translational PKC-mediated phosphorylation is the NMDA receptor itself (Chen and Huang, 1992). When the receptor is phosphorylated, it loses the magnesium block normally present at resting membrane potentials. The cell can now respond maximally to glutamate without a prior depolarization – the gain of the cell is increased and as a consequence it begins to respond to previously subthreshold inputs (Fig. 11.5). Other forms of phosphorylation, particularly those mediated by tyrosine kinases, may be equally important in modulating the activity of the NMDA receptor (Yu et al., 1997).

There are, then, a number of ways in which central sensitization can be induced: by release of either glutamate (acting on AMPA, NMDA, and mGluR receptors) or substance P acting on NK_1 receptors, by activation of voltage-dependent ion channels, and by activation of intracellular signaling pathways. Thus, there are multiple opportunities for pharmacologic intervention. NMDA and NK_1 receptor antagonists, voltage-gated ion channel blockers, and protein kinase C inhibitors have all been shown to be effective in eliminating central sensitization in preclinical laboratory experiments (King et al., 1988; Woolf and Thompson, 1991; Xu et al., 1991, 1992; Coderre, 1992; Coderre and Melzack, 1992a, 1992b; Dougherty et al., 1992; Dougherty and Willis, 1992; Ren, Hylden et al., 1992; Ren, Williams et al., 1992; Chapman and Dickenson, 1993a, 1993b; Laird et al., 1993; Meller et al., 1993; Ma and Woolf, 1995a, 1995b).

Central Sensitization and Opioids

Opioids acting on μ receptors offer a powerful approach for preventing the establishment of central sensitization. They act both pre- and postsynaptically, reducing transmitter release by calcium channel blockade and increasing potassium channel activity, respectively (Duggan and North, 1984) (Fig 11.6). Together, they act to reduce release of those transmitters that generate slow synaptic potentials (Yaksh et al., 1980) while preventing depolarization of the postsynaptic neuron such that neither NMDA receptor nor calcium channels are opened. The consequence is a reduction in the amplitude and duration of the C-fiber–evoked slow synaptic potentials and temporal summation (Sivilotti et al., 1995) (Fig. 11.7). This, in turn, reduces the effectiveness of C-fiber inputs to induce central sensitization, as evidenced by the lack of increased excitability generated in spinal neurons by a brief C-fiber conditional input following a moderate dose of systemic morphine (Woolf and Wall, 1986b) (Fig. 11.7).

Pre- versus Post-Treatment with Opioids

Surgical injury contributes to postoperative pain both by inducing central sensitization in spinal neurons such that normally innocuous inputs become painful and by generating inflamed tissue, which maintains a low level of nociceptor input to the central nervous system. These two phenomena are not independent; central sensitization is not autonomous but requires peripheral input to sustain it. The treatment of postoperative pain must be viewed, therefore, as a continuum starting before the surgical intervention and continuing until injured tissue has healed. In the initial excitement over the possibility that central sensitization may contribute to postoperative pain, a misunderstanding of the underlying biology occurred, which led to unrealistic expectations for the pre-emptive approach. The misunderstanding was the assumption that pre-emptive therapy required targeting only the afferent input generated intra-operatively, without any appreciation that postoperative afferent C-fiber input would be substantial from the inflamed site and would continue to initiate central sensitization. The demand for pre-emptive trials simply to compare pre-incisional

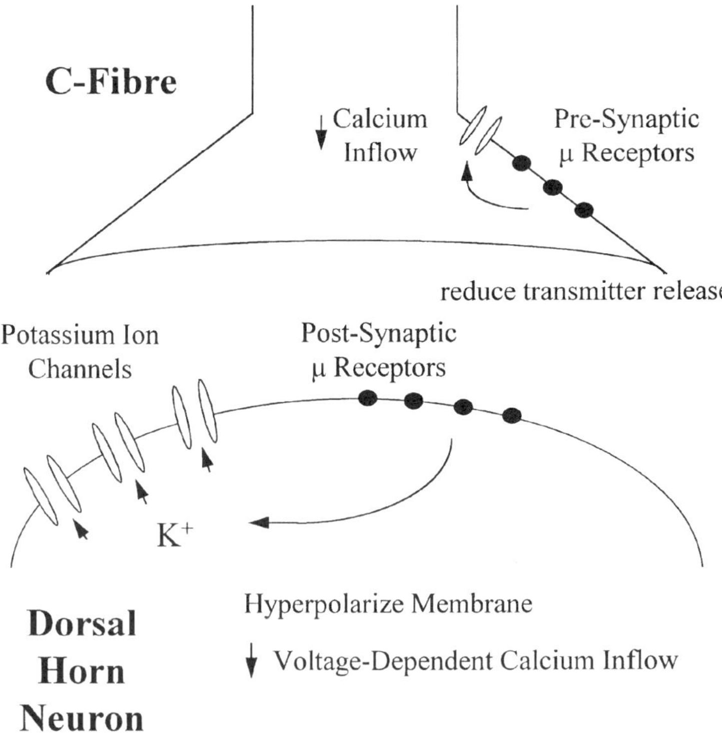

Figure 11.6. Mu receptors are located both presynaptically on C-fiber terminals and postsynaptically on spinal neurons and can both decrease transmitter release and hyperpolarize the postsynaptic membrane. Both actions will decrease the capacity of C-fibers to induce central sensitization and explain the pre-emptive action of opioid agonists. The postsynaptic hyperpolarizing action can suppress abnormal excitability, explaining how these compounds can also suppress pre-existing hyperexcitability and normalizing sensitivity.

versus immediate postoperative therapy as a measure of the contribution of central excitability changes to postoperative pain was, therefore, misguided. A more sophisticated approach is required, one aimed at pre-empting the effects of inputs generated during and after the surgery.

There is, nevertheless, some rationale for pre- versus post-treatment with opioids. Pretreatment with opioids, by blocking synaptic transmitter release and preventing postsynaptic voltage-dependent calcium influx, will dampen the induction of activity-dependent excitability increases (Chapman et al., 1994; Dickenson and Sullivan, 1987b), leading to a reduction in the phosphorylation of NMDA receptors and the generation of central sensitization. Once central sensitization has been generated, however, opioids can continue to have efficacy by virtue of their postsynaptic action, producing hyperpolarization and thereby minimizing the manifestation of abnormal hypersensitivity. This postsynaptic action, which normalizes sensibility, may require a higher dose than pretreatement, thereby preventing increased sensitivity. In animal

Morphine and C-fiber Function

Decreased Slow Synaptic Potentials

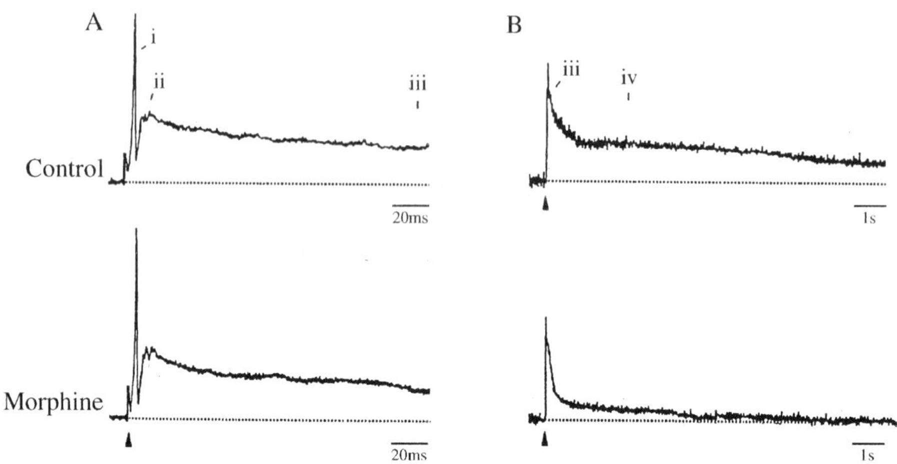

Decreased Temporal Summation

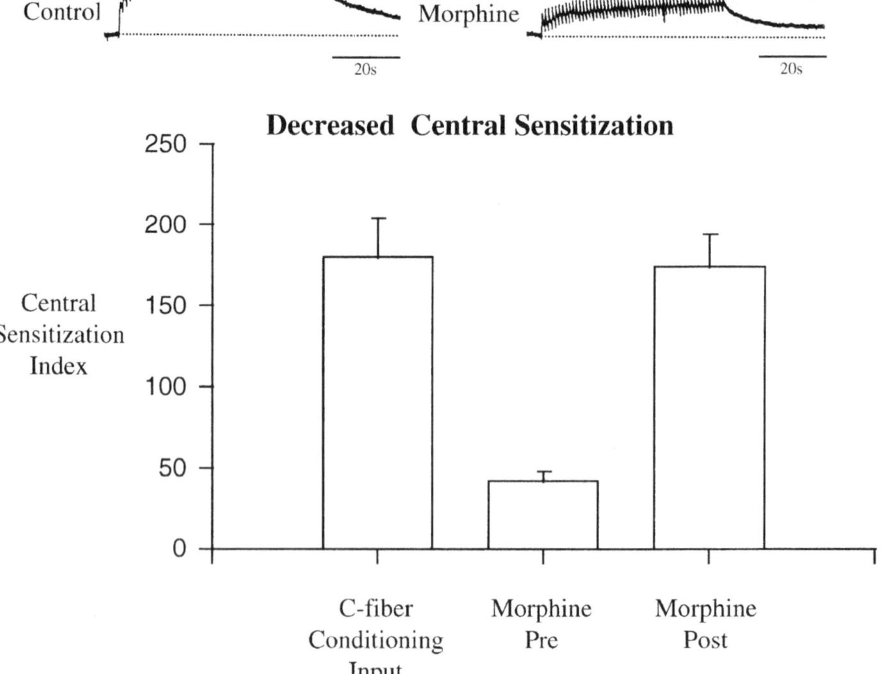

experiments, for example, a higher dose of morphine is required to block established central sensitization than to prevent its induction (Woolf and Wall, 1986b) (Fig. 11.7).

The powerful antihypersensitivity action of μ receptor opioids needs to be differentiated from their analgesic action. The former involves blocking central sensitization and the latter nociceptive transmission. The efficacy of opioids in preventing central sensitization stems from their multiple pre- and postsynaptic sites of action and the fact that their effect is independent either of the specific transmitters (excitatory amino acid or neuropeptide) or their multiple ligand-gated or metabotropic G-protein–coupled receptors, providing a broader spectrum of action than postjunctional receptor antagonists such as NK_1 receptor antagonists. There are, therefore, two optimal approaches to block pharmacologically central sensitization. The first is a broad-acting compound with a presynaptic action such as opioids; the second is to target the NMDA receptor, the convergent mechanism by which multiple inputs can modulate membrane excitability. At present, we have only the former: Ketamine and dextrorphan, although having NMDA blocking action, are not suitable for routine clinical pain control, but drugs targeted at the glycine site of the NMDA receptor are being developed that may have fewer of the psychotropic actions of competitive NMDA receptor antagonists.

Clinical Evidence

A large number of clinical studies have been carried out in recent years in an attempt to demonstrate a clinical difference in postoperative pain or analgesic requirements between various treatments given pre- or postsurgery. The results of a few of these studies have been conflicting for a number of reasons, including poor design and a misunderstanding of the basic science. As a result, some controversy has arisen over the clinical implications of the pre-emptive strategy and of the role of central sensitization in postoperative pain. Nevertheless, it is now fair to state that there is unequivocal evidence of pre-emptive clinical effects, including the use of opioids, and that the emphasis of clinical studies should now be on optimizing this therapeutic approach. Based on the improved understanding of the mechanisms that operate

---

Opposite

Figure 11.7. Morphine has a selective effect on the slow synaptic potentials generated by C-fibers, and this explains its effect on central sensitization. The top panels illustrate the effect of morphine on C-fiber–evoked slow potentials at a fast time base (A) and at a slow time base (B). Note the selective decrease in the slow potentials. This effect, in turn, results in decreased temporal summation, as illustrated in the middle panel. The bottom panel illustrates that the central sensitization included by a C-fiber conditioning input is reduced by pretreatment with 0.5mg/kg morphine (Morphine Pre). The same dose given after the C-fiber input has no effect on the established excitability, so that a much higher dose is required. (Adapted from Woolf and Wall [1986] and Sivilotti et al. [1994].)

to produce pain, a new approach, continous pre-emption, needs to be evaluated in further trials.

The concept of pre-emptive analgesia was first widely introduced to clinicians by Patrick Wall in an editorial in 1988 (Wall, 1988). Subsequent to this editorial, many studies were performed using different analgesic drugs and techniques. A number of the earliest papers compared preoperative analgesic treatment with either regional local anaesthetics, nonsteroidal anti-inflammatory drugs, or opioids with no treatment (McQuay et al., 1988; Koskinen et al., 1991). In several of these studies the authors demonstrated long-lasting analgesia after the pre-emptive treatment, but the finding was not always consistent (Harrison et al., 1994; Johansson et al., 1994). Nevertheless, compared with general anesthesia alone, pre-emptive analgesia has considerable benefits (Wang et al., 1996). An indication of the importance of the issue is the recent finding that acute pain after major surgery predicts long-term pain (Katz et al., 1996). Postoperative pain needs to be controlled, not only to reduce suffering but to prevent long-term sequaelae.

To specifically test the hypothesis that a treatment started before surgery is more effective in the reduction of postoperative pain than a treatment given immediately on recovery from anesthesia, the identical analgesic strategy needs to be compared in two groups of patients where the only difference is timing of the analgesic strategy. This model was proposed by McQuay (1992) and became the basis of the design of many subsequent studies. This design tests only for pre-emptive analgesia in its narrowest sense – that is, what is the influence of nociceptive activity generated during surgery on postoperative pain. Unfortunately, in addition, a number of these studies suffered from design flaws that incorporated confounding factors that negated their findings. Frequently the confounding factors were simple matters such as giving both pre- and postemptive groups an opioid premedication (Pryl et al., 1993) or starting surgery before the onset time of the pre-emptive drug was given (Rice et al., 1990). Nevertheless, pre-emptive effects can be demonstrated both clinically (Woolf and Chong, 1993) and in volunteers (Pedersen et al., 1996).

In such clinical studies the outcome measures of pre-emptive treatment need to be carefully chosen. They must be selected to be as objective as possible, without interference by factors other than a difference in analgesic effect. In many early studies, the time to first analgesic demand after the end of surgery was used (Hill et al., 1987; Pavy et al., 1995). This measure can be confounded, among other things, by variation in individual responses to general anesthesia; if the patient is slow to wake because of residual anesthesia, this will influence time to analgesic request. The patient must have free access to analgesia, a condition not easily met in many postoperative recovery wards. In many studies the patients were given patient-controlled analgesia (PCA) in the form of intravenous morphine boluses as the method of postoperative pain control after their pre- or postoperative treatments. It is then possible to compare total morphine used in a given period of time between the pre-emptive and postemptive treatment groups as a measure of outcome. In this case pain scores recorded over the same period should not, if free access to morphine is available, differ between the groups. Instead, the idea is to see if the patients achieved the same pain relief with less postoperative morphine self-administration (Richmond et al., 1993; Collis et al., 1995). This outcome measure also has limitations because there are factors other than pain that influence the use of PCA by an individual patient. Patient personality factors, anxiety, and expectations of recovery can all influence PCA usage. Analgesic consumption may reflect not only pain intensity but postoperative distress (Jamison et al., 1993). For this reason the study design needs careful thought to ensure that the patients included are a homogeneous group. An indication that pre-emptive effects are not dependent on patient reports comes from a veterinary study showing a pre-emptive effect of pethidine in rats undergoing ovariohysterectomy (Lascelles et al., 1995). The challenge, then, is to find the least subjective, most sensitive, and most clinically relevant outcome measure.

Analgesic consumption as an outcome measure also predicates studying groups of patients undergoing surgery which is sufficiently painful that all patients will require some postoperative analgesia. Some studies have been conducted in patients undergoing surgery in which a significant number of subjects required no postoperative analgesia. This complicates interpretation of these studies because it is difficult to show any improvement using small groups of patients in which some patients have no or minimal pain. For this reason studies involving abdominal and thoracic surgery (Katz et al., 1992; Richmond et al., 1993; Sabanathan, 1995) have tended to prove more useful to demonstrate pre-emptive efficacy than operations such as inguinal herniaorraphy.

Improvements in study design in clinical research, particularly an understanding of the statistical power of studies, has led to a clearer understanding of why negative results are found. Many studies can be criticized for the small numbers of patients studied in each group, and if rigorous statistical standards are applied, some studies that are often cited in this field should not have entered the literature.

Opioids and Pre-emptive Analgesia

A number of studies have been conducted using opioid administration as the analgesic strategy to investigate the efficacy of pre-emptive analgesia. Katz et al. (1992) produced evidence for pre-emptive analgesia in a study that compared the effect of giving fentanyl 4 μg/kg via an epidural catheter either before or 15 minutes after surgical incision. They found that the postoperative consumption of morphine by PCA was significantly less at 12 and 24 hours in the pre-emptive group. Opioid drugs given intravenously have been examined for a pre-emptive effect in several studies, and there appear to be different effects with different opioids. Alfentanil, a synthetic opioid with a rapid onset and offset, has been used in two studies (Mansfield et al., 1994; Wilson et al., 1994). In both of these studies alfentanil given either at induction or 1 minute after skin incision was tested, and all patients were then given morphine. The researchers were unable to demonstrate any difference in postoperative analgesic consumption. These studies serve to illustrate some of the problems of clinical studies in pre-emptive analgesia, as discussed by Kissin (1996), in which insufficient differences between the control and pre-emptive groups can be accounted for by insufficient duration of action of the antinociceptive protection, alfentanil having a very short half-time in the brain. In addition, the use of morphine immediately after the incision would be expected to produce a pre-emptive effect on the nociceptive input generated in the postincisional surgery in the control group.

In two other studies, morphine, which has a longer duration of action, was administered either at the induction of anesthesia or at the very end of the surgery. Richmond et al. (1993) demonstrated a significant reduction in morphine consumption over the first 24 hours postoperatively in a group of women undergoing total abdominal hysterectomy who received a single dose of 10 mg of morphine intravenously at induction compared with a group given the same dose at the end of the surgery. This study has two additional interesting findings. The authors tested the skin around the wound for touch and pain sensitivity using Von Frey hairs. These calibrated filaments were used to test sensitivity of the skin just above the incision, and the group given morphine after the surgery was demonstrated to have an area of wound hyperalgesia not present in the pre-emptive group. This is supportive evidence that pre-emptive analgesia operates by preventing central sensitization in patients. The authors measured pain scores at 24 hours, after free access to morphine, and at 48 hours after a second 24 hours with only simple analgesics. At 48 hours the group that had the pre-emptive morphine had more pain than the control group. The researchers suggested the hypothesis that the additional morphine used in the postgroup had a pre-emptive effect in the second 24-hour period. This effect of more pain in the second 24 hours was also seen in the Katz et al. (1992) study, but the difference there did not reach significance.

A second study using the same surgical procedure, abdominal hysterectomy (Mansfield et al., 1996), compared two different doses of morphine administered pre-emptively with a dose given at the end of surgery. The investigators gave doses of 0.15 mg/kg (10 mg in a 70-kg patient) at induction, 0.3 mg/kg (21 mg in a 70-kg patient) at induction, and 0.15 mg/kg at the end of surgery. In this study no difference between pre- and post-treatment in the lower-dose group was detected, but a significant difference was found with the higher dose. In contrast, Collis et al. (1995) compared two groups, one that received 20 mg of morphine at induction of anesthesia and another that was given 10 mg at the induction and 10 mg at the end of surgery, but they could not demonstrate any difference in postoperative morphine consumption. In this study the authors noted a very high incidence of nausea and vomiting in the patients, indicating both that this side effect of morphine limits its use beyond certain dose levels and that there appears to be a ceiling effect of the pre-emptive action of morphine. Postoperative nausea and vomiting associated with opioids is a substantial problem, with patients often stating that they do not use the PCA because they would rather experience pain than nausea. In designing new opioids for postoperative pain, a reduction in the incidence of postoperative nausea and vomiting is imperative. Intramuscular morphine is not a useful route of administration, although some pre-emptive effect can be seen (Richmond et al., 1993; Hendolin et al., 1996), and either systemic (Richmond et al., 1993) or intraspinal/epidural (Choe et al., 1997) administration is necessary.

There is, then, some evidence for a pre-emptive effect with morphine, but less or none with single boluses of short-acting opioids. The extent of the pre-emptive effect with opioids is perhaps less dramatic than that shown with effective local anesthetic block (Sabanathan, 1995). The reason may be related to the duration of the nociceptive input after a surgical procedure, since the initial postoperative period is characterized by an acute inflammatory reaction, which itself generates nociceptive input. The pre-emptive treatment needs to be maintained into the postoperative period to ensure that significant nociceptive input either does not reach the spinal cord or does not induce central sensitization. This would be pre-emptive analgesia in its broader sense, incorporating prevention in surgical and postoperative periods. Where a local anesthetic block that is sufficiently dense to prevent conduction in C-fibers can be established before surgery, a clinically significant pre-emptive effect can be demonstrated (Shir et al., 1994). Unfortunately, producing this density of block under general anesthesia can be difficult to achieve in practice. This result has led to attempts to demonstrate pre-emptive effects with a balanced or multimodal approach to analgesia (Kavanagh et al., 1994; Rockemann et al., 1996).

The question remains – can effective, continuous pre-emption be provided with opioids? Combinations of continuous infusions of morphine combined with PCA have been reported not to reduce the number of demands from the pump in one study (Doyle et al., 1993). In another study, however, an intraoperative infusion of fentanyl, compared with an intraoperative infusion of ketamine and a control group, demonstrated a markedly reduced requirement for postoperative analgesia in both of the infusion groups compared with the control (Tverskoy et al., 1994). The authors also demonstrated reduced wound hyperalgesia over a period that outlasted the duration of action of the opiate and ketamine. A more recent study using a combination of 2 mg morphine and 60 mg ketamine epidurally for upper abdominal surgery before the operation, versus the same treatment at the end of surgery, found a longer-lasting analgesia with a reduced requirement for supplemental analgesia in the first group with no difference in adverse effects (Choe et al., 1997). Until an opioid without side effects is available, opioid sparing strategies need to be adopted to ensure sufficient analgesia without sedation and nausea to enable ambulatory surgery, accelerated surgical stay programs, and early organ recovery (Kehlet et al., 1996).

Summary

In conclusion, pre-emptive analgesia with opioids can be demonstrated. Morphine given as an IV bolus before surgery reduces postoperative analgesic consumption and eliminates wound hypersensitivity compared with the same dose given at the end of surgery. Short-acting synthetic opioids given in a bolus dose are not effective, but intraoperative infusions at a reasonable dose are effective and have long-lasting actions. Pre-emptive analgesia strategy must now be designed to cover the period of postoperative inflammation as well as during direct surgical intervention. When this is achieved with local anesthetic regional block, the effects are clinically impressive (Wang et al., 1996). The challenge of opioid pre-emptive analgesia is to provide effective continuous pre-emption, either by infusion of short-acting compounds or by long-acting drugs, to generate pain relief as effective as regional blocks but without producing unacceptable sedation, confusion, nausea, or constipation.

REFERENCES

Chapman, V., and Dickenson, A.H. (1993a). Enhanced responses of rat dorsal horn neurones after ultraviolet irradiation of the hindpaw; roles of the NMDA receptor. *Neurosci. Lett.* **176,** 41–44.

Chapman, V., and Dickenson, A.H. (1993b). The effect of intrathecal administration of RP 67580, a potent neurokinin 1 antagonist on nociceptive transmission in the rat spinal cord. *Neurosci. Lett.* **157,** 149–152.

Chapman, V., Haley, J.E., and Dickenson, A.H. (1994). Electrophysiological analysis of pre-emptive effects of spinal opioids on NMDA mediated events. *Anesthesiology.* **81,** 1429–1435.

Chen, L., and Huang, L.-Y.M. (1992). Protein kinase C reduces Mgx^+ block of NMDA-receptor channels as a mechanism of modulation. *Nature.* **356,** 521–523.

Choe, H., Choi, Y.S., Kim, Y.H., Ko, S.H., Choi, H.G., Han, Y.J., and Song, H.S. (1997). Epidural morphine plus ketamine for upper abdominal surgery: Improved analgesia from preincisional versus postincisional administration. *Anesth. Analg.* **84,** 560–563.

Coderre, T.J. (1992). Contribution of protein kinase C to persistent nociception following tissue injury in rats. *Neurosci. Lett.* **140,** 181–184.

Coderre, T.C., and Melzack, R. (1985). Increased pain sensitivity following heat injury involves a central mechanism. *Behav. Brain Res.* **15,** 259–262.

Coderre, T.J., Katz, J., Vaccarino, A.L., and Melzack, R. (1993). Contribution of central neuroplasticity to pathological pain: Review of clinical and experimental evidence. *Pain.* **52,** 259–285.

Coderre, T.J., and Melzack, R. (1992a). The role of NMDA receptor-operated calcium channels in persistent nociception after formalin-induced tissue injury. *J. Neurosci.* **12**(9), 3671–3675.

Coderre, T.J., and Melzack, R. (1992b). The contribution of excitatory amino acids to central sensitization and persistent nociception after formalin-induced tissue injury. *J. Neurosci.* **12,** 3665–3670.

Collis, R., Brandner, B., Bromley, L.M., and Woolf, C.J. (1995). Is there any clinical advantage of increasing the pre-emptive dose of morphine or combining pre-incisional with post-operative morphine administration? *Br. J. Anaesth.* **74,** 396–399.

Cook, A.J., Woolf, C.J., Wall, P.D., and McMahon, S.B. (1987). Dynamic receptive field plasticity in rat spinal cord dorsal horn following C primary afferent input. *Nature.* **325,** 151–153.

Davis, K.D., Meyer, R.A., and Campbell, J.N. (1993). Chemosensitivity and sensitization of nociceptive afferents that innervate the hairy skin of monkey. *J. Neurophysiol.* **69,** 1071–1081.

Dickenson, A.H., and Sullivan, A.F. (1987a). Evidence for a role of the NMDA receptor in the frequency dependent potentiation of deep rat dorsal horn nociceptive neurones following C-fibre stimulation. *Neuropharmacology.* **26,** 1235–1238.

Dickenson, A.H., and Sullivan, A.F. (1987b). Subcutaneous formalin-induced activity of dorsal horn neurones in the rat: Differential responses to an intrathecal opiate administered pre or post formalin. *Pain.* **30,** 349–360.

Dolphin, A.C., Menon-Johansson, A., Campbell, V., Berrow, N., and Sweeney, M.I. (1994). Modulation of voltage dependent calcium channels by $GABA_B$ receptors and G proteins in cultured rat dorsal root ganglion neurons: Relevance to transmitter release and its modulation. In *Cellular mechanisms of sensory processing,* ed. L. Urban. Berlin: Springer-Verlag, pp. 49–61.

Dougherty, P.M., Palecek, J., Paleckova, V., Sorkin, L.S., and Willis, W.D. (1992). The role of NMDA and non-NMDA excitatory amino acid receptors in the excitation of primate spinothalamic tract neurons by mechanical, chemical, thermal and electrical stimuli. *J. Neurosc.* **12,** 3025–3041.

Dougherty, P.M., and Willis, W.D. (1992). Enhanced responses of spinothalamic tract neurons to excitatory amino acids accompany capsaicin-induced sensitization in the monkey. *J. Neurosci.* **12,** 833–894.

Doyle, E., Robinson, D., and Morton, N.S. (1993). Comparison of patient controlled analgesia with and without background infusion after lower abdominal surgery in children. *Br. J. Anaesth.* **71,** 670–673.

Dubner, R., and Ruda, M.A. (1992). Activity-dependent neuronal plasticity following tissue injury and inflammation. *Trends Neurosci.* **15** (3), 96–103.

Duggan, A.W., and North, R.A. (1984). Electrophysiology of opioids. *Pharmacol. Rev.* **35,** 219–281.

Harrison, C.A., Morris, S., and Harvey, J.S. (1994). Effect of illioinguinal and illiohypogastric block and wound infiltration with 0.5% bupivacaine on post operative pain after inguinal hernia repair. *Br. J. Anaesth.* **72,** 691–693.

Heath, M.J., Womack, M.D., and MacDermott, A.B. (1994). Substance P elevates intracellular calcium in both neurons and glial cells from the dorsal horn of the spinal cord. *J. Neurophysiol.* **72,** 1192–1198.

Hendolin, H., Nuutinen, L., Kokki, H., and Tuomisto, L. (1996). Does morphine premedication influence the pain and consumption of postoperative analgesics after total knee arthroplasty? *Acta Anaesthesiol. Scand.* **40,** 81–85.

Hill, C.M., Carroll, M.J., Giles, A.D., and Pickvance, N. (1987). Ibuprofen given pre and post operatively for the relief of pain. *Internat. J. Oral Maxillofac. Surg.* **16,** 420–424.

Jamison, R.N., Taft, K., O'Hara, J.P., and Ferrante, F.M. (1993). Psychosocial and pharmacologic predictors of satisfaction with intravenous patient controlled analgesia. *Anesth. Analg.* **77,** 121–125.

Johansson, B., Glise, H., Hallerback, B., Dalman, P., and Kristoffersson, A. (1994). Preoperative local infiltration with ropivacaine for postoperative pain relief after cholecystectomy. *Anesth. Analg.* **78,** 210–214.

Katz, J., Jackson, M., Kavanagh, B.P., and Sandler, A.N. (1996). Acute pain after thoracic surgery predicts long-term post-thoracotomy pain. *Clin. J. Pain.* **12,** 50–55.

Katz, J., Kavanagh, B.P., Sandler, A.N., Nierenberg, H., Boylan, J.F., Friedlander, M., and Shaw, B.F. (1992). Preemptive analgesia. Clinical evidence of neuroplasticity contributing to postoperative pain. *Anesthesiology.* **77,** 439–446.

Kavanagh, B.P., Katz, J., Sandler, A.N., Nierenberg, H., Roger, S., Boylan, J.F., and Laws,

A.K. (1994). Multimodal analgesia before thoracic surgery does not reduce post operative pain. *Br. J. Anaesth.* **73,** 184–189.

Kehlet, H., Rung, G.W., and Callesen, T. (1996). Postoperative opioid analgesia: Time for a reconsideration? *J. Clin. Anesth.* **8,** 441–445.

King, A.E., Thompson, S.W.N., Urban, L., and Woolf, C.J. (1988). An intracellular analysis of amino acid induced excitations of deep dorsal horn neurones in the rat spinal cord slice. *Neurosci. Lett.* **89,** 286–292.

Kissin, I. (1996). Pre-emptive analgesia: Why its effect is not always obvious. *Anesthesiology.* **84,** 1015–1019.

Koltzenburg, M., Lundberg, L.E.R., and Torebjork, H.E. (1992). Dynamic and static components of mechanical hyperalgesia in human hairy skin. *Pain.* **51,** 207–220.

Koltzenburg, M., Torebjork, H.E., and Wahren, L.K. (1994). Nociceptor modulated central sensitization causes mechanical hyperalgesia in acute chemogenic and chronic neuropathic pain. *Brain.* **117,** 579–591.

Koskinen, R., Tigerstedt, I., and Tammisto, T. (1991). The effect of preoperative alfentanil on the need for immediate postoperative pain relief. *Acta Anaesthesiol. Scand.* **35,** O21.

Laird, J.M.A., Hargreaves, R.J., and Hill, R.G. (1993). Effects of RP 67580, a non-peptide neurokinin 1 receptor antagonist, on facilitation of a nociceptive spinal flexion reflex in the rat. *Br. J. Pharmacol.* **109,** 713–718.

LaMotte, R.H., Lundberg, L.E.R., and Torebjork, H.E. (1992). Pain, hyperalgesia and activity in nociceptive C units in humans after intradermal injection of capsaicin. *J. Physiol. (London).* **448,** 749–764.

Lascelles, B.D., Waterman, A.E., Cripps, P.J., Livingston, A., and Henderson, G. (1995). Central sensitization as a result of surgical pain: Investigation of the pre-emptive value of pethidine for ovariohysterectomy in the rat. *Pain.* **62,** 201–212.

Levine, J.D., and Taiwo, Y.O. (1994). Inflammatory pain. In *Textbook of pain,* ed. Wall, P.D., and Melzack, R. Edinburgh: Churchill Livingstone, 45–56.

Ma, Q.-P., and Woolf, C.J. (1995a). Noxious stimuli induce an N-methyl-D-aspartate receptor dependent hypersensitivity of the flexion withdrawal reflex to touch – implications for the treatment of mechanical allodynia. *Pain.* **61,** 383–390.

Ma, Q.-P., and Woolf, C.J. (1995b). Involvement of neurokinin receptors in the induction but not the maintenance of mechanical allodynia in the rat flexor motoneurones. *J. Physiol. (London).* **486** (3), 769–777.

MacDermott, A.B., Mayer, M.L., Westbrook, G.L., Smith, S.J., and Baker, J.L. (1986). NMDA-receptor activation increases cytoplasmic calcium concentration in cultured spinal cord neurons. *Nature.* **321,** 519–522.

Mansfield, M.D., James, K.S., and Kinsella, J. (1996). Influence of dose and timing of administration of morphine on postoperative pain and analgesic requirements. *Br. J. Anaesth.* **76,** 358–361.

Mansfield, M., Meikle, R., and Miller, C. (1994). A trial of pre-emptive analgesia. Influence of timing of preoperative alfentanil on postoperative pain and analgesic requirements. *Anaesthesia.* **49,** 1091–1093.

Mayer, M.L., Westbrook, G.L., and Guthrie, P.B. (1984). Voltage-dependent block by MG^{2+} of NMDA responses in spinal cord neurones. *Nature.* **309,** 261–263.

McMahon, S.B., Lewin, G.R., and Wall, P.D. (1993). Central hyperexcitability triggered by noxious inputs. *Curr. Opin. Neurobiol.* **3,** 602–610.

McQuay, H.J. (1992). Pre-emptive analgesia. *Br. J. Anaesth.* **69,** 1–3.

McQuay, H.J., Carroll, D., and Moore, R.A. (1988). Post-operative orthopaedic pain – the effect of opiate premedication and local anesthetic blocks. *Pain.* **33,** 291–295.

Meller, S.T., Dykstra, C., and Gebhart, G.F. (1993). Acute mechanical hyperalgesia is produced by coactivation of AMPA and metabotropic glutamate receptors. *Neuroreport.* **4,** 879–882.

Mendell, L.M., and Wall, P.D. (1965). Responses of dorsal cord cells of peripheral cutaneous unmyelinated fibres. *Nature.* **206,** 97–99.

Miller, B.A., and Woolf, C.J. (1996). Glutamate-mediated slow synaptic currents in neonatal rat deep dorsal horn neurons in vitro. *J. Neurophysiol.* **76,** 1465–1476.

Nagy, I., Maggi, C.A., Dray, A., Woolf, C.J., and Urban, L. (1993). The role of neurokinin and N-methyl-D-aspartate receptors in synaptic transmission from capsaicin sensitive primary afferents in the rat spinal cord in vitro. *Neuroscience.* **52,** 1029–1037.

Nagy, I., Miller, B.A., and Woolf, C.J. (1994). NK_1 and NK_2 receptors contribute to C-fibre evoked slow potentials in the rat spinal cord. *Neuroreport.* **5,** 2105–2108.

Pavy, T.J., Gambling, D.R., Merrick, P.M., and Douglas, M.L. (1995). Rectal morphine potentiates spinal morphine analgesia after cesarean delivery. *Anaesth. Intensive Care.* **23,** 555–559.

Pedersen, J.L., Crawford, M.E., Dahl, J.B., Brennum, J., and Kehlet, H. (1996). Effect of preemptive nerve block on inflammation and hyperalgesia after human thermal injury. *Anesthesiology.* **84,** 1020–1026.

Pryl, B.J., Vanner, R.G., Enriquez, N., and Reynolds, F. (1993). Can pre-emptive lumbar epidural blockade reduce postoperative pain following lower abdominal surgery? *Anesthesia.* **48,** 120–123.

Reeh, P.W. (1994). Chemical excitation and sensitization of nociceptors. In *Cellular mechanisms of sensory processing. NATO ASI series. Cell Biology; vol 79,* ed. Urban, L. Berlin and Heidelberg: Springer-Verlag, 119–131.

Ren, K., Hylden, J.L.K., Williams, G.M., Ruda, M.A., and Dubner, R. (1992). The effects of a non-competitive NMDA receptor antagonist, MK-801, on behavioural hyperalgesia and dorsal horn neuronal activity in rats with unilateral inflammation. *Pain.* **50,** 331–344.

Ren, K., Williams, G.M., Hylden, J.L.K., Ruda, M.A., and Dubner, R. (1992). The intrathecal administration of excitatory amino acid receptor antagonists selectively attenuated carrageenan-induced behavioral hyperalgesia in rats. *Eur. J. Pharmacol.* **219,** 235–243.

Rice, L.J., Pudimat, M.A., and Hannallah, R.S. (1990). Timing of caudal block placement in relation to surgery does not affect duration of postoperative analgesia in paediatric ambulatory patients. *Can. J. Anesthesiol.* **37,** 429–431.

Richmond, C.E., Bromley, L.M., and Woolf, C.J. (1993). Preoperative morphine pre-empts postoperative pain. *Lancet.* **342,** 73–75.

Rockemann, M.G., Seeling, W., Bischof, C., Borstinghaus, D., Steffen, P., and Georgieff, M. (1996). Prophylactic use of epidural mepivacaine/morphine, systemic diclofenac, and metamizole reduces postoperative morphine consumption after major abdominal surgery. *Anesthesiology.* **84,** 1027–1034.

Sabanathan, S. (1995). Has postoperative pain been eradicated? *Ann. Royal Coll. Surg., England.* **77,** 202–209.

Shir, Y., Raja, S.N., and Frank, M. (1994). The effect of epidural versus general anesthesia on postoperative pain and analgesic requirements in patients undergoing radial prostatectomy. *Anesthesiology.* **80,** 49–56.

Simone, D.A., Sorkin, L.S., Oh, U., Chung, J.M., Owens, C.M., LaMotte, R.H., and Willis,

W.D. (1991). Neurogenic hyperalgesia: Central neural correlates in responses of spinothalamic tract neurons. *J. Neurophysiol.* **66,** 228–246.

Sivilotti, L.G., Gerber, G., Rawat, B., and Woolf, C.J. (1995). Morphine selectively depresses the slowest, NMDA-independent component of C-fibre evoked synaptic activity in the rat spinal cord in vitro. *Eur. J. Neurosci.* **7,** 12–18.

Sivilotti, L.G., Thompson, S.W.N., and Woolf, C.J. (1993). The rate of rise of the cumulative depolarization evoked by repetitive stimulation of small-calibre afferents is a predictor of action potential windup in rat spinal neurones in vitro. *J. Neurophysiol.* **69,** 1621–1631.

Thompson, S.W.N., King, A.E., and Woolf, C.J. (1990). Activity-dependent changes in rat ventral horn neurones in vitro: Summation of prolonged afferent evoked postsynaptic depolarizations produce a D-APV sensitive windup. *Eur. J. Neurosci.* **2,** 638–649.

Thompson, S.W.N., Woolf, C.J., and Sivilotti, L.G. (1993). Small caliber afferents produce a heterosynaptic facilitation of the synaptic responses evoked by primary afferent A fibres in the neonatal rat spinal cord in vitro. *J. Neurophysiol.* **69,** 2116–2128.

Torebjork, H.E., Lundberg, L.E.R., and LaMotte, R.H. (1992). Central changes in processing of mechanoreceptor input in capsaicin-induced sensory hyperalgesia in humans. *J. Physiol. (London).* **448,** 765–780.

Treede, R.-D., Meyer, R.A., Raja, S.N., and Campbell, J.N. (1992). Peripheral and central mechanisms of cutaneous hyperalgesia. *Prog. Neurobiol.* **38,** 397–421.

Tverskoy, M., Oz, Y., Isakson, A., Finger, J., Bradley, E.L., and Kissin, I. (1994). Preemptive effect of fentanyl and ketamine on postoperative pain and wound hyperalgesia. *Anesth. Analg.* **78,** 205–209.

Urban, L., and Randic, M. (1984). Slow excitatory transmission in rat dorsal horn: Possible mediation by peptides. *Brain Res.* **290,** 336–341.

Wall, P.D. (1988). The prevention of post operative pain. *Pain.* **32,** 289–290.

Wall, P.D., and Woolf, C.J. (1984). Muscle but not cutaneous C-afferent input produces prolonged increases in the excitability of the flexion reflex in the rat. *J. Physiol. (London).* **356,** 443–458.

Wang, J.J., Ho, S.T., Liu, H.S., Tzeng, J.I., Tze, T.S., and Liaw, W.J. (1996). The effect of spinal versus general anesthesia on postoperative pain and analgesic requirements in patients undergoing lower abdominal surgery. *Reg. Anesth.* **21,** 277–280.

Wilson, R.J.T., Leith, S., Jackson, I.J.B., and Hunter, D. (1994). Pre-emptive analgesia from intravenous administration of opioids. *Anesthesia.* **49,** 591–593.

Woolf, C.J. (1983). Evidence for a central component of post-injury pain hypersensitivity. *Nature.* **306,** 686–688.

Woolf, C.J. (1994). A new strategy for the treatment of inflammatory pain: Prevention or elimination of central sensitization. *Drugs.* **47,** 1–9.

Woolf, C.J. (1995). Somatic pain: Pathogenesis and prevention. *Br. J. Anaesth.* **75,** 169–176.

Woolf, C.J., and Chong, M.-S. (1993). Pre-emptive analgesia: Treating postoperative pain by preventing the establishment of central sensitization. *Anesth. Analg.* **77,** 1–18.

Woolf, C.J., and King, A.E. (1989). Subthreshold components of the cutaneous mechanoreceptive fields of dorsal horn neurons in the rat lumbar spinal cord. *J. Neurophysiol.* **62,** 907–916.

Woolf, C.J., and King, A.E. (1990). Dynamic alterations in the cutaneous mechanoreceptive fields of dorsal horn neurons in the rat spinal cord. *J. Neurosci.* **10,** 2717–2726.

Woolf, C.J., Shortland, P., and Sivilotti, L.G. (1994). Sensitization of high mechanothreshold superficial dorsal horn and flexor motor neurons following chemosensitive primary afferent activation. *Pain.* **58** (2), 141–155.

Woolf, C.J., and Thompson, S.W.N. (1991). The induction and maintenance of central sensitization is dependent on N-methyl-D-aspartic acid receptor activation: Implications for the treatment of post-injury pain hypersensitivity states. *Pain.* **44,** 293–299.

Woolf, C.J., and Wall, P.D. (1986a). The relative effectiveness of C primary afferent fibres of different origins in evoking a prolonged facilitation of the flexor reflex in the rat. *J. Neurosci.* **6,** 1433–1443.

Woolf, C.J., and Wall, P.D. (1986b). Morphine-sensitive and morphine-insensitive actions of C-fibre input on the rat spinal cord. *Neurosci. Lett.* **64,** 221–225.

Xu, X.-J., Dalsgaard, C.-J., and Wiesenfeld-Hallin, Z. (1992). Intrathecal CP-96,345 blocks reflex facilitation induced in rats by substance P and C-fiber-conditioning stimulation. *Eur. J. Pharmacol.* **216,** 337–344.

Xu, X.-J., Maggi, C.M., and Wiesenfeld-Hallin, Z. (1991). On the role of NK_2 tachykinin receptors in the mediation of spinal reflex excitability in the rat. *Neuroscience.* **44,** 483–490.

Yaksh, T.L., Jessell, T.M., Gamse, R., Mudge, A.W., and Leeman, S.E. (1980). Intrathecal morphine inhibits substance P release from mammalian spinal cord in vivo. *Nature.* **286,** 155–157.

Yoshimura, M., and Jessell, T.M. (1989). Primary afferent evoked synaptic responses and slow potential generation in rat substantia gelatinosa neurons in vitro. *J. Neurophysiol.* **62,** 96–108.

Yoshimura, M., and Nishi, S. (1992). Excitatory amino acid receptors involved in primary afferent-evoked polysynaptic EPSPs of substantia gelatinosa neurons in the adult rat spinal slice. *Neurosci. Lett.* **143,** 131–134.

Yu, X.M., Askalan, R., Keil II, G.J., and Salter, M.W. (1997). NMDA channel regulation by channel-associated protein tyrosine kinase Src. *Science.* **275,** 674–678.

CHAPTER TWELVE

Intraoperative Use of Opioids

CARL C. HUG, JR.

Introduction

Since the discovery of general anesthesia in the 1840s, opium and its principal analgesic component morphine have been used in conjunction with general anesthetics to produce surgical anesthesia. As preanesthetic medication, morphine-type drugs provided sedation, reduction of anxiety, and analgesia, facilitating the patient's toleration of preanesthetic preparations, including vascular cannulation. Premedication with an opioid facilitates the induction of general anesthesia, and Claude Bernard in 1869 demonstrated that morphine premedication reduced the amount of chloroform required to anesthetize dogs.

In the 1890s, Schneiderlein and other German physicians attempted to produce surgical anesthesia by combining morphine and scopolamine, both in very large doses. The patients had to be restrained for the surgeon to operate, and many died postoperatively from ventilatory depression because mechanical ventilation was unknown at that time. Then, in the 1960s, Lowenstein et al. (1969) combined morphine with d-tubocurarine to produce general anesthesia in critically ill patients undergoing valvular heart surgery. When this anesthetic technique was later extended to physically fit individuals undergoing coronary artery bypass surgery, there was an unacceptably high incidence of hypertension and tachycardia as well as intraoperative awareness and recall of intraoperative events. Because of its side effects, especially those related to histamine release, there were limitations on the doses of morphine that human patients could tolerate.

During World War II, intense efforts were made to discover synthetic morphine-like drugs (i.e., opioids). Many of these drugs were investigated and used for preoperative medication and intraoperative supplementation of general and regional anesthesia. Meperidine (pethidine, Demerol) was one of the more popular totally synthetic opioids used in the practice of anesthesia, but its side effects were even more restrictive than those of morphine with respect to the maximally tolerated dose (histamine release, negative inotrope, and metabolites producing seizures). Stanley and Webster (1978) drew attention to another totally synthetic opioid, fentanyl, and began to explore its use as a primary anesthetic drug for patients undergoing all types of cardiac surgery. Because of its relatively minor effects on hemodynamics and the

Christoph Stein, ed., *Opioids in Pain Control: Basic and Clinical Aspects*. Printed in the United States of America.

ease with which it could be used in enormous doses, fentanyl became the most widely used opioid in large doses for general anesthesia in patients undergoing cardiac and all other types of major surgery. When its U.S. patent expired, fentanyl became available at relatively low cost, and it continues to be the most popular opioid for intraoperative use. The demands for rapid recovery from general anesthesia in the 1990s era of managed care reduced the frequency of use of so-called "high-dose narcotic anesthesia" in favor of more modest opioid doses used in conjunction with inhaled anesthetics and intravenous hypnotics. Today, fentanyl and other opioids continue to be used for preanesthetic medication, as the analgesic component of intraoperative sedation during procedures done with monitored anesthesia care, as supplements to regional and general anesthetics, for extended analgesia and sedation in the intensive care setting, and for control of postoperative pain. High-dose opioid anesthesia is still used in critically ill patients who cannot tolerate the cardiac depressant effects of inhaled and intravenous anesthetics and for whom prolonged intensive care with mechanical ventilation is anticipated.

The Opioid Drugs

Although multiple types of opioid receptors have been described and numerous compounds synthesized to interact with these receptors, the μ-agonists are the only ones that are widely used intraoperatively by anesthesiologists. The μ-opioid receptor is the one responsible for virtually all of the desirable effects of opioids used in anesthetic regimens and, for the most part, mediate the undesirable side effects and toxicity as well. Although there are marked differences in analgesic potency, the pure μ-receptor agonists do not differ substantially in their efficacy (i.e., maximum effect achievable in laboratory experiments), but side effects limit the maximum dose that is tolerated by human patients for morphine, meperidine, and their congeners. The major differences among the pure μ-opioid agonists have to do with their side effects and with their pharmacokinetics (see later in this chapter).

In addition to pure μ-receptor agonists, there are drugs characterized as mixed agonist-antagonists (e.g., butorphanol, nalbuphine), which have a relatively low efficacy (i.e., low maximum effect or ceiling), and their use is largely restricted to substitution for analgesic doses of morphine (5–15 mg) in the perioperative period. Antagonistic actions of some of the agonist-antagonists further limit their usefulness in the perioperative setting. Pure μ-receptor antagonists (e.g., naloxone) are useful in differential diagnosis (e.g., opioid-induced biliary colic vs. angina pectoris) and in the resuscitation of patients demonstrating severe respiratory depression due to overdoses of opioids. Antagonists are rarely needed in the perioperative period since they antagonize analgesia and the other desirable effects of the opioids along with their antagonism of ventilatory depression. Therefore, most practitioners prefer to avoid unmasking pain and perhaps inducing other side effects (e.g., startle response, hypertension, and tachycardia) in favor of supporting the patient's ventilation mechanically until the residual effects of perioperatively administered opioids decline as the opioid is eliminated from the body.

Intraoperatively Useful Effects of Opioids

Opioids act within the central nervous system (CNS) to produce analgesia and sleep (i.e., narcotic analgesics). Obviously, it is these effects that are generally desirable in all of the perioperative uses of opioids. Mental clouding may be appreciated by some patients, especially those with pain and anxiety, but it can lead to dysphoria in patients without pain, especially in those who fear losing control. CNS actions of opioids that are of particular interest to the anesthesiologist include their antitussive effect, which facilitates the patient's tolerance of airway manipulation and tracheal intubation; ventilatory depression, which facilitates controlled mechanical ventilation; and the suppression of sympathetic and somatic reflex responses to noxious stimulation. The latter is probably an extension of the basic analgesic action of opioids.

Undesirable effects produced by opioids acting within the CNS include nausea, retching and vomiting,[1] bradycardia, miosis, skeletal muscle rigidity, physical dependence, and tolerance to the opioids (but not cross tolerance to other types of CNS drugs). Undesirable peripheral actions of the opioids are mediated primarily by their direct effects on smooth muscle found in the gastrointestinal and genitourinary tracts, which result in colic (pain due to smooth muscle spasm and distention of the biliary tract or ureters), constipation, and urinary retention. Morphine and most of its congeners, meperidine, and several of the synthetic opioids (but not fentanyl or its derivatives) release histamine from mast cells and thereby can produce flushing, hypotension, and bronchospasm. The flushing and hypotension are often inconsequential and relatively easily treated. The intensity of these side effects, especially bronchospasm, can vary considerably among patients. Since bronchospasm can be life threatening, opioids releasing histamine are best avoided in patients with a history of reactive airway diseases. The pruritus associated with systemic or spinal (intrathecal, epidural) administration of opioids is primarily a CNS-mediated autonomic response; histamine release is inconsistent in patients suffering from severe pruritus secondary to opioid administration.

The popularity of opioids in anesthetic plans derives from both the desirable effects they produce and the things they do *not* do (Table 12.1).

Limitations of Opioids as "Anesthetics"

The opioids are capable of inducing sleep from which many patients can be aroused by a sufficiently intense noxious stimulation that exceeds their analgesic efficacy. None of the currently available opioids reliably induce and maintain unconsciousness and satisfactory anesthetic conditions (i.e., suppression of sympathetic and somatic reflex responses to intense noxious stimulation) in all patients even when

[1]Low (analgesic) doses of opioids stimulate the chemoreceptor trigger zone to produce nausea, retching, and vomiting; high doses depress the vomiting center and suppress these side effects.

Table 12.1. *Advantages of Opioids*

- Minimal direct cardiac depression (with the exception of meperidine, which is a negative inotrope in doses approximating 5 mg/kg).
- Preservation of autoregulation of blood flow in the CNS, heart, and kidneys.
- No significant interactions with autonomic or cardiovascular drugs.
- No sensitization of the heart to cathecholamines.
- Minimal changes in evoked potentials within the CNS.
- Arousable patient in the absence of hypnotics and anesthetics.
- Specific antagonists available.
- Postoperative analgesia.
- Increased toleration of an endotracheal tube and airway manipulation.
- Facilitation of controlled mechanical ventilation.
- Do not trigger malignant hyperpyrexia.
- No direct toxicity to any organ or tissue (as long as hypoxemia is prevented).
- Not teratogenic, but newborn depression occurs after maternal dose, and fetal/neonatal physical dependence occurs with chronic maternal use.

administered in enormous doses (e.g., fentanyl in doses exceeding 50 μg/kg) (Hug, 1990). Moreover, the loss of responsiveness (unconsciousness?) induced by opioids is often associated with the production of skeletal muscular rigidity, which can be manifested in a variety of ways (e.g., glottic closure, rigidity of the chest and abdomen, flexion of the extremities, flapping movement of the feet). Glottic closure and truncal rigidity interfere with positive pressure ventilation in these uniformly apneic patients. Rigidity also impairs the surgeon's ability to perform the operation. Prevention or treatment of opioid-induced rigidity is most reliably accomplished with a skeletal muscle relaxant, which in turn obscures somatic signs of intraoperative awakening of the patient. The risks of intraoperative awakening and subsequent recall of intraoperative events leads many, if not most, anesthesiologists to administer amnesic drugs (e.g., benzodiazepines, scopolamine, nitrous oxide) to patients who are managed with an opioid used in a large dose as the primary anesthetic agent. Prevention of recall does not guarantee prevention of intraoperative awakening with its associated fear and anxiety, even in the absence of pain. Hence, the most common opioid-based anesthetic regimen includes supplementation with intravenous hypnotics or inhaled anesthetics to minimize the risks of intraoperative arousal and awareness, to enhance the suppression of sympathetic and somatic reflex responses to noxious stimuli, and to reduce greatly the total dose of opioid required by the patient in order to achieve an appropriately rapid recovery postoperatively. In some patients, the control of intraoperative hypertension and tachycardia requires the administration of vasodilator and β-adrenergic receptor blocking drugs, especially when a potent inhaled or intravenous anesthetic is not included in the anesthetic regimen.

Interaction of Opioids with Inhaled Anesthetics and Intravenous Hypnotics

The opioids interact synergistically with intravenous hypnotics and inhaled anesthetics in regard to "anesthetic depth," ventilatory depression, and hypotension. Analgesic doses of opioids clearly reduce the requirements for inhalational anesthetics (e.g., MAC reduction) and for intravenous hypnotics (e.g., propofol) by 30–60% in both human patients and experimental animals. In humans, it has been demonstrated that opioids and natural sleep, and presumably drugs producing sleep, interact synergistically to depress spontaneous ventilation as well as the ventilatory responses to hypercarbia and hypoxemia.

In regard to hypotension, the following observations are noteworthy. It is possible to maintain stable blood pressure during induction of unconsciousness by a benzodiazepine or etomidate, whereupon administration of a small dose of an opioid (e.g., a 50 μg total dose of fentanyl) can produce hypotension, which is mild in most patients but sometimes severe. After induction with inhaled or intravenous anesthetics that are known to produce hypotension, the subsequent administration of an opioid can intensify the hypotension. Conversely, large doses of opioids (e.g., fentanyl up to 150 μg/kg) can be administered with relatively small hemodynamic changes, perhaps mild bradycardia and slight reductions in blood pressure. Then, with the subsequent administration of a very low dose of hypnotic (e.g., 2 mg midazolam, 5 mg diazepam, 50 mg thiopental), hypotension occurs, again usually of minor degree but sometimes to a marked degree. The unifying feature in these interactions is a reduction of sympathetic tone emanating from the CNS, leading to decreased sympathetic tone to vascular smooth muscle in the arteries and veins. Venodilation increases venous capacitance and reduces blood return to the heart, leading to a reduction in cardiac output, and peripheral arterial dilation leads to a reduction in total peripheral resistance, with both effects contributing to the observed hypotension. In the vast majority of patients, the hypotension is readily treated by administration of a vasopressor (e.g., phenylephrine).

Pharmacokinetics and Dynamics

The most important differences among the pure μ-receptor agonists are in their pharmacokinetic characteristics. From the viewpoint of the anesthesiologist using these drugs intraoperatively, the three most important differences relate to (1) latency to peak effect, (2) volume of distribution, and (3) recovery time.

Latency to peak effect refers to the time it takes for equilibration of drug concentrations between the blood (plasma) and the site(s) of drug action; in the case of the opioids the sites are located principally in the CNS. Equilibration half-time ($t\frac{1}{2}_{keo}$) is the term used to characterize this pharmacokinetic feature. As with any half-time, the equilibration is one-half complete in one half-time, and it takes approximately three half-times for the equilibration to approach 90% completion. The opioids used most frequently intraoperatively include alfentanil and remifentanil with a brief latency to peak effect ($t\frac{1}{2}_{keo}$ 1–2 minutes), fentanyl and sufentanil with somewhat longer latencies ($t\frac{1}{2}_{keo}$ 4–6 minutes), and morphine with a long latency ($t\frac{1}{2}_{keo}$ not measured but estimated to exceed 15 minutes). The practical implications of a very short latency to peak effect (and achievement of the maximum drug concentration in the CNS from a given dose) are that suppression of responses to noxious stimuli can be achieved rapidly utilizing the minimum required doses and that the relationship between dose and effect is easily recognized. With prolonged latency, there is delay in suppressing responses to noxious stimulation, so there is a tendency to use larger than necessary doses in order to compensate for the slower equilibration half-time, and the relationship between dose and effect is less easily recognized. Larger than necessary doses of the highly lipophilic opioids (e.g., fentanyl, sufentanil) lead to their accumulation in the body and a corresponding lengthening of recovery time. A delay of 4 or more minutes in controlling a response to a noxious stimulation intraoperatively is often unacceptable and sometimes embarrassing to the anesthetist. Alternatives to administering larger than ultimately necessary doses of fentanyl and sufentanil include utilization of drugs with a brief latency to peak effect (e.g., alfentanil, thiopental, propofol).

Latency to peak effect should be distinguished from the initial onset of drug action, which occurs almost immediately with the highly lipophilic fentanyl-type opioids. In the case of fentanyl, for example, the onset of ventilatory depression becomes apparent during a 30-second injection, whereas the peak effect of that injection may require 4 to 8 minutes or more to be achieved.

Also, the latency to peak effect should be distinguished from the delay in reaching the intended effect due to a gradual buildup of drug concentrations in plasma during the early phases of a constant-rate drug infusion in the absence of loading dose.

Volume of distribution is a pharmacokinetic term that provides an indication of how extensively a drug is taken up by body tissues. Highly lipophilic drugs (e.g., fentanyl, thiopental, isoflurane) have enormous volumes of distribution, indicating their extensive sequestration in all body tissues, especially those with a high lipid content (e.g., adipose tissue). Because the blood flow to adipose tissue is slow relative to the capacity of the tissue to take up highly lipophilic drugs, there is progressive accumulation of the drug in adipose tissue over time as long as there is a free-drug (i.e., not bound to protein or other tissue components) concentration gradient from blood (plasma) to tissue. Such a gradient is maintained by administering very large doses, repeated doses, or a continuous infusion. A drug that accumulates in tissues during drug administration slowly diffuses out of those tissues after administration of the drug is discontinued, and the free-drug concentration gradient reverses in

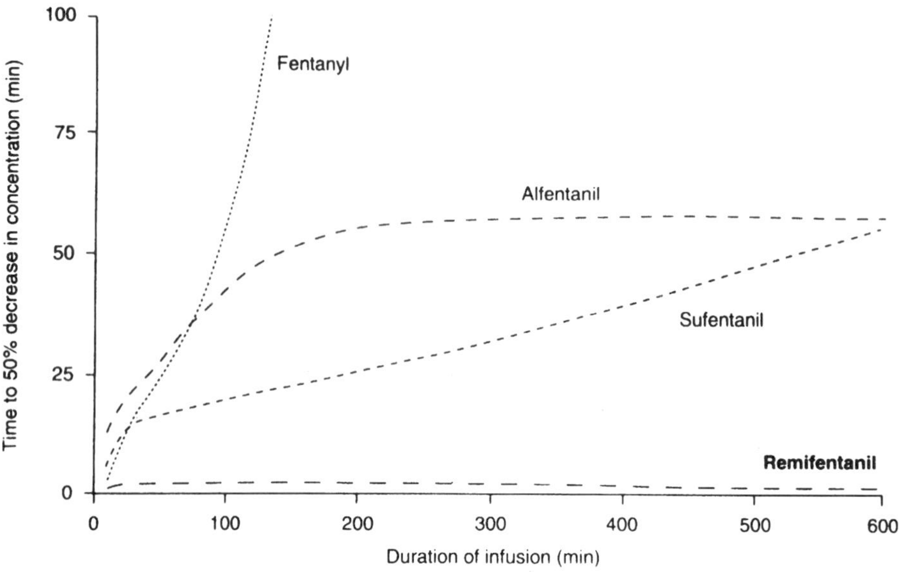

Figure 12.1. Simulation of the time required for a 50% reduction in the effect site concentration of four opioids after infusions designed to maintain constant effect site concentrations for up to 10 hours. (Reproduced with the permission of the author and ADIS from Egan, 1996.)

the direction of tissue to blood (plasma). Depending on the actual amount of the drug accumulated in those tissues, its slow release serves to maintain the blood (plasma) concentration and to prolong the duration of drug effect (i.e., recovery time), even for drugs with a high clearance rate by organs of elimination (e.g., the liver). Because the release of the drug is slow, its clearance from the blood by organs of elimination is correspondingly slow. The overall impact of drug accumulation and the comparison of different drugs can be represented by the so-called context-sensitive half-time (CSt½) of recovery (Hughes et al., 1992). That is, in the context of a continuous infusion to steady state, the time required for any level of drug concentration to decline by 50% is referred to as the context-sensitive half-time (CSt½). As can be seen in Figure 12.1, there is a progressive lengthening of the CSt½ as the duration of fentanyl administration is prolonged. In contrast, alfentanil, with a lesser volume of distribution (and interestingly enough, lower clearance rate by the liver), reaches a plateau CSt½ of approximately 50–60 minutes. This reflects the fact that alfentanil accumulates to a lesser degree in body tissues, redistribution from sites of action to nonresponsive tissues is limited, and its ultimate CSt½ reflects its actual elimination half-time (t½β, the classic pharmacokinetic term). Remifentanil is unique among the fentanyls in undergoing esterase hydrolysis in multiple body tissues and organs so that accumulation does not occur (Egan, 1996). All of the other opioids are cleared primarily by hepatic biotransformation, which requires that the drug be transported from sites of its accumulation through the blood to the liver in order to be inactivated. Morphine, which has a relatively small volume of distribution, is readily cleared from the body by its biotransformation in the liver, but morphine's effect is determined by its rate of diffusion out of the CNS, which is slower than its rate of elimination from the body as a whole. Hence, in the case of morphine, the dose can be titrated to the intensity of its effects without concern about progressive accumulation with repeated doses or sustained infusions.

Recovery time reflects not only the pharmacokinetic characteristics of the drug but also the extent to which drug concentrations exceed the concentrations at which recovery will occur in each patient. The latter concept is best illustrated by an example. When ventilation is supported mechanically, there is no known dose-related side effect or toxicity to indicate the presence of an excessive level of fentanyl. This effect is in stark contrast to many of the intravenous and inhalational anesthetics, which produce hypotension in a dose-related fashion, and unacceptable degrees of hypotension limit the doses that are administered. Suppose that the concentration of fentanyl required to suppress an individual patient's response to skin incision in combination with 0.5% isoflurane in end-tidal gas is 4 ng/ml. Suppose further that the patient would resume spontaneous ventilation when the concentration of fentanyl in plasma declined to 1 ng/ml. Because there is no way to predict the exact dose and concentration required for any individual patient (see "Variability" later in the chapter), suppose the anesthesiologist maintained a fentanyl concentration in plasma of 8 ng/ml. If the CSt½ for the duration of fentanyl administration in this example was 30 minutes, the patient would require 90 minutes, or three times the CSt½, to recover from the 8 ng/ml level, whereas the recovery time would be 60 minutes (two times the CSt½) if the concentration had been maintained at the minimally required level of 4 ng/ml.

To summarize, the factors affecting the recovery time for the highly lipophilic fentanyl-type opioids include the total dose of opioid, the time over which the opioid has been administered, the extent to which its concentrations at μ-receptors exceeds the minimum requirements of the patient, drug distribution and elimination processes, and a variety of variables affecting pharmacodynamics (the concentration-effect relationship; see the next section).

Pharmacodynamics

Understanding the pharmacology of a drug includes knowing the relationship between a drug's dose and its effect. This relationship may be divided into the relationship between dose and drug concentration in blood (plasma) – *pharmacokinetics* – and the relationship between drug concentration in blood (plasma) and the intensity of its effect – *pharmacodynamics.* For the opioids, the intensities of their desirable effects as well as their side effects and toxicity are proportional to the concentration produced at opioid receptors. It is not possible in human beings and it is very difficult in animals to measure drug concentrations at receptor sites. However, the relationship between drug concentration in blood (plasma) and intensity of effect can be determined reliably in two ways: measuring the different intensities of drug effect at different stable levels of drug concentration in blood (plasma) and administering a constant-rate infusion of a drug to produce progressively increasing concentrations in plasma and correlating those concentrations with progressively increasing intensities of drug effect.

Variability among Patients

Studies of the concentration versus effect relationship for opioids clearly demonstrate that a number of important factors contribute to variability among patients in their responses to the same dose or concentration of an opioid. In addition to age (both chronologic and physiologic), disease state, presence of other drugs, and so on, there are two important variables that are frequently not mentioned in regard to anesthetic drugs, including the opioids. (1) There appear to be intrinsic (genetic?) differences among patients who are matched for all of the known variables affecting pharmacokinetics and dynamics. (2) In the case of drugs used primarily to suppress responses to noxious stimuli, the intensity of the stimuli is an important variable that affects the dose and concentration of drug required to suppress responses to the stimuli. Experienced and careful observers among anesthesiologists generally agree that there is a hierarchy of intensities among different types of noxious stimuli. For example, insertion of an intravenous cannula or a urethral catheter rarely produces a response in lightly anesthetized patients, whereas a skin incision at the same level of anesthesia might induce hypertension, tachycardia, and body movement. Compared to a skin incision, tracheal intubation, rigidity bronchoscopy, and invasion of periosteum (e.g., sternotomy) appear to be more intense stimuli than a skin incision in that they typically require a higher concentration of anesthetic drugs to prevent or suppress sympathetic and somatic reflex responses.

Generally speaking, except for extremes of hepatic impairment, renal failure, hypoproteinemia, and hemodynamic aberrations, pharmacokinetic variability among patients explains only a minor portion of the variability observed in the dose versus response relationships reported in clinical practice. Pharmacodynamic variability, however, ranges from two- to sixfold even among closely matched patients treated identically (intrinsic variability) (Ausems et al., 1988) and even more so in regard to drug interactions, intensity of noxious stimulation, and certain disease states. Some indications of the degrees of variability attributed to intrinsic differences and to different types of noxious stimuli (Ausems et al., 1986) are evident in Figures 12.2 and 12.3.

There are two fundamentally different ways of dealing with this overall variability among patients in clinical anesthesiology. The first is to produce and to maintain a drug concentration in blood (plasma) that will suppress 90+ percent of responses to all types of noxious stimuli in all patients. This is easy to do with fentanyl-type opioids, which

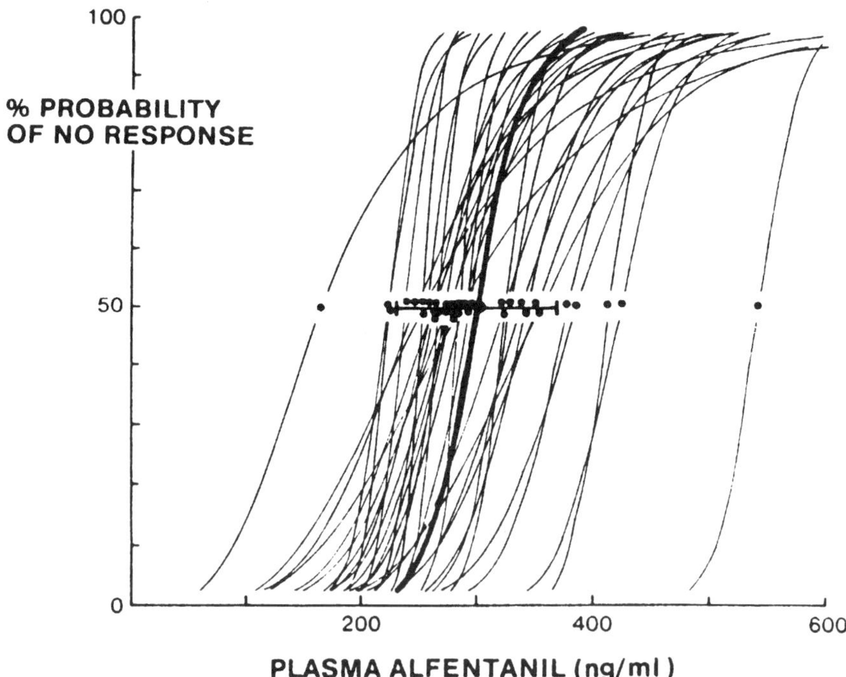

Figure 12.2. Alfentanil plasma concentration versus effect curves for each of 34 healthy young women during the intra-abdominal phase of lower abdominal gynecologic surgery for infertility problems. Patients received alfentanil and 66% nitrous oxide in oxygen. The Cp_{50} (dots) and slope of each curve were defined from multiple quantal responses or nonresponses of each patient using logistic regression. The heavy dark line represents the average data for all 34 patients, and the bracket indicates ±SD of the mean Cp_{50}. (Reproduced with the permission of Lippincott-Raven Publishers from Ausems et al., 1988.)

have no known toxicity to limit the concentrations tolerated by patients whose ventilation is supported mechanically, but it leads to excessive dosage, drug accumulation, and prolonged recovery times (see the discussion of context-sensitive half-time earlier in the chapter) (Hall et al., 1993). The second approach is to titrate the drug dose or concentration to the individual patient's need under the particular circumstances (Ausems et al., 1986, 1988). This is a challenging and work-intensive task, which generally requires limiting the use of muscle relaxants to the degree and time actually required in order to allow somatic responses indicative of inadequate anesthesia. It also requires that the drug concentration be progressively reduced in the absence of any response to ongoing noxious stimulation until the patient actually responds, thereby providing an indication of the minimal drug level required to suppress responsiveness. This procedure takes time and effort and requires the anesthesiologist to educate surgeons, nurses, technicians, and others about the rationale for allowing the patient to respond. It is most easily accomplished with drugs having a

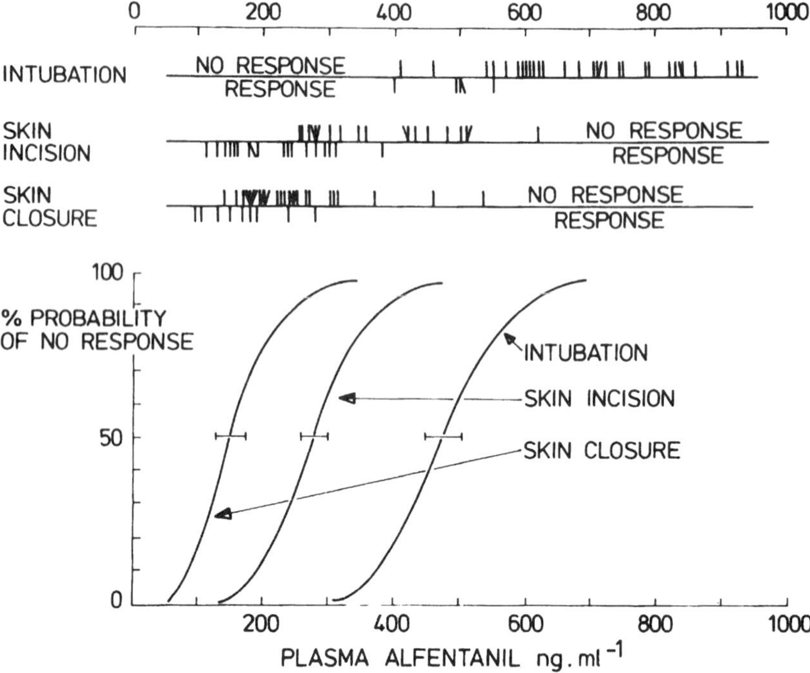

Figure 12.3. Relationship between plasma concentrations of alfentanil combined with 66% nitrous oxide and their effects on the responses of 57 patients to three specific noxious stimuli of short duration. The plasma concentration-effect curves for these three stimuli were defined from quantal data (response or no response) using logistic regression. The brackets indicate ±SE of the Cp_{50} value for each stimulus. (Reproduced with the permission of Lippincott-Raven Publishers from Ausems et al., 1986.)

short latency to peak effect and employing computer-controlled infusion devices that can quickly and reliably achieve stable drug levels in blood (plasma)[2] and rapidly make proportional changes (up and down) so that the anesthesiologist can define the individual patient's therapeutic window (effective concentration range of the drug) (Ausems et al., 1988). Drugs with a short latency to peak effect and a short context-sensitive half-time (e.g., sevoflurane, desflurane, alfentanil, and remifentanil) facili-

[2]Computers programmed with average pharmacokinetic values typically produce actual drug concentrations in blood (plasma) within ±20% of the concentration chosen by the anesthesiologist. In practice, these differences between the actual concentration produced and the concentration chosen by the anesthetist are not a problem because the computer allows rapid changes in the concentration if the concentration proves excessive or inadequate. The real benefit of computer control is (1) rapid achievement of a stable drug concentration, the effects of which can be evaluated by the anesthesiologist; and (2) rapid changes in the actual concentration in direct proportion to the changes in the target concentration entered into the computer. In addition, the computer can keep track of the total amount of drug used and simulate the rate of decline of drug concentrations and recovery time once drug administration is discontinued.

tate the up-and-down titration of drug concentration to meet the individual patient's needs under the particular circumstances.

Dosing Guidelines

Given the high degree of variability among individual patients in the doses and concentrations of opioids required to relieve pain and suffering in the awake patient and to prevent unwanted responses to noxious stimulation in the anesthetized patient, only very broad and generalized guidelines can be offered. It is extremely important for the practitioner to keep in mind the factors that contribute to alterations in the dosage requirements for opioids. Among the numerous factors that have been identified, the most important in practical terms are the intensity and duration of noxious stimulation, the presence of other drugs, and the patient's physiologic age and degree of functional impairment produced by the disease.

In terms of intraoperative use of the opioids, the most commonly used drugs are fentanyl, morphine, and their congeners. In addition, there is the new ultrashort-acting fentanyl derivative remifentanil (Michelsen and Hug, 1997). Guidelines for these drugs can be interpolated to their congeners on the basis of comparative analgesic potencies.

In terms of intraoperative use, two major dose ranges may be considered. So-called "high dose opioid anesthesia" employs an opioid as the primary anesthetic agent along with a skeletal muscle relaxant, and the opioid is supplemented with small intravenous doses of a hypnotic (e.g., barbiturate, benzodiazepine, etomidate, propofol) or major tranquilizer (e.g., droperidol). Alternatively, nitrous oxide or relatively low-inspired concentration of a volatile anesthetic (e.g., isoflurane) can be used to minimize the risk of arousal, awareness, and postoperative recall of intraoperative events. This type of anesthesia is generally reserved for critically ill patients who are expected to require postoperative intensive care, including mechanical ventilation. However, the availability of the ultrashort-acting remifentanil may broaden the use of this high-dose opioid technique to other types of patients undergoing a broader variety of surgical operations. Typical dose ranges for "opioid anesthesia" for morphine are 0.5–3 mg/kg (duration of approximately 4 hours), for fentanyl 10–20 μg/kg loading dose plus 1–4 μg/kg/hours, and for remifentanil 1–3 μg/kg/minute.

Much lower dose levels, usually close to the dosage range used to produce analgesia in the conscious patient, are needed when the opioids are used as supplements to general anesthetic agents (e.g., isoflurane, propofol). Typical opioid dosages used for preanesthetic medication, monitored anesthesia care in conjunction with an intravenous hypnotic, and supplementation of general, regional, or local anesthesia are as follows: morphine 2–10 mg IV to start and an average of 2–3 mg/hour, fentanyl 25–150 μg IV to start and an average of 0.5–2 μg/kg/hour for maintenance, and remifentanil 0.25–1 μg/kg/minute for maintenance with or without a loading dose.

Again, the key issue is to titrate the dose of each individual drug to each patient's needs in order to avoid risky degrees of ventilatory depression in the spontaneously breathing patient and prolonged recovery times in the patient maintained with mechanical ventilation. One practical guideline is to maintain a respiratory frequency greater then 10 breaths per minute in the spontaneously breathing patient. At this spontaneous ventilatory rate, the analgesic effect of the opioid is usually satisfactory because analgesia and respiratory depression go together.

REFERENCES

Ausems, M.E., Hug, C.C., Jr., Stanski, D.R., and Burm, A.G.L. (1986). Plasma concentrations of alfentanil required to supplement nitrous oxide anesthesia for general surgery. *Anesthesiology.* **65,** 362–373.

Ausems, M.E., Vuyk, J., Hug, C.C., Jr., and Stanski, D.R. (1988). Comparison of a computer-assisted infusion versus intermittent bolus administration of alfentanil to supplement nitrous oxide for lower abdominal surgery. *Anesthesiology.* **68,** 851–861.

Egan, T.D. (1996). Remifentanil pharmacokinetics and pharmacodynamics. A preliminary appraisal. *Clin. Pharmacokinet.* **29,** 80–94.

Hall, R.I., Moldenhauer, C.C., and Hug, C.C., Jr. (1993). Fentanyl plasma concentrations maintained by a simple infusion scheme in patients undergoing cardiac surgery. *Anesth. Analg.* **76,** 957–963.

Hug, C.C., Jr. (1990). Does opioid "anesthesia" exist? *Anesthesiology.* **73,** 1–4.

Hughes, M.A., Glass, P.S.A., and Jacobs, J.R. (1992). Context-sensitive half-time in multi-compartment pharmacokinetic models for intravenous anesthetic drugs. *Anesthesiology.* **76,** 334–341.

Lowenstein, E., Hallowell, P., Levine, F.H., et al. (1969). Cardiovascular response to large doses of intravenous morphine. *N. Engl. J. Med.* **281,** 1389–1393.

Michelsen, L.G., and Hug, C.C., Jr. (in press). The pharmacokinetics of remifentanil. *J. Clin. Anesth.*

Stanley, T.H., and Webster, L.R. (1978). Anesthetic requirements and cardiovascular effects of fentanyl-oxygen and fentanyl-diazepam-oxygen in man. *Anesth. Analg.* **57,** 411–416.

CHAPTER THIRTEEN

Opioids in Acute Pain

NARINDER RAWAL

Introduction

Despite many advances in our understanding of pain pathophysiology, development of new drugs, and sophisticated drug-delivery systems, a majority of surgical patients continue to receive inadequate therapy for postoperative pain. Historically, the treatment of postoperative pain has been given low priority by both surgeons and anesthesiologists, so that patients have accepted pain as a necessary part of the postoperative experience (Spence, 1980; Mitchell and Smith, 1989; Warfield and Kahn, 1995).

Ineffective pain management has significant implications for patient well-being. Patients in pain suffer more complications, which can lead to longer hospital stays. Although much remains to be done, specialists find that improvements are taking place gradually. Anesthesiology based acute pain services (APS) are playing an increasingly important role in these developments (Ready et al., 1988; Rawal and Berggren, 1994). Evidence is growing that improved analgesia may be associated with less morbidity and mortality and with lower hospitalization costs (Rawal et al., 1984; Yeager et al., 1987; Tuman et al., 1991).

Opioid-Analgesic Drugs

Opioids are the most extensively used analgesics in the management of moderate to severe acute pain and in pain related to malignant disease. Opioids produce their effect by binding to specific opioid receptors located in the brain, spinal cord, and other areas of the body. They have been shown to have specific antinociceptive receptor effects at several sites within the brain, including periaqueductal gray, rostral ventral medulla, and substantia nigra and also within the dorsal horn of the spinal cord. Additionally, opioids have antinociceptive effects mediated through peripheral μ and κ receptors in inflamed tissue (Stein et al., 1989). Several receptor populations have been identified, for example, μ, κ, and δ. It has been proposed that these receptors have their subpopulations – for example, that the μ receptor has two subtypes, μ_1, which mediates analgesia, whereas μ_2 is responsible for respiratory depression and physical dependence. Understandably, much research is focused on

Christoph Stein, ed., *Opioids in Pain Control: Basic and Clinical Aspects*. Printed in the United States of America.

Table 13.1. *Pharmacologic Profiles of Opioid Receptors*

Mu-1 (μ_1)	**Mu-2** (μ_2)	**Kappa** (κ)	**Delta** (δ)
Analgesia	Analgesia	Analgesia	Analgesia
Supraspinal	—	Supraspinal	Supraspinal
Spinal	Spinal	Spinal	Spinal
—	Respiratory depression	Sedation	Respiratory depression
Euphoria	—	Dysphoria	—
Low addiction potential	Addiction risk	Low addiction potential	Addiction risk
—	Constipation	—	Constipation (minimal risk)
Bradycardia	—	—	—
Hypothermia	—	—	—
Urinary retention	—	Diuresis	—

developing pure μ_1 agonists (Table 13.1). Based on their effects on opioid receptors, opioid drugs may be agonists, antagonists, partial agonists, or agonist-antagonists.

Opioids are still the main drugs for relief of pain. Morphine-3-glucuronide (M3G) and morphine-6-glucuronide (M6G) are the main metabolites of morphine. The relative importance of these metabolites to the pharmacologic characteristics and clinical effects of morphine continues to be debated. Animal studies have demonstrated that M6G binds to μ receptors, whereas M3G has very low affinity for opioid receptors and does not possess analgesic activity. Indeed, M3G has been shown to antagonize morphine and M6G-induced analgesia and respiratory depression in the rat. This is the basis of the hypothesis that M3G is associated with tolerance development. M3G is also believed to be responsible for conditions such as hyperalgesia, allodynia, and myoclonus, which are seen after high-dose morphine treatment (Yaksh and Harty, 1987; Christup, 1997).

Recent research related to opioids has concentrated on developing new drugs based on increased knowledge of opioid receptors and developing newer drug-delivery systems for old drugs based on increasing knowledge of their pharmacokinetics and pharmacodynamics.

Opioid Agonists

Several new agonist (alfentanil, sufentanil, remifentanil), antagonist (naltrexone, nalmefene), and agonist-antagonist (nalbuphine, buprenorphine, butorphanol, meptazinol, dezocine) drugs have been introduced recently. The pure agonist opioids alfentanil and sufentanil act on μ receptors, and their analgesic effects are intense and dose related. Both opioids are highly lipophilic and have a short onset of action and fast elimination and are, therefore, well suited for administration by infusion. However, these drugs have not been used much by intravenous route for treating postoperative pain. In contrast, the combination of high receptor affinity and high lipid solubility makes these opioids particularly attractive for epidural administration. Both drugs have been used for treating postoperative pain either alone or in combination with local anesthetic drugs. Many new agonist opioids are more potent, but they may not represent an advance because a wider margin between analgesia and respiratory depression has not been demonstrated.

Opioids in Ambulatory Surgery

The rate of recovery following opioid administration is determined by the duration of drug administration as well as by the rate of distribution and elimination. Adverse effects such as prolonged respiratory depression are avoided by drug titration and use of adjustable infusion. Appropriate titration with the newest opioid, remifentanil, an ultrashort-acting opioid that hydrolyzes rapidly by esterases, may eliminate the concern over residual respiratory depression. However, rapid recovery has to be balanced against the need for additional postoperative analgesics.

Agonist-Antagonist Opioids

The agonist-antagonist opioids are a heterogeneous group that differ considerably from pure antagonists. These differences are invaluable in understanding opioid action, pain, and addiction. With pure agonists, increasing the dose generally causes an increase in analgesia and respiratory depression. Measurement of efficacy is difficult with agonist-antagonist opioids mainly because dose-response relationships for these drugs are not linear. In low drug concentration the agonist effect predominates, whereas in higher concentrations the antagonist effect is predominant. Thus, the drug may have low efficacy at higher doses.

Much has been written about the decreased risk of respiratory depression exhibited by these drugs. A "ceiling effect" on respiration has been demonstrated for nalbuphine, buprenorphine, dezocine, and meptazinol. Increasing the dose of an opioid will not increase respiratory depression after a certain point, since the respiratory depression is believed to reach a plateau. Some of the agonist-antagonist opioids may be safer because of a ceiling effect for respiratory depression, but the ceiling also applies to analgesia. In general, these drugs have good adverse effect profiles; serious respiratory depression is uncommon; and nausea, constipation, and urinary retention occur less frequently than with morphine. However, serious respiratory depression has been reported with agonist-antagonist drugs (Sekar and Mimpriss, 1987; Thörn et al., 1988; Rosow, 1989).

Table 13.2. *Adverse Effects of Opioids*

Organ System	Possible Adverse Effects
Central nervous system	Sedation, miosis, euphoria, nausea and vomiting, addiction risk
Respiratory system	Respiratory depression, apnea
Gastrointestinal system	Delayed gastric emptying, constipation
Cardiovascular system	Bradycardia, myocardial depression
Genitourinary system	Urinary retention
Other	Pruritus, allergy

Of the currently available agonist-antagonists, buprenorphine is probably the most widely used. It is a lipophilic agent with high receptor affinity. Its potency is about 25–50 times that of morphine, and its duration of action is about 5–6 hours after intramuscular injection. The drug has excellent absorption by sublingual route and has been used extensively for the management of postoperative and cancer pain. Although a ceiling effect for respiratory depression has been demonstrated in animals, significant respiratory depression may occur with doses used clinically. The nonreversibility of buprenorphine-induced respiratory depression by naloxone has been reported by many investigators (Sekar and Mimpriss, 1987; Thörn et al., 1988). The respiratory stimulant doxapram may be more suitable if respiratory depression occurs after buprenorphine.

In the literature many studies have demonstrated the successful use of systemic agonist-antagonist drugs such as nalbuphine to reduce the risk of spinal opioid-induced adverse effects such as pruritus, urinary retention, and respiratory depression.

Adverse Effects of Opioids

Table 13.2 shows the possible adverse effects of opioids. With short-term, moderate-dose opioid treatment, as in postoperative pain management, the CNS and gastrointestinal side effects predominate. Sedation, dizziness, miosis, respiratory depression, nausea, and vomiting appear to be dose dependent. Biliary colic as a result of spasm of sphincter of Oddi tends to occur more frequently after morphine as compared with pethidine administration. Opioids may increase sphincter tone and release antidiuretic hormone resulting in urinary retention. Opioid tolerance and physical dependence are unusual in the postoperative setting but can be a problem with chronic opioid treatment. Excessive opioid doses may lead to respiratory depression, apnea, circulatory collapse, coma, and death. The equianalgesic doses of different opioids are shown in Table 13.3. The two most feared side effects of opioid administration are respiratory depression and addiction risk.

Table 13.3. *Analgesic Doses of Opioids That Are Equianalgesic with IM Dose of 10 mg Morphine*

Opioid	IM Dose (mg)	Oral Dose (mg)
Pethidine	100	400
Methadone	8–10	15–20
Morphine	10	30–60
Heroin	3–5	50–60
Codeine	130	200
Hydromorphone	1.5	6–8
Buprenorphine	0.3–0.4	0.4 (sublingueal)
Nalbuphine	10	—
Butorphanol	2	—

Methods of Postoperative Analgesia

Opioids remain the most useful drugs for treating moderate to severe pain. Table 13.4 shows the methods available to treat postoperative pain. Opioids can be administered by several routes, each offering advantages and disadvantages (Table 13.5).

Intramuscular Administration of Analgesics

Postoperative pain has been traditionally managed with intermittent injection of intramuscular opioids. Often a standard dose is prescribed on an "as needed" basis. The standard practice of injecting intramuscular opioids on demand yields poor results for several reasons. Among the reasons are difficulties in quantifying pain, widely varying analgesic requirements depending on type of surgery and location of surgical incision, and varying pharmacokinetics among individuals. Failure to recognize the extent of pain and fear of precipitating respiratory depression may lead to analgesia being withheld, resulting in irregular administration, fluctuating plasma levels, and, hence, inadequate pain relief. Intramuscular injections are painful, and the technique induces a feeling of dependency on the nursing staff.

Despite these disadvantages, intermittent intramuscular opioids remain the most common method of administering postoperative analgesia. The technique of injecting intramuscular opioids on demand represents familiar practice – generations of nurses have used the technique, and it may therefore be safe because of accumulated experience. Since no special equipment is required, the technique is simple and inexpensive. Gradual onset of analgesia allows observation of gradual onset of possible overdose.

Table 13.4. *Postoperative Analgesia Techniques*

I.	**Administration of opioids**
	Intramuscular injection
	Subcutaneous (intermittent bolus injection, continuous infusion)
	Oral (tablets, mixture)
	Patient-controlled analgesia (PCA)
	Rectal
	Intravenous (intermittent bolus, continuous infusion)
	Epidural (intermittent bolus, continuous infusion)
	Sublingual
	Oral transmucosal (Oralet) ("lollipop")
	Transdermal (regular "patch," iontophoresis "patch")
	Intranasal
II.	**Administration of nonopioid analgesics**
	Paracetamol (oral, rectal)
	Nonsteroidal anti-inflammatory drugs (NSAIDs) (oral, rectal, IM, IV, intra-articular)
	Dipyrone (Novalgin) (oral, rectal, IM, IV)
III.	**Regional techniques**
	Epidural (local anesthetics and/or opioids, and/or clonidine)
	Spinal (local anesthetics and/or opioids, and/or clonidine)
	Paravertebral
	Peripheral nerve blocks
	Wound infiltration
	Interpleural
	Intra-articular (local anesthetic and/or opioid)
IV.	**Nonpharmacologic methods**
	Transcutaneous electrical nerve stimulation (TENS)
	Cryoanalgesia
	Acupuncture
V.	**Psychological methods**

However, too frequently adequate analgesia is not achieved by this approach. Pain is not necessarily constant throughout the postoperative period, and an increase in pain may follow movement and physiotherapy. The goal of opioid administration is to find the often narrow therapeutic window between unrelieved pain and excessive sedation and respiratory depression. Drug and dose selection as well as dosing frequency should be individualized. Frequent evaluation of the adequacy of pain therapy is

Table 13.5. *Advantages and Disadvantages of Different Routes of Opioid Administration*

Method of Administration	Advantages	Disadvantages
Oral	• Convenient for staff and patients • Inexpensive • Simple	• Absorption slow and variable • Impractical after surgery due to risk of vomiting and delayed gastric emptying • Problem with first-pass metabolism of morphine
Intramuscular	• Convenient for staff • Inexpensive	• Absorption slow and variable • Uncomfortable for patients
Rectal	• Feasible when oral or parenteral administration not possible • Useful for children	• Absorption slow and variable • Cultural objections in some countries
Intravenous infusion	• Administration simple • Guaranteed absorption	• Risk of respiratory depression and hypoxia • Risk of malfunction with infusion pump • Requires careful monitoring
IV bolus (titrated to effect)	• Enables individualization of therapy • Inexpensive	• Staff training required
Patient-controlled analgesia (PCA)	• High patient satisfaction • Enables individualization of therapy	• Expensive equipment • Risk of malfunction/error • Staff training required • Strict monitoring (labor intensive)
Epidural opioids	• Excellent analgesia at small doses • Superior to other methods • Improves postoperative outcome in high-risk patients	• Requires skilled anesthesiologist • Risk of delayed respiratory depression • Strict monitoring (labor intensive)
Peripheral nerve blocks	• Excellent analgesia • Superior to other methods • No cardiovascular or respiratory problems	• Requires skilled anesthesiologist

important. It should be recognized that properly administered opioids can provide excellent analgesia. With attentive nursing care, appropriate drug and dosing selection, and frequent pain assessment, conventional intramuscular opioid therapy can become “on demand” and may be as effective as PCA.

Intravenous Analgesic Administration

Intravenous Infusions

To achieve rapid analgesia in the early postoperative period small boluses of intravenous opioids are commonly administered. Intravenous administration of analgesics delivers a more predictable maximum concentration as compared to oral or intramuscular administration because the absorption process is eliminated. The main advantage is the rapid onset of pain relief. However, intermittent injections will result in wide fluctuations of plasma concentration. Due to rapid decline of plasma levels the analgesic effect may be of short duration, and continuous intravenous infusions have been used. Lipophilic opioids with rapid onset of action (fentanyl, alfentanil, pethidine) are preferable to morphine for this route of opioid administration. There is always a risk of respiratory depression, and periods of apnea associated with arterial desaturation have been reported. The technique should therefore be used only in high-dependency areas. It has been developed further by the additional demand bolus analgesia and is better known as patient-controlled analgesia (PCA) (see Chapter 14 this volume).

Intravenously Titrated Bolus Injections

This is an excellent method to obtain rapid pain relief and is commonly used in postanesthesia recovery rooms, neonatal units, and burns units. The method is also recommended to manage episodes of "breakthrough pain" or "incident pain" experienced during physiotherapy, dressing changes, and cancer pain therapy. Small doses of opioids are titrated to effect, thus achieving the most important goal of pain management – individualized analgesia. At our institution, ward nurses administer 1–2 mg morphine every 4–5 minutes until the pain score is 3 or below on the 10-grade visual analog scale (VAS). The technique is used when PCA is not indicated or there is a shortage of PCA pumps. The patient is monitored for 30 minutes (bedside nurse presence is not necessary); a sedation score below 2 (on a 4-grade score) and respiratory rate above 10/minute are aimed for. At our institution, this technique has replaced IM opioid injection as the most common analgesic technique on all surgical wards. Although pain management by IV-titrated bolus opioid injections is labor intensive, our nursing staff have accepted this technique because they have experienced that the advantages outweigh the problems due to the somewhat increased workload. Since 1991, pain has been assessed every 3 hours in all patients undergoing surgery; the hospital policy is to maintain a VAS ≤3 at all times.

Subcutaneous Administration

As with other routes of opioid administration, morphine is still the most common opioid for intermittent or continuous subcutaneous administration. Drugs given by this route should be in such concentrations that large volumes are avoided because they may be a cause of local pain. The dosage, uptake of morphine into circulation, clinical effects, and adverse effects are also similar to those following intramuscular morphine administration. A more comfortable alternative for the patient is subcutaneous administration via an indwelling, fine plastic cannula fixed with a transparent dressing below the clavicle or close to the umbilicus. Injections through this indwelling cannula eliminate the need for painful, repeated injections. This technique is commonly used in the treatment of cancer pain; it is also recommended as a more humane alternative to repeated IM injections for management of postoperative pain.

Oral Administration

Oral administration is generally regarded as unsuitable for administering opioids in early postoperative period because of the delay in gastric emptying and consequently the lack of absorption of the drug from the small intestine. Oral opioids have low bioavailability because of first-pass metabolism in the liver. How ever, these drugs may be useful in treating pain after outpatient surgery and in the late postoperative period when the gastrointestinal function has recovered after major surgery.

Slow-release morphine is believed to achieve more sustained blood concentrations than intramuscular morphine and offers the advantage of ease of administration. It is commonly used for the treatment of cancer pain, but it has no role in postoperative pain because of its slow onset of action. The equianalgesic doses of some of the commonly used analgesics are shown in Table 13.3.

Rectal Administration

Treatment of postoperative pain by rectal-administered drugs depends greatly on traditions and routines in various countries. Thus, it is a common method in Scandinavian countries and in France, but almost taboo in Greece, Portugal, and Ireland (Rawal et al., 1996). The technique is useful in children who dislike the pain and discomfort of intramuscular injection. Absorption of drugs is unaffected by nausea, vomiting, or delay in gastric emptying.

As compared to oral administration, the rectal route has the advantage of possible avoidance of the first-pass effect, since the portal system is bypassed. Morphine and NSAIDs such as diclofenac, ibuprofen, and naproxen have been successfully employed as postoperative analgesics. Oral NSAIDs may cause dyspepsia, gastric erosions, or bleeding; however, the use of suppositories may reduce these adverse effects. Although the risks are not completely eliminated because gastric irritation is not a local effect only, plasma concentrations of the drug also play an important role. At our institution, about 20,000 patients undergo surgery annually; unless there is a contraindication (liver disease, rectal disease), all patients receive a paracetamol suppository as "base analgesia" every 6 hours. Adults and older children administer the drug themselves. The dosage is 1 g for adults and 15–20 mg/kg for children.

Sublingual Administration

Buprenorphine is a potent synthetic agonist-antagonist opioid with a high receptor affinity and a slow dissociation constant of drug-receptor complex, which permits a prolonged drug effect in the presence of low plasma concentrations. Tablets may be removed from the mouth in the event of overdosage, and accidental swallowing does not result in toxicity because of high first-pass hepatic metabolism and resultant low bioavailability. The major disadvantages are the relatively high degree of sedation and nausea. Respiratory depression when it occurs can be severe and prolonged and is not reversible by naloxone (Sekar and Mimpriss, 1987; Thörn et al., 1988).

Oral Transmucosal Route

Fentanyl incorporated into a candy matrix and formulated in a lollipop is a novel method of opioid administration. Studies in adult volunteers have shown that oral transmucosal fentanyl produces dose-dependent increases in sedation and analgesia. These fentanyl lollipops have also been used successfully for premedication in children. Doses around 15–20 mg/kg appear satisfactory. However, the incidence of adverse effects, such as facial pruritus and nausea, was high. Larger doses were associated with considerable respiratory depression and an extremely high incidence of pruritus, nausea, and vomiting (Feld et al., 1989; Stanley et al., 1989). The concept of administering opioids via a nonthreatening and psychologically appealing delivery system appears attractive. Data from the studies just cited suggest that the palatable lollipops were readily accepted by the children. In the United States the lollipops are marketed under the name Oralet. Further studies are necessary to confirm that this novel method has a wider application for premedication and postoperative analgesia.

Intranasal Administration

The nasal route is less traumatic than intramuscular injection and is more aesthetic than rectal administration, and it may be particularly acceptable to children. Butorphanol, fentanyl, and sufentanil have been administered intranasally to treat moderate to severe pain. Both drugs have also been used for premedication. Intranasal cocaine has been known to drug addicts for a long time. In recent years other drugs, such as midazolam, ketamine, and nitroglycerine, have been used in anesthesiology. Sufentanil is preferred to fentanyl because smaller volumes are required due to the higher potency of the drug. Sufentanil in total dose of 10–20 μg and doses of 1.5–3 μg/kg has been shown to provide effective preoperative sedation of rapid onset. However, in children receiving larger doses (4.5 μg/kg) intranasal sufentanil was associated with vomiting, marked decrease in ventilatory compliance, muscular rigidity, and convulsive activity (Henderson et al., 1988; Vercauteren et al., 1988). At our institution, fentanyl 1 μg/kg is frequently used to treat pain in the recovery room in situations in which the child has pulled out the intravenous line. Intranasal fentanyl is not associated with the burning sensation that is reported with other drugs such as sufentanil and midazolam. A patient-controlled intranasal analgesia (PCINA) device has been described (Striebel et al., 1996).

Transdermal (PCA) Iontophoresis

Currently available PCA devices are expensive and require ongoing maintenance. Some devices are bulky, which may delay early ambulation. Many are perceived as complex to program, increasing the risk of dose error. There is a great potential for developing PCA techniques that are more flexible and easier to use. One approach under investigation is the transdermal administration of opioids by electro-transport. Pressing a button on a skin patch starts active transdermal transport of the opioid by iontophoresis. Transfer of ionized drugs can be facilitated by a small current across two electrodes, one above the drug reservoir and the other at a distal skin site. The dose can be adjusted by the delivery current to avoid a depot effect; drug delivery can be stopped by switching off the current (Gangarosa, 1993). Preliminary results with fentanyl and morphine are encouraging, and the product is expected to be on the market soon. By offering an important alternative to traditional approaches to PCA, this modality has the potential to make the PCA technique more widely available.

Spinal Opioids and Postoperative Pain

Unless specified otherwise, the term *spinal* has been employed as a generic equivalent to both epidural and intrathecal (subarachnoid) in this chapter.

The discovery of spinal opioid receptors has opened new horizons in pain management. By bypassing the blood and the blood-brain barrier, small doses of opioids administered in either the subarachnoid or epidural spaces provide profound and prolonged segmental analgesia. This approach undoubtedly represents a major breakthrough in pain management. Since their introduction into clinical practice in 1979, spinal opioids have achieved great international popularity in a variety of clinical settings, either as sole analgesic agents or in combination with low-dose local anesthetics. Numerous studies have shown that spinal opioids can provide profound postoperative analgesia with less central and systemic adverse effects than opioids administered systematically. Segmental analgesia induced by intraspinal opioids has a role in the management of a wide variety of surgical and nonsurgical painful conditions. The technique has been employed successfully to treat intraoperative, postoperative, traumatic, obstetric, chronic, and cancer pain (Cousins and Mather, 1984; Vercauteren, 1993).

Management of postoperative pain is the commonest indication for spinal opioid analgesia. The techniques have been used to provide pain relief following a wide variety of surgeries such as upper and lower abdominal and thoracic surgery, including cardiac, perineal, and orthopedic surgery. Spinal opioids have also been used to provide analgesia in different age groups including children and are considered particu-

Table 13.6. *Lipid Solubility, Doses, Onset, and Analgesia Duration of the Most Common Opioids for Epidural Administration*

Opioid	Lipid Solubility**	Bolus Dose†	Onset (minutes)	Duration (hours)
Morphine	1	2–5 mg	30–60	12–24
Hydromorphone	1.4	1.0–1.5 mg	20–30	6–12
Diamorphine	10.0	2–6 mg	10–15	6–12
Pethidine	28.0	25–75 mg	10–20	4–8
Methadone	82.0	6–8 mg	10–20	4–8
Fentanyl	580	50–100 μg	10–15	2–4
Sufentanil	1,270	20–50 μg	5–10	2–4

*Data are from different studies and therefore are not strictly comparable.
**Octanol partition coefficient in relation to morphine.
†Doses should be reduced for elderly and high-risk patients.

larly beneficial in elderly high-risk patients. A large number of controlled studies have documented the efficacy of the technique for postoperative pain. In terms of analgesia and restoration of postoperative pulmonary function following abdominal or thoracic surgery, the technique has been found to be superior to alternative methods such as intermittent IM injection of opioids, PCA with IV opioids, intercostal block, and epidural block with local anesthetics. The technique has been applied for treating pain from fractured ribs and in ICU patients with multiple injuries. It should be emphasized that most of these impressive results are seen when the opioid used is morphine.

The unique feature of spinal opioid analgesia is the lack of sensory, sympathetic, or motor block, which allows patients to ambulate without the risk of orthostatic hypotension or motor incoordination usually associated with local anesthetics administered epidurally or opioids administered parenterally. These advantages of spinal opioids are particularly beneficial in high-risk patients undergoing major surgery, patients with compromised pulmonary or cardiovascular function, grossly obese patients, and elderly patients (Rawal et al., 1984; Yeager et al., 1987; Tuman et al., 1991).

When an opioid is administered in the epidural space it has to cross the dura before reaching the opioid receptors in the spinal cord. In addition to the physical barrier presented by the dura, the epidural space is highly vascularized and also contains variable amounts of fat and connective tissue. These factors influence the pharmacokinetics of epidurally administered opioids. Depending on the lipophilicity of the opioid, a certain portion of the drug enters the CSF and spinal cord after crossing the dura, a certain portion enters the systemic circulation via epidural veins, and a certain portion binds to epidural fat. Lipophilicity facilitates systemic absorption of opioids.

In general, highly lipid-soluble drugs such as fentanyl and sufentanil have a more rapid onset and shorter duration of effect than hydrophilic drugs such as morphine (Table 13.6). The hydrophilic opioids are cleared slowly from CSF, resulting in high concentrations of the drug spreading rostrally with bulk flow of CSF and saturating the entire length of the spinal cord. Thus, administration of epidural morphine at the caudal or lower lumbar level will provide analgesia for upper abdominal or thoracic surgery. In contrast, lipophilic opioids such as fentanyl and sufentanil provide a more segmental analgesic effect; therefore, the efficacy of these opioids is dependent on the siting of the epidural catheter.

The long duration of analgesia of epidural morphine allows it to be used as an intermittent bolus twice a day whereas opioids such as fentanyl and sufentanil are better suited for continuous infusion because of their short duration of analgesia.

Adverse Effects of Epidural Opioids

Some of the reported adverse effects of epidural opioids such as nausea, vomiting, somnolence, and early respiratory depression are dose dependent and are believed to be due to the vascular uptake into systemic circulation. The characteristic adverse effects of epidural opioids are pruritus, urinary retention, and late-onset respiratory depression.

Pruritus

The reported incidence of itching following opioids is quite variable; the probable reason is that if not asked specifically, the majority of patients do not complain about this complication because of its mild nature. The risk of severe, distressing itching is extremely low. Pregnant patients appear more at risk whatever opioid is administered. Patients treated for malignant or chronic pain with epidural or intrathecal opioids do not experience pruritus after the first or second day, presumably because of rapid development of tolerance.

The exact mechanism for epidural opioid-induced pruritus is unclear, but it is presumed to be centrally mediated due to activation of μ receptors. Small doses of naloxone can be used to treat pruritus without reversing analgesia. Other opioid antagonists such as naltrexone and nalmefene, antihistaminic drugs, agonist-antagonist opioids such as butorphanol and nalbuphine, and subhypnotic doses of the anesthetic induction agent propofol have all been successfully used to treat pruritus (Wittels et al., 1993; Kendrick et al., 1996; Warwick et al., 1997).

Urinary Retention

It is difficult to establish the incidence of urinary retention since a majority of patients who receive epidural analgesia are patients undergoing major surgery who are usually catheterized. Cystometric studies have demonstrated that whatever the dose epidural morphine reduces the strength of detrusor contraction, leading to a corresponding increase in bladder volume. These changes can be prevented and reversed by naloxone (Rawal et al., 1983). However, if naloxone is given in large doses, the reversal of urodynamic effects of epidural morphine will be achieved at the cost of partial or complete reversal of analgesia (Rawal et al., 1986). In general, if patients are unable to void 6 hours after surgery, a single in-and-out catheterization is indicated to prevent myogenic bladder damage because of prolonged overdistention.

Respiratory Depression

One major advantage of epidural versus parenteral opioid administration is the greatly reduced risk of respiratory depression. Indeed, the most common indication for epidural opioids is the management of postoperative pain in high-risk patients undergoing major surgery. However, delayed respiratory depression occurring several hours after opioid administration is the most serious side effect of this technique. Delayed respiratory depression is believed to result from rostral spread of opioids in the CSF to the brainstem and respiratory center (Cousins and Mather, 1984; Morgan, 1989; Etches et al., 1989).

Today we have a better understanding of the pattern of respiratory depression. It is slow and progressive in onset rather than a sudden apneic event. It should be noted that respiratory rate alone is unreliable for establishing the presence or lack of respiratory depression. Monitoring of level of consciousness (usually on a four-grade scale) is important because increasing sedation is associated with advancing respiratory depression. The belief that lipophilic opioids (fentanyl, sufentanil, pethidine) are safer than morphine because they do not spread rostrally in the CSF is being increasingly questioned (Etches et al., 1989; Rawal, 1992). Delayed respiratory depression after epidural opioids is extremely rare (0.1% to 1%), is unpredictable, and can occur with any opioid. As with opioids administered by any route, the risk of respiratory depression after epidural opioids in large doses is increased with advanced age, with concomitant use of systemic opioids and/or sedatives, in high-risk patients, and in opioid-naive patients (Table 13.7). It is generally accepted that all patients receiving epidural opioids should be monitored for at least 12 hours after epidural morphine, less time after lipophilic opioids. If trained staff can monitor respiratory rate and sedation frequently (every hour), there is no reason why the patients cannot be nursed on regular surgical wards. In addition, pulse oximetry can also be used if available.

Combination of Local Anesthetics and Opioids

The rationale for the combination technique is that these two types of drugs eliminate pain by acting at two distinct sites, the local anesthetic at the nerve axon and the opioid at the receptor site in the spinal cord. Spinal opioids alone provide good pain

Table 13.7. *Risk Factors for Respiratory Depression Following Epidural or Intrathecal Opioid Administration*

- Large doses (>5 mg epidural morphine, >0.3–0.4 mg intrathecal morphine)
- Advanced age
- High-risk patients (according to ASA classification)
- Opioid-naive patients
- Concomitant administration of other analgesics or sedatives
- Thoracic opioid administration (vs. lumbar)?

relief at rest but may not be adequate during physiotherapy and mobilization. Patients receiving a combination of low-dose local anesthetic and opioid have a more rapid onset of analgesia, more profound and longer-lasting pain relief, and less motor blockade than patients receiving either drug alone (Mourisse et al., 1992; Ferrante et al., 1993). For example, patients undergoing knee replacement surgery are not immediately ambulatory in the early postoperative period, making these patients uniquely suited for an analgesic regimen that includes some degree of neural blockade that facilitates vigorous physical therapy and continuous passive motion of the operated knee. Although combination therapy is used for postoperative and labor pain, the results are more impressive in labor pain because it is well recognized that labor pain is different from postoperative pain because it is not relieved by epidural opioids alone. Combination therapy as continuous infusion or as epidural PCA ("walking epidural") has been extensively studied in the obstetric population.

Despite convincing animal and clinical data, several controlled studies comparing combination therapy with opioids alone have questioned the practice of adding bupivacaine to opioid. Bupivacaine has the potential to cause local anesthetic–related side effects such as hypotension, motor weakness, urinary retention, and pressure sores due to skin sensory loss. The use of bupivacaine may delay mobilization in some patients. The optimum combination that has opioid-sparing synergistic effect without delaying mobilization is yet to be established. In some studies the combination of local anesthetic drugs and opioids did not improve analgesia and in fact was associated with increased morbidity. This has been reported for fentanyl-bupivacaine combination after orthopedic surgery and abdominal or thoracic surgery and for hydromorphone-bupivacaine combination after cesarean section (Badner et al., 1991; Badner and Westmore, 1992; Parker and White, 1992; Peach and Westmore, 1994).

A variety of factors influence the rate of epidural opioid infusion that is necessary for effective analgesia. These include the site and type of surgery, type of pain (labor vs. postsurgery), choice of opioid and its loading dose, volume of the injectate, concentration of the local anesthetic, and patient characteristics that influence epidural pharmacokinetics and pharmacodynamics of the given opioid. Siting of the catheter tip in the epidural space is also important; thus, bupivacaine 0.1% with fentanyl given through a lumbar catheter was associated with a high incidence of lower limb weakness whereas motor weakness was insignificant when local anesthetic (0.1–0.2% bupivacaine) was administered at the thoracic level (Dahl et al., 1992).

Patient-Controlled Epidural Analgesia (PCEA)

The increasing popularity of the IV PCA technique in pain management has generated interest in the use of epidural opioids via a PCA pump. This technique allows the patient to self-titrate an epidural opioid or opioid-local anesthetic combination to a desired level of analgesia. Epidural PCA can be expected to combine the flexibility and convenience of PCA with the superior analgesia of epidural opioids (Parker and White, 1992; Curry et al., 1994; Eagan and Ready, 1994). It has also been suggested that epidural PCA with opioids results in a more rapid recovery and shorter hospitalization than IV PCA or IM opioids (Bellamy et al., 1989; Lamer, 1990).

However, results from other studies of epidural PCA are less impressive. A high incidence of numbness and leg weakness during epidural infusion of 0.1% bupivacaine with opioid (fentanyl or morphine) has been reported.

Although the concept of PCA ensures adequate analgesia the selection of drug concentrations, combinations, bolus doses, lock-out intervals and basal infusion rates are often arbitrary, making comparisons between different studies difficult. It is also difficult to draw meaningful conclusions because of factors such as small patient populations with multiple surgical procedures, comparisons of different drugs and modes of delivery, and use of combinations consisting of a large variety of local anesthetic concentrations and opioid drugs and dosages (Boudreault et al., 1991; Ferrante et al., 1991; Glass et al., 1992; Cohen et al., 1993). The issues become more complicated by use of techniques in which the added drug may be a low-dose local anesthetic given to patients receiving continuous infusion of opioids, or vice versa – for example, epidural PCA with opioid to supplement a continuous infusion of local anesthetic. Another problem with epidural PCA is the role of the basal infusion mode. The mode has been questioned on the grounds that basal infusion leads to higher drug use without decreasing pain scores or the number of patient demands for analgesic medication. It has also been suggested that a programming error may have more serious consequences with a basal infusion mode than with the conventional intermittent dosing technique.

In general, there is a lack of randomized studies to identify the best lipophilic opioid. Appropriate dosage regimens for epidural PCA after different types of surgeries also need to be defined. Studies are also necessary to evaluate the cost-benefit ratio of this technique. These issues need to be addressed before the role of PCEA in pain management can be established.

Route Selection – Epidural or Intrathecal?

Whereas the efficacy, optimal dose, duration of analgesia, and adverse effects profile of epidural opioids have been extensively documented, there is a paucity of similar information for intrathecal opioids. The intrathecal route is a direct one because there is no dura to be penetrated and the drug is deposited close to its site of action – the opioid receptors.

Compared with the intrathecal route, epidural administration is complicated by the pharmacokinetics of dural penetration, epidural fat deposition, and systemic opioid absorption. Additionally, it is believed that the analgesia following intrathecal morphine administration is more predictable, more intense, and longer lasting than that following epidural morphine. This observation is particularly valid in multitrauma ICU patients (Rawal and Tandon, 1985) and in laboring parturients (Abboud et al., 1984). Intrathecal sufentanil has been shown to provide better and longer-lasting analgesia than epidural sufentanil for labor pain (Camann et al., 1993). Numerous reports have documented the excellent and prolonged analgesia following intrathecal administration of morphine.

Intrathecal administration of opioids has the advantages of simplicity, reliability, and low dose requirements. To compensate for the effects of systemic uptake and fat sequestration, the epidural dose of morphine is about 10–20 times greater than that required for intrathecal injection (Stoelting, 1989). Since excellent analgesia is achieved by a very small dose, the patients can be expected to be less sedated, more cooperative, and more mobile with all the attendant advantages.

In recent years reports of intrathecal administration of nonmorphine opioids have appeared in the literature. A technique that is simple and quick and that provides reliable and prolonged postoperative pain relief has obvious attraction.

The reasons for the limited popularity of the intrathecal as compared to the epidural route may be (1) catheter technology is unreliable at present; (2) there is risk of postdural puncture headache; (3) lipid-soluble opioids do not provide as prolonged analgesia as hydrophilic morphine (over 20 hours) after a single injection; (4) there is greater risk of adverse effects, including the dreaded late-onset respiratory depression; and (5) there is greater risk of spinal cord neurotoxicity.

Drug Selection

Opioids

The European survey showed that a variety of opioids are being used epidurally and intrathecally. Morphine and fentanyl are the commonest opioids in Europe (Table 13.8).

On the basis of pharmacologic models proposed for spinal opioid transport, the risk of late-onset respiratory depression is high with hydrophilic morphine. In contrast, lipophilic opioids such as fentanyl, sufentanil, and meperidine are considered

Table 13.8. *Choice of Opioids for PCA in Europe**

Austria	M > Pir
Belgium	M, Pir > F
Denmark	M
Finland	O > M, F
France	M
Germany	Pir
Greece	—
Iceland	—
Ireland	M
Italy	M > B
Netherlands	M > N
Norway	M
Portugal	M
Spain	M
Sweden	M
Switzerland	M > T
UK	M > D
Mean	**M > Pir > O > F > B, D, N, T**

*Data from a 17-nation survey of 105 hospitals.
M = morphine, Pir = piritramide, F = fentanyl,
O = oxycodone, B = buprenorphine, N = nicomorphine,
T = tramadol, D = diamorphine.
Source: Rawal, N. (1995). Patient controlled analgesia (PCA) for postoperative pain – A European survey. *Br. J. Anaesth.* **74,** 134 (abstract).

safe because of segmental localization such that minimal drug is available for rostral migration in CSF to reach medullary respiratory centers by diffusion and bulk flow. This has led to the widespread use of fentanyl as a safe opioid for epidural administration. However, the earlier belief that continuous infusions of epidural fentanyl do not cause late-onset respiratory depression has been shown to be incorrect (Brockway et al., 1990; Weightman, 1991) (Table 13.9).

The potency of epidural opioids is believed to be inversely related to lipophilicity. Fentanyl, sufentanil, meperidine, and buprenorphine are more lipophilic than morphine and therefore less potent. Reviewing the literature Chrubasik et al. (1993) conclude that currently there are no arguments that justify the placement of an epidural catheter if lipophilic opioids such as sufentanil, buprenorphine, or methadone are to

Table 13.9. *Incidence of Respiratory Depression Following Epidural Opioids*

Total Number of Patients	Number	Incidence	Authors	Reference
6,000–9,000*	23	0.25–0.4%	Gustafsson et al., 1982	*Br. J. Anaesth.* **54,** 479
1,085*	10	0.9%	Stenseth et al., 1985	*Acta Anaesthesiol. Scand.* **29,** 148
14,000*	13	0.09%	Rawal et al., 1987	*Br. J. Anaesth.* **59,** 791
4,880*	12	0.25%	Fuller et al., 1990	*Can. J. Anaesth.* **37,** 636–640
2,378	19	0.13%	Zimmermann and Stewart, 1993	*Can. J. Anaesth.* **40,** 568–575.
49,183**	45	0.09%	Rawal et al., 1995	*Reg. Anesth.* **20,** A45

* Morphine.
** Morphine (n = 33), fentanyl (n = 4), oxycodone (n = 4), diamorphine (n = 4).

be used postoperatively. Dosage requirements and quality of analgesia are similar whether these drugs are administered IV or epidurally. Furthermore, plasma or serum concentrations during continuous epidural administration of these opioids are indistinguishable from those during continuous IV infusion. The authors believe that the risk of respiratory depression may be higher during continuous epidural than continuous IV treatment because of the dual distribution of epidural opioids to the brainstem via blood and CSF (Chrubasik et al., 1993). However, this is questioned by some workers (Camann et al., 1992; Benzon et al., 1993; Solamäki et al., 1993). Thus, it would seem that the early onset of analgesia following lipophilic opioids may not be enough to justify the dangers, inconvenience, and additional cost of the epidural over the parenteral route (Nagle and McQuay, 1990; Camu and Debucquoy, 1991). It appears that morphine is the only opioid that fulfills the requirements of prolonged, sedation-free segmental analgesia. A few studies have shown that morphine is cost effective in high-risk patients. There is a need for similar controlled outcome studies using lipophilic opioids.

Nonopioids

Inhibition of afferent nociceptive transmission by mechanisms other than those acting on spinal opioid receptors has been demonstrated in several neurophysiologic studies. Nonopioid receptor selective agents such as serotinergic, muscarinic, adenosinergic, γ-aminobutyric acid (GABA), somatostatin agonists, and substance P antagonists are believed to inhibit pain modulation at the spinal level. In clinical practice analgesic effects have been demonstrated following epidural or intrathecal administration of nonopioid drugs such as clonidine, somatostatin, octreotide, ketamine, calcitonin, midazolam, neostigmine, and droperidol. However, the role of spinal nonopioids is beyond the scope of this chapter.

Summary

Opioids are extensively used in the management of moderate to severe acute pain and pain related to malignant disease and remain the most important drugs in pain management. Although it is well recognized that pain management by intermittent injection of opioids is woefully inadequate, most patients continue to receive IM opioids because of the simplicity of, and familiarity with, this technique. However, the introduction of simple methods of pain scoring and a greater degree of flexibility in the administration of opioids would lead to considerable improvement in the management of postoperative pain.

The discovery of opioid receptors has opened new horizons in pain management. Spinal opioid analgesia is the most important development in pain treatment in several decades. Numerous studies have demonstrated the profound analgesic effects of spinal opioids, and the technique is frequently used to treat intraoperative, postoperative, traumatic, obstetric, chronic, and cancer pain.

In recent years many new agonist and agonist/antagonist opioids have been developed based on increased knowledge of opioid receptors. Similarly, increased knowledge of pharmacokinetics and pharmacodynamics of opioids has led to the development of a variety of new drug-delivery systems for old opioids such as fentanyl and morphine. The concept of PCA allows flexibility, convenience, and excellent patient satisfaction. It is not surprising, therefore, that in addition to IV administration opioids are also being studied subcutaneously, spinally, and intranasally and by the transdermal route. Opioids also have many disadvantages. The use of opioids is associated with adverse effects on several organ systems and with considerable morbidity. In recent years several nonopioid analgesics have been introduced. However, in general these drugs have "opioid-sparing" rather than "opioid-eliminating" effects for moderate to severe pain. Although many attempts have been made by the pharmaceutical industry to develop newer analgesic drugs that may possess the analgesic efficacy of morphine but with fewer adverse effects – a "safer morphine" – success has not been achieved so far.

REFERENCES

Abboud, T.K., Shnider, S.M., Raya, J.A., Grobler, N.M., Sadri, S., Khoo, S.S., De Souza, B., Baysinger, C.L., and Miller, F. (1984). Intrathecal administration of hyperbaric morphine for the relief of pain in labour. *Br. J. Anaesth.* **56,** 1351–1360.

Badner, N.A., Reimer, E.J., Komar, W.E., and Moote, C.A. (1991). Low-dose bupivacaine does not improve postoperative epidural fentanyl analgesia in orthopedic patients. *Anesth. Analg.* **72,** 337–341.

Badner, N.H., and Komar, W.E. (1992). Bupivacaine 0.1% does not improve postoperative epidural fentanyl analgesia after abdominal or thoracic surgery. *Can. J. Anaesth.* **39,** 330–336.

Bellamy, C.D., McDonnell, F.J., and Colclough, G.W. (1989). Postoperative epidural pain management results in shorter hospital stay than IV PCA morphine: A comparison in anterior cruciate ligament repair (abstract). *Anesthesiology.* **71,** A686.

Benzon, H.T., Wong, H.Y., and Belavic, A.M., Jr. (1993). A randomized double-blind comparison of epidural fentanyl infusion versus patient-controlled analgesia for postthoracotomy pain. *Anesth. Analg.* **76,** 316–322.

Boudreault, D., Brasseur, L., Samii, K., and Lemoing, J. (1991). Comparison of continuous epidural bupivacaine infusion plus either continuous epidural infusion or patient-controlled epidural injection of fentanyl for postoperative analgesia. *Anesth. Analg.* **73,** 132–137.

Brockway, M.S., Noble, D.W., Sharwood-Smith, G.H., and McClure, J.H. (1990). Profound respiratory depression after extradural fentanyl. *Br. J. Anaesth.* **64,** 243–245.

Camann, W.R., Loferski, B.L., Fancinllo, G.J., Stone, M.L., and Datta, S. (1992). Does epidural administration of butorphanol offer any clinical advantage over intravenous route? *Anesthesiology.* **76,** 216–220.

Camann, W.R., Mintzer, B.H., Denney, R.A., and Datta, S. (1993). Intrathecal sufentanil for labor analgesia. Effects of added epinephrine. *Anesthesiology.* **78,** 870–874.

Camu, F., and Debucquoy, F. (1991). Alfentanil infusion for postoperative pain: A comparison of epidural and intravenous routes. *Anesthesiology.* **75,** 171–178.

Christrup, L.L. (1997). Morphine metabolites. *Acta Anaesth. Scand.* **41,** 116–122.

Chrubasik, J., Chrubasik, S., and Martin, E. (1993). Benefits and risks of epidural opioids in the treatment of postoperative pain. In *Advances in pain therapy II,* eds. Chrubasik, J., Cousins, M., and Martin, E. Berlin: Springer-Verlag, 94–113.

Cohen, S., Amar, D., Pantuck, C.B., Pantuck, E.J., Goodman, E.J., Widroff, J.S., Kanas, R.J., and Brady, J.A. (1993). Postcesarean delivery epidural patient-controlled analgesia. *Anesthesiology.* **78,** 486–491.

Cousins, M.J., and Mather, L.E. (1984). Intrathecal and epidural administration of opioids. *Anesthesiology.* **61,** 276–310.

Curry, P.D., Pacsoo, C., and Heap, D.G. (1994). Patient-controlled epidural analgesia in obstetric anaesthetic practice. *Pain.* **57,** 125–128.

Dahl, J.B., Rosenberg, J., Hansen, B.L., Hjortsø, N.-C., and Kehlet, H. (1992). Differential analgesic effects of low-dose epidural morphine-bupivacaine at rest and during mobilization after major abdominal surgery. *Anesth. Analg.* **74,** 362–365.

Egan, K.J., and Ready, L.B. (1994). Patient satisfaction with intravenous PCA or epidural morphine. *Can. J. Anaesth.* **41,** 6–11.

Etches, R.C., Sandler, A.N., and Daley, M.D. (1989). Respiratory depression and spinal opioids. *Can. J. Anaesth.* **36,** 165–185.

Feld, L.H., Champeau, M.W., van Steennis, C.A., and Scott, J.C. (1989). Preanesthetic medication in children: A comparison of oral transmucosal fentanyl citrate versus placebo. *Anesthesiology.* **71,** 374–377.

Ferrante, F.M., Fanciullo, G.J., Grichnik, K.P., Vaisman, J., Sacs, G.M., and Concepcion, M.A. (1993). Regression of sensory anesthesia during continuous epidural infusions of bupivacaine and opioid for total knee replacement. *Anesth. Analg.* **77,** 1179–1184.

Ferrante, F.M., Lu, L., Jamison, S.B., and Datta, S. (1991). Patient-controlled epidural analgesia: Demand dosing. *Anesth. Analg.* **73,** 547–552.

Gangarosa, L.P. (1993). Iontophoresis in pain control (Review). *Pain Digest.* **3,** 162–174.

Glass, P.S.A., Estok, P., Ginsberg, B., Goldberg, J.S., and Sladen, R.N. (1992). Use of patient-controlled analgesia to compare the efficacy of epidural to intravenous fentanyl administration. *Anesth. Analg.* **74,** 345–351.

Henderson, J.M., Brodsky, D.A., Fisher, D.M., Brett, C.M., and Hertzka, R.E. (1988). Pre-induction of anesthesia in pediatric patients with nasally administered sufentanil. *Anesthesiology.* **68,** 671–675.

Kendrick, W.D., Woods, A.M., Daly, M.Y., Birch, R.F.H., and DiFazio, C. (1996). Naloxone versus nalbuphine infusion for prophylaxis of epidural morphine-induced pruritus. *Anesth. Analg.* **82,** 641–647.

Lamer, T.J. (1990). Postoperative pain management with epidural narcotics results in shorter hospital stay than IV or IM narcotics (abstract). *Reg. Anesth.* **15,** 83.

Mitchell, R.W.D., and Smith, G. (1989). The control of acute postoperative pain. *Br. J. Anaesth.* **63,** 147–158.

Morgan, M. (1989). The rational use of intrathecal and extradural opioids. *Br. J. Anaesth.* **63,** 165–188.

Mourisse, J., Hasenbos, M.A.W.M., Gielen, M.J.M., Moll, J.E., and Cromheecke, G.J.E. (1992). Epidural bupivacaine, sufentanil or the combination for post-thoracotomy pain. *Acta Anaesth. Scand.* **36,** 70–74.

Nagle, C.J., and McQuay. (1990). Extradural pethidine. *Br. J. Anaesth.* **65,** 730–732.

Paech, M.J., and Westmore, M.D. (1994). Postoperative epidural fentanyl infusion – is the addition of 0.1% bupivacaine of benefit? *Anaesth. Int. Care.* **22,** 9–14.

Parker, R.K., and White, P.F. (1992). Epidural patient-controlled analgesia: An alternative to intravenous patient-controlled analgesia for pain relief after cesarean delivery. *Anesth. Analg.* **75,** 245–251.

Rawal, N. (1992). Spinal opioids. In *Practical management of pain,* ed. Raj, P.P. St. Louis: Mosby Year Book, 829–851.

Rawal, N., and Allvin, R. (1996). EuroPain Study Group on Acute Pain. Paediatric premedication and postoperative pain management in Europe. A 17-nation survey. *Br. J. Anaesth.* **76,** 96–97.

Rawal, N., and Berggren, L. (1994). Organization of acute pain services – a low cost model. *Pain.* **57,** 117–123.

Rawal, N., and Tandon, B. (1985). Epidural and intrathecal morphine in intensive care units. *Intens. Care Med.* **11,** 129–133.

Rawal, N., Möllefors, K., Axelsson, K., et al. (1983). An experimental study of urodynamic effects of epidural morphine and of naloxone reversal. *Anesth. Analg.* **62,** 641–647.

Rawal, N., Schött, U., Tandon, B., et al. (1986). Influence of i.v. naloxone infusion on analgesia and untoward effects of epidural morphine. *Anesthesiology.* **64,** 194–201.

Rawal, N., Sjöstrand, U., Christoffersson, E., et al. (1984). Comparison of intramuscular and epidural morphine for postoperative analgesia in the grossly obese: Influence on postoperative ambulation and pulmonary function. *Anesth. Analg.* **63,** 583–592.

Ready, L.B., Oden, R., Chadwick, H.S., Benedetti, C., Rooke, G.A., Caplan, R., and Wild, L.M. (1988). Development of an anesthesiology-based postoperative pain management service. *Anesthesiology.* **68,** 100–106.

Rosow, C. (1989). Newer opioid analgesics and antagonists. *Anesth. Clin. N. Am.* **7,** 319–333.

Salomäki, T.E., Leppaluoto, J., Laitinen, J.O., Vuolteenho, O., and Nuutinen, L.S. (1993). Epidural versus intravenous fentanyl for reducing hormonal, metabolic and physiological responses after thoracotomy. *Anesthesiology.* **79,** 672–679.

Sekar, M., and Mimpriss, T.J. (1987). Buprenorphine, benzodiazepines and prolonged respiratory depression. *Anaesthesia.* **42,** 567–568.

Spence, A.A. (1980). Editorial: Relieving acute pain. *Br. J. Anaesth.* **52,** 245–246.

Stanley, T.H., Leiman, B.C., Rawal, N., Marcus, M.A., van den Nieuwenhuyzfen, W.A., Cronau, L.H., and Pace, N.L. (1989). The effects of oral transmucosal fentanyl citrate premedication on preoperative behavioral responses and gastric volume and acidity in children. *Anesth. Analg.* **69,** 328–335.

Stein, C., Millan, M.J., Shippenberg, T.S., Peter, K., and Herz, A. (1989). Peripheral opioid receptors mediating antinociception in inflammation. Evidence for involvement of mu, delta and kappa receptors. *J. Pharmacol. Exp. Ther.* **248,** 1269–1275.

Stoelting, R.K. (1989). Intrathecal morphine – an underused combination for postoperative pain management (editorial). *Anesth. Analg.* **68,** 707–709.

Striebel, H.W., Oelmann, T., Spies, C., Rieger, A., and Schwagmeier, R. (1996). Patient-controlled intranasal analgesia: A method for noninvasive postoperative pain management. *Anesth. Analg.* **83,** 548–551.

Thörn, S.E., Rawal, N., and Wennhager, M. (1988). Prolonged respiratory depression caused by sublingual buprenorphine. *Lancet.* **i,** 179–180.

Tuman, K.J., McCarthy, R.J., March, R.J., DeLaria, G.A., Patel, R.V., and Ivankovich, A.D. (1991). Effects of epidural anesthesia and analgesia on coagulation and outcome after major vascular surgery. *Anesth. Analg.* **73,** 696–704.

Vercauteren, M., Boeckx, E., Hanegreefs, G., Noorduin, H., and van den Bussche, G. (1988). Intranasal sufentanil for pre-operative sedation. *Anaesthesia.* **43,** 270–273.

Vercauteren, M.P. (1993). The role of perispinal route for postsurgical pain relief. *Ballières Clin. Anaesth.* **7,** 769–792.

Warfield, C.A., and Kahn, C.H. (1995). Acute pain management. Programs in U.S. hospitals and experiences and attitudes among U.S. adults. *Anesthesiology.* **83,** 1090–1094.

Warwick, J.P., Kearns, C.F., and Scott, W.E. (1997). The effect of subhypnotic doses of propofol on the incidence of pruritus after intrathecal morphine for Caesarean section. *Anaesthesia.* **52,** 265–275.

Weightman, W.M. (1991). Respiratory arrest during fentanyl infusion of bupivacaine and fentanyl. *Anaesth. Intens. Care.* **19,** 282–284.

Wittels, B., Glosten, B., Faure, E.A.M., Moawad, A.H., Ismail, M., Hibbard, J., Amundsen, L., Binstock, W., Senal, J.A., Cox, S.M., Blacksam, S.C., Karl, L., and Thisted, R.A. (1993). Opioid antagonist adjuncts to epidural morphine for postcesarean analgesia: Maternal outcomes. *Anesth. Analg.* **77,** 925–932.

Yaksh, T.L., and Harty, G.J. (1987). Pharmacology of the allodynia in rats evoked by high dose intrathecal morphine. *J. Pharmacol. Exp. Ther.* **244,** 501–507.

Yeager, M.P., Glass, D.D., Neff, R.K., et al. (1987). Epidural anesthesia and analgesia in high-risk surgical patients. *Anesthesiology.* **66,** 729–736.

CHAPTER FOURTEEN

Patient-Controlled Analgesia with Opioids

KLAUS A. LEHMANN

Introduction

Opioids have a long history in the clinical setting. Being old, however, does not necessarily mean being well known or even liked by the majority of clinicians. Opioids are usually prescribed in too low doses, and physicians' prescriptions are often even more reduced by the nursing staff (Atchison et al., 1991; Juhl et al., 1993; McCormack et al., 1993; Stratton Hill, 1993; Oates et al., 1994; Stevens et al., 1995; Whipple et al., 1995). In the author's experience, there are mainly two reasons for the hesitation of health-care personnel to use adequate opioid dosages, and, interestingly, they differ, whether one deals with general practitioners or hospital doctors. The first group is concerned with tolerance and addiction (which is not justified in pain patients; however, the subject is beyond the scope of this chapter) and the second with the vital risk of respiratory depression. It is hard to understand why two groups of medical experts share the same concern but for different reasons. The only explanation is that both groups have hardly ever had an adequate education in the field of pain and/or opioid analgesics. It was the development of a new analgesic technique, patient-controlled analgesia (PCA), that greatly increased our knowledge of the clinical effects of opioids, particularly in patients suffering from painful conditions, a group that differs quite obviously from the volunteers from whom most older pharmacology textbooks derived their conclusions.

PCA was first described for laboring patients in the 1960s, but became widely recognized only after its introduction to the field of postoperative pain in the mid-1980s. Until then, there were many reasons for inadequate treatment. Doctors usually had to delegate pain relief to the nursing staff, who were also overloaded with work. As a consequence, rigid intramuscular doses were (and often still are) administered at fixed intervals or only on (urgent) request, without adapting the types of analgesics or application modes to the patient's individual requirements, despite the unpredictability of pain intensity and tolerance. So far it has been virtually impossible to establish the role played by age, sex, anaesthetic, or surgical technique, proba-

Christoph Stein, ed., *Opioids in Pain Control: Basic and Clinical Aspects*. Printed in the United States of

bly because psychological factors, such as previous experience, anxiety, depression, neuroticism, and self-discipline on the part of the patient, can seldom be satisfactorily standardized or recorded in an objective manner (Chapman, 1992).

The therapeutic concept of PCA is an attempt to solve many of the problems just discussed all at once. If the patient can decide how much pain he or she is experiencing or is prepared to suffer, self-administration of potent analgesics should satisfy the need for analgesia and reduce the nursing staff workload. Recent evidence shows that many patients prefer to tolerate some pain (as long as they can help themselves immediately) and thus accept higher pain scores with less drug consumption; but there are others who will never be satisfied even with virtually free access to an opioid (Kluger and Owen, 1990).

At present, more than 950 papers and some handbooks (Harmer et al., 1985; Ferrante et al., 1990; Lehmann and Klaschik [eds.], 1991) have been published on the uses and problems of PCA. The most important studies are discussed in newer reviews (Lehmann, 1991, 1993, 1994a, 1995). Although opioids are by far the most frequently used analgesics for PCA, they are not the only drugs for self-administration. So far, there is limited experience with local anaesthetics for peripheral nerve blocks (Gouverneur and Singelyn, 1992) and more with epidural analgesia in labor (Gambling et al., 1990; Viscomi and Eisenach, 1991; Purdie et al., 1992; Vercauteren, 1992; Curry et al., 1994; Lubenow et al., 1994), often in combination with epidural opioids (Ferrante et al., 1991; Paech, 1992; Cohen et al., 1993; Gambling et al., 1993; Yu and Gambling, 1993). Recently, patient-controlled sedation during minor surgical procedures has been reported (Cook et al., 1993; Osborne et al., 1994; Rodrigo and Tong, 1994; Bernard et al., 1996; Cork et al., 1996; Dell, 1996; Hamid et al., 1996; Herrick, Gelb et al., 1996), but more studies are required to evaluate its clinical benefit.

PCA Devices

Early devices, which simply allowed patients in labor to adjust flow rates of analgesic dilutions, were soon followed by electronically controlled systems. Except for technical details, most PCA machines differ only slightly. They consist of electronically controlled infusion pumps supervised by microprocessors. Whenever the patient feels pain relief is necessary, he or she can activate the system. The unit dispenses a preprogrammed amount of analgesic into an intravenous infusion, intramuscularly, subcutaneously, or even into the spinal space. Unauthorized alteration of dosing parameters or overdose is prevented by a number of safety factors. Recently, disposable PCA devices have been introduced, which can be used for about three days (Lehmann, 1985).

There are slight differences between the systems regarding the use of concurrent infusions (Lehmann, 1995). Some provide tail doses, which are fixed-rate infusions for a certain period of time following patient demand. Some devices allow a baseline infusion, either at a fixed or an adaptive rate. In the latter the actual infusion is calculated from the dose administered during the last 60-minute interval; that is, high analgesic consumption as expressed by high demand frequencies increases the baseline infusion. This application mode leads to a significant reduction of total demand, which many patients appreciate (Lehmann et al., 1992). Even more sophisticated delivery strategies have been proposed. At present, the concept of pharmacokinetically tailored PCA (PKPCA) is the most promising one. Patient demands are used to trigger suitable infusion rates, based on pharmacokinetic principles (Hill and Mather, 1993), for maintaining stable plasma concentrations (Hill et al., 1992; Irwin et al., 1996; Mies et al., 1994).

Clinical Experience

Among possible areas for PCA use, postoperative pain treatment remains the most frequently reported. PCA during labor or for the treatment of chronic pain has so far been reported only sporadically (Bruera et al., 1988; Ferrell et al., 1992; Hill et al., 1992; Jadad et al., 1992; Zech et al., 1992; Zech et al., 1993; Ferrante et al., 1995). Good results were indicated with sickle cell–related pain (Gonzalez et al., 1991; Shapiro et al., 1993). Intraoperative self-administration was tried in extracorporal shock wave lithotripsy (Schelling et al., 1992; Dickert et al., 1993; Irwin et al., 1996).

Most papers describe intravenous self-administration; subcutaneous or intramuscular PCA has seldom been used (Harmer et al., 1983; Bruera et al., 1988; White, 1990; Bruera et al., 1991; Zech et al., 1993; Doyle, Morton et al., 1994; Kalso et al., 1996). Spinal application has recently gained wide interest. So far, the epidural route is favored (Ferrante et al., 1991; Vercauteren, 1992; Grass et al., 1994; Brown and McCarthy, 1995; Kalso et al., 1996), but only a few controlled studies performed direct comparisons with intravenous PCA. Paech et al. (1994) found that IV and epidural pethidine had a similar onset of action after cesarean section, but the spinal route provided better pain relief and patient acceptance (Paech, 1992). Chauvin et al. (1993), however, could not verify that alfentanil was superior after spinal application. There are similar controversies regarding the best spinal application site. With sufentanil, no difference was found between thoracic or lumbar epidural administration (Swenson et al., 1994), although Caudle et al. (1993) preferred the thoracic route for epidural fentanyl in children (Caudle et al., 1993). Even intrathecal PCA has been tried (Domsky and Tarantino, 1992; Cohen et al., 1994), but more studies are necessary before conclusive recommendations can be made.

More recently, noninvasive application modes for PCA have been introduced. Sublingual buprenorphine was first tried with good results (Carl et al., 1987; Chraemmer Jorgensen et al., 1988; Witjes et al., 1992), followed by oral morphine, hydromorphone, or methadone (Säwe et al., 1981; Litman and Shapiro, 1992). Fentanyl lollipops – that is, transmucosal delivery – was suggested as an alternative, not only for premedication but also for the management of acute or chronic pain (Ashburn et al., 1993; Fine et al., 1991). The latest development is intranasal PCA

Table 14.1. *Equipotency Studies*

Analgesic	Demand Dose (μg)	Hourly Maximum Dose (mg/hour)	Consumption (μg/kg/hour)	Consumption (mg/70 kg/d)	RPS* (0–5)	Relative Equipotent Dose (product)
Sufentanil**	6	0.04	0.10	0.2	1.85	0.004
Fentanyl	34	0.25	0.46	0.8	1.07	0.01
Buprenorphine	40	0.32	0.63	1.1	1.57	0.02
Alfentanil	212	1.5	4.96	8.3	1.37	0.15
Hydromorphone	566	2.94	6.60	11.1	2.25	0.33
l-Methadone	1,145	5.95	14.20	23.9	1.60	0.50
Piritramide	1,990	15.0	30.44	51.1	1.42	0.96
Morphine	1,920	14.8	29.60	49.7	1.52	1
Nalbuphine	3,846	28.5	117.52	197.4	1.82	4.75
Pentazocine	7,980	60.0	135.57	227.8	1.60	4.82
Nefopam	3,846	28.5	132.75	223.0	2.90	8.56
Pethidine	9,615	100.0	175.10	294.2	2.22	8.63
Tramadol	9,615	100.0	203.12	341.2	2.27	10.24
Metamizol	50,000	500.0	1804.21	3031.0	3.02	121.09

Note: Results as arithmetic means; relative equipotent dose was calculated from the product of consumption and retrospective pain score (Lehmann, 1993, 1994).
*Retrospective pain scores: 0, no pain at all; 1, sometimes moderate pain; 2, always moderate pain; 3, sometimes severe pain; 4, always moderate and sometimes severe pain; 5, discontinuation due to inefficiency.
**Sufentanil: 40 patients recovering from major gynecologic surgery; other drugs: patients after major abdominal and orthopedic surgery.

(Striebel et al., 1995); patient-controlled iontophoresis is imminent (Ashburn et al., 1992; Nimmo, 1992).

Almost every opioid has been administered by PCA in the postoperative period. Initially, it was considered an advantage that PCA not only helped to improve the quality of analgesia but also reduced total dosage when compared with conventional regimens. This conclusion proved to be rash, however. The observations of these investigations are confirmed by the author's own results. Groups of 40 patients recovering from elective major abdominal or orthopedic surgery were treated with different analgesics for about 24 hours after extubation. Dosing parameters are given in Table 14.1; lock-out time was 1 minute. Demand rate and analgesic consumption were documented, as were retrospective verbal pain scores obtained in standardized interviews on the following day. The product of mean opioid consumption and retrospective pain score was used for equipotency comparisons. As can be seen in Figure 14.1, individual variability in analgesic requirements was extremely high. Although the patients had virtually free access to the dose, the therapeutic outcome was often

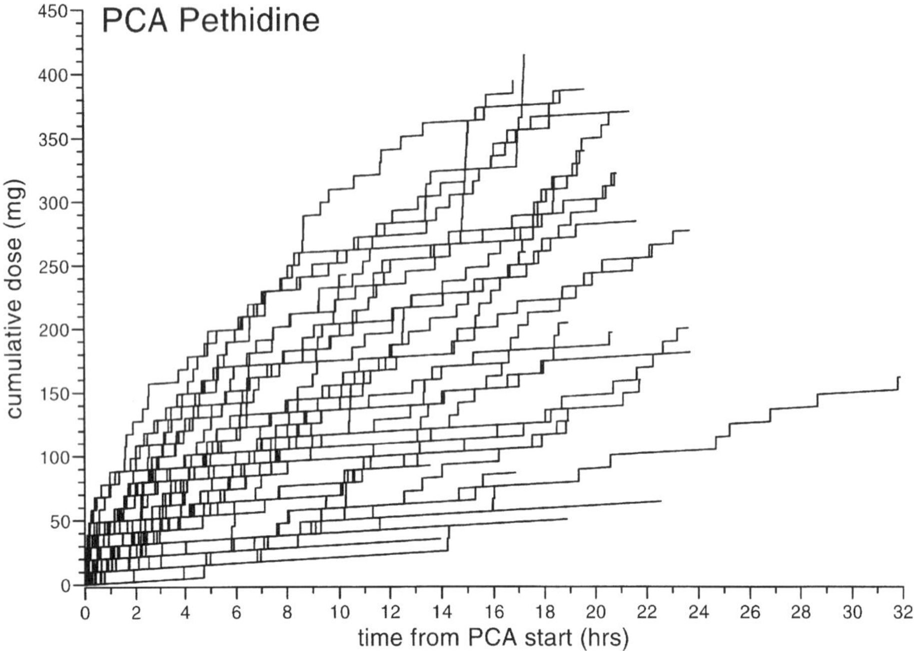

Figure 14.1. Cumulative dose-time plots of 40 patients recovering from major abdominal or orthopedic surgery who were allowed to self-administer pethidine (see also Table 14.1). Each step is indicative of a valid demand.

different: the self-administered dosage was not always correlated with overall efficacy. Some patients requested rather low dosages, even after upper abdominal interventions, and felt quite comfortable, whereas others recovering from minor surgery experienced comparatively little pain relief despite high analgesic consumption. Even strict standardization (for sex, type of surgery, anaesthesia, and so on) led to only minor reductions of variability (Lehmann, 1993, 1994a).

Altogether, acceptance was excellent. Of 1,454 patients, 76% preferred PCA to previously experienced conventional pain therapy. And 57% wished to remain connected to the PCA pump at the end of the observation period. Only 9% of patients would have preferred personal treatment by the nursing staff, which confirms data from other studies (Ballantyne et al., 1993; Boulanger et al., 1993; Egan and Ready, 1994). Difficulties in handling the device were reported in 13%, mostly elderly patients. Tables 14.2 and 14.3 compare acceptance with retrospective pain scores and the incidence of side effects. It is reasonable to assume that such results are interrelated, and this area must be investigated systematically in the future.

The ideal drug should have an immediate onset and medium duration of effect and be potent (i.e., not exert an early ceiling effect). Side effects should be minor and abuse potential minimal. Although these options exclude, in the opinion of some authors, all agonist-antagonists and both short- and long-acting analgesics, Tables

Table 14.2. *Side Effects during Intravenous Postoperative PCA*

Analgesic	n	Male/Female	NAU	EM	H	SE	EU	DYS	PR	SW
Alfentanil	40	(21/ 19)	30	15	0	30	13	5	0	20
Buprenorphine	139	(67/ 72)	42	17	0	0	4	6	11	37
Fentanyl	295	(28/273)	47	37	6	1	3	2	4	23
Hydromorphone	120	(60/ 60)	18	7	0	0	7	2	8	21
l-Methadone	120	(22/ 98)	38	22	0	0	2	0	3	16
Metamizol	40	(16/ 24)	35	30	0	3	0	0	0	73
Morphine	141	(47/ 94)	26	11	0	5	4	4	3	18
Nalbuphine	40	(19/ 21)	18	8	0	0	3	8	0	13
Nefopam	40	(20/ 20)	3	3	0	0	0	0	0	0
Pentazocine	40	(19/ 21)	20	15	0	0	5	5	3	35
Pethidine	40	(20/ 20)	8	5	0	13	0	0	0	8
Piritramide	160	(73/ 87)	26	12	0	12	1	3	2	14
Sufentanil	40	(0/ 40)	50	33	3	3	5	8	0	40
Tramadol	199	(61/138)	41	16	2	2	0	0	0	6
Σ	1,454	(473/981)	34	20	2	3	3	3	3	21

Note: Results as %; NAU = nausea, EM = emesis, H = headache, SE = heavy sedation, EU = euphoria, DYS = dysphoria, PR = pruritus, SW = sweating.

14.2 and 14.3 suggest that the best guideline is for the staff to be comfortable using the drug (Woodhouse et al., 1996).

Several attempts were made to decrease the relatively high incidence of postoperative nausea and vomiting. Transdermal scopolamin was effective in children (Doyle, Byers et al., 1994). Recently, combinations of analgesics and antiemetics (droperidol, metoclopramide, ondansetron), concomitantly delivered by PCA, were found to be interesting alternatives (Alexander et al., 1995; Gan et al., 1995; Lehmann, 1995; McKenzie et al., 1995; Roberts et al., 1995; Walder and Aitkenhead, 1995; Russel et al., 1996; Wrench et al., 1996).

An important factor that may influence PCA efficacy is the size of the demand dose. Patients will trust the concept only if they notice a direct connection between demand and effect. Of course, this will not be the case if too small a demand dose is chosen. It was thought that high demand frequencies would obviate this problem and finally result in a sufficient cumulative effect. Investigations of tramadol showed, however, that doubling the demand dose resulted in significantly higher efficacy without doubling analgesic intake (Lehmann, 1994b). It can be concluded that, on the one hand, patients are able to *reduce* their demand frequency as soon as they feel

Table 14.3. *Patient Acceptance after Intravenous Postoperative PCA*

		Comparison of PCA with Earlier Conventional Pain Treatment			Continuation of PCA Desired				
Analgesic	**RPS**	+	=	–	+	=	–	**Preferred Nurse**	**Difficult to Handle**
Alfentanil	1.37	80.0	13.3	6.7	67.5	25.0	7.5	15.0	2.5
Buprenorphine	1.37	87.8	10.8	1.3	67.6	19.4	12.9	3.6	13.7
Fentanyl	1.84	80.1	9.9	9.9	68.1	13.6	18.3	7.5	11.2
Hydromorphone	2.25	91.3	8.7	0	70.8	25.8	3.3	0	5.0
l-Methadone	1.49	91.1	4.5	4.5	45.0	24.2	30.8	6.7	11.7
Metamizol	3.02	11.1	37.0	51.9	20.0	37.5	22.5	22.5	37.5
Morphine	1.36	76.3	17.5	6.3	34.0	31.9	34.0	7.1	9.2
Nalbuphine	1.82	56.5	26.1	17.4	37.5	27.5	35.0	7.5	5.0
Nefopam	2.90	46.2	7.7	46.2	27.5	15.0	57.5	15.0	7.5
Pentazocine	1.60	68.4	15.8	15.8	40.0	35.0	25.0	5.0	7.5
Pethidine	2.22	47.1	35.3	17.6	52.5	30.0	17.5	5.0	30.0
Piritramide	1.51	82.2	9.6	8.2	65.0	21.9	52.5	11.3	17.2
Sufentanil	1.85	57.5	27.3	15.2	75.0	10.0	15.0	55.0	7.5
Tramadol	1.25	70.1	12.6	17.2	58.8	29.1	12.1	8.5	19.1
Mean	1.69	75.8	13.1	11.1	57.2	23.1	23.5	9.0	13.1

Note: Results as %; RPS = mean retrospective pain score; + better/positive, = comparable/uncertain, – worse/negative.

comfortable, but, on the other, that they are not willing to approach the permitted maximal doses by *raising* their demand frequency (Lehmann, 1990). The reasons remain to be clarified, but the phenomenon suggests that there are optimum demand doses for all analgesics (Owen et al., 1989; Doyle, Mottard et al., 1994). Some authors feel that doses should be adjusted to patients' weight and body surface or to therapeutic efficacy. Recently, a device was introduced that lets patients choose among different demand doses (Owen et al., 1995). Another now widely accepted strategy to improve the efficacy of PCA is an intravenous loading dose, which is increased stepwise (usually in the recovery room) until the patient reports sufficient pain relief. With this approach, PCA itself is used to maintain analgesia rather than to establish it. Although this concept is appealing, comparative investigations are still rare (Lehmann et al., 1986; Demartini et al., 1995; Macintyre and Jarvis, 1996). The excellent effect of loading dosages confirms the general observation that analgesic intake is highest during the first few hours after an operation and then tends to

Table 14.4. *PCA Settings for Some Frequently Used Postoperative Opioids*

	Demand Dose*		Lock-out Time (minutes)	
Analgesic	**Mean**	**Median**	**Mean**	**Median**
Morphine	1.6	1.4	7.9	6.0
Pethidine	20.2	17.5	11.1	10.0
Nalbuphine	4.0	3.9	5.5	5.0
Fentanyl	23.7	20.0	3.5	5.0
Alfentanil	116.5	100.0	3.3	1.0
Sufentanil	5.2	6.0	8.0	8.0
Buprenorphine	62.5	60.0	3.0	3.0

Note: Averaged from 70 studies.
*Morphine to nalbuphine: mg; fentanyl to buprenorphine: µg.

decrease slowly. PCA is thus most valuable during the early postoperative period, and treatment for more than two to three days is seldom necessary.

There has been only little concern so far regarding the duration of the lock-out time period (Black et al., 1990; Gambling et al., 1993; Ginsberg et al., 1995). If individual loading doses are titrated, lock-out times in the range of 5–10 minutes should be appropriate in most cases, as long as optimum demand doses are prescribed. Table 14.4 gives typical PCA settings from the literature.

Successful use of PCA requires that the concept be understood and accepted by the patient, nursing staff, and physician. Pre- and postoperative information should not only address appropriate handling of the device (there was one case of oversedation when a patient misunderstood the ready indicator of his PCA device as a signal to request the next dose [Johnson and Daugherty, 1992]) but also predict that partial relief, rather than complete *freedom* from pain, may be expected. With this in mind, PCA can also be used successfully in children (from about 6 years on [Irwin et al., 1992; Doyle et al., 1993; Dunbar et al., 1995; Lehmann, 1995; Sittl et al., 1995; Sümpelmann et al., 1996]) and in frail elderly patients (Egbert et al., 1990; Fredman et al., 1996; Herrick, Ganapathy et al., 1996; Herrick, Gelb et al., 1996; Macintyre and Jarvis, 1996). To our knowledge, tolerance or even dependence does not occur in pain patients if opioids are individually titrated.

Safety Aspects and Mishaps

The respiratory centers in the brainstem are triggered by several mechanisms. Any increase in cerebrospinal fluid pCO_2 or decrease of pH leads to chemoreceptor activation. Opioids depress this reflex in a dose-dependent manner. However, because the respiratory centers are part of the reticular formation, they are also triggered in an activity-dependent manner. Brainstem stimulation by whatever mechanism (i.e., any input from the exterior or interior milieu, and therefore – most importantly – pain) compensates to a certain degree the chemoreceptor reflex depression. It is now generally accepted that a clinically relevant respiratory depression is connected with overdose, which in turn reduces the problem to finding adequate dosages. If one admits that 10–30% of surgical patients do not need any postoperative analgesic, then even 5 mg of morphine intramuscularly may mean overdose. Thus, the general rule to prevent opiate-induced respiratory depression must be to administer only the dosage that is individually necessary; this administration is best performed by intravenous titration. Any reduction of vigilance should be avoided thereafter. Several studies have reported that patients ceased breathing during pain management with opioids and concomitant benzodiazepines or barbiturates or that well-tolerated dosages turned out to be dangerous after additional analgesic techniques were used (e.g., regional blockade or spasmolytic agents [Lehmann, 1993, 1994a; Etches, 1994]).

Our own recent results using continuous monitoring of transcutaneous blood gases and pulse oxymetry revealed that respiratory depression occurs during routine use of PCA, but is not generally caused by PCA. Table 14.5 shows the incidence of hypercapnia and desaturation following various types of anesthesia; there were no significant differences between patients receiving conventional pain management and those using PCA (Lehmann and Klaschik, 1991; Lehmann et al., 1993), or between those receiving active drug and placebo (Grond et al., 1995), which confirms previous findings from the literature (Fleming and Coombs, 1992; Wheatley et al., 1992).

In view of the preceding remarks, it is not astonishing that clinically relevant respiratory depression during adequate use of intravenous postoperative PCA is extremely rare (Kluger and Owen, 1991; Fleming and Coombs, 1992). Several available case reports, however, can be explained by the overdose hypothesis as just outlined. Some authors reported patients with initially quite normal respiratory patterns, which deteriorated as a consequence of postoperative bleeding, but could be managed by fluid substitution (Dahlström et al., 1982; Fleming and Coombs, 1992; Owen et al., 1992). Low respiratory rates were caused by dislocation of the intravenous catheter, which led to a subcutaneous depot into which further demands were applied without immediate pain relief; after complete absorption, the patient was then overdosed. Mismanagement by the nursing staff was the reason for some incidents (Looi-Lyons et al., 1996). In patients with renal insufficiency, the pharmacologically active metabolites morphine-6-glucuronide or norpethidine can accumulate (Fleming and Coombs, 1992; Geller, 1993; Lehmann and Zech, 1993; Stone et al., 1993). Most respiratory depressions were recognized early enough to be successfully treated (Lehmann, 1995). So far, one near-fatal and one fatal outcome was reported, in which technical defects caused fast infusions of high dosages of papaveretum or pethidine (Kreitzer et al., 1989; Grover and Heath, 1992).

Table 14.5. *Continuous Postoperative Respiratory Monitoring Following Various Types of Anaesthesia: Extremes of Observation Hours 1–4*

	pct CO_2 > 50 mm	pct CO_2 > 55 mm	sO_2 < 90%	sO_2 < 85%
Volunteers	0.06	0	0.24	0
Halothane	9.95	3.59	7.49	0.20
Halo-PCA	2.38	0	11.85	1.25
Enflurane	15.77	11.83	4.43	0.11
Enfl-PCA	7.38	6.46	2.52	0.33
Isoflurane	7.24	0.30	7.99	0.61
Isofl-PCA	24.97	15.97	8.06	1.68
NLA	9.69	0.61	11.00	0
NLA-PCA	7.90	1.09	5.82	0.04

Note: Results as percents of all data, measured in 30-second intervals, from a total of 214 patients.

PCA is now often used routinely on wards (Lehmann and Klaschik 1991; Stehr-Zirngibl et al., 1995). The value of continuous monitoring of oxygen saturation or apnea alarms remains to be established. Most authors recommend that no concurrent infusion be used because the result would be overdose in some patients (Lehmann et al., 1992; Parker et al., 1992; Doyle et al., 1993; Schug and Torrie, 1993), but some newer studies have reached different conclusions (Doyle et al., 1993; McCoy et al., 1993). Similarly, a warning was given against "spouse-controlled" analgesia in sleeping patients (Wakerlin, 1990; Lam, 1993; Ashburn et al., 1994; Stehr-Zirngibl, 1995). Patients suffering from sleep apnea syndromes should be carefully monitored (VanDerCar et al., 1991).

Although so far rare, some mishaps may have been masked by PCA and may have led to serious complications. The author knows of a patient who died from myocardial infarction after routine surgery, who had not complained of ischemic pain but instead increased his demand rate. This case was not documented by the nursing staff, and no clinical conclusions were drawn from the increased analgesic intake. Meyer and Eagle (1992) reported a similar situation in which a pulmonary embolus was not recognized early enough as a function of PCA; fortunately, this patient survived (Meyer and Eagles, 1992). The conclusion to be drawn from such incidents is that regular monitoring of pain intensity, analgesic consumption, respiratory rate, and sedation scores must be guaranteed for safe performance of PCA (and of all other effective pain management strategies). Most authorities recommend that naloxone be available near the patient. Written orders for ward physicians and nursing staff are required. An acute pain service seems to be the best option for dealing with all organizational problems (Fleming and Coombs, 1992; Schug and Torrie, 1993; Ashburn et al., 1994; Schug and Fry, 1994).

Recently, questions have arisen concerning whether the generous application of relatively high opioid doses could favor the development of postoperative ileus (Petros et al., 1995; Nitschke et al., 1996). Conclusive answers are still missing.

Is PCA Cost Effective?

The question of the cost effectiveness of PCA cannot be easily answered. Some researchers argue that PCA saves nursing time, whereas others state that the monitoring workload will increase. Unfortunately, only a few papers have dealt with cost-effectiveness relationships (Hecker and Albert, 1980; Smith et al., 1991; Schug and Large, 1993; Cohen et al., 1994; Koh and Thomas, 1994; Chan et al., 1995). That good pain relief itself shortens the hospital stay (and thus saves money) is another controversial topic; most studies do not support this idea. In the author's opinion, the greatest merit of PCA is that it has highlighted the importance of individual pain management. The more we realize what has been wrong in the past, the more we can improve daily practice, even without PCA devices. Good experience has been reported with nurse-controlled analgesia (NCA), an approach in which the nursing staff is allowed to inject small opioid doses intravenously with the same limits that are used in PCA devices (Murphy and Opie, 1991; Purdie et al., 1992; Weldon et al., 1993; Sumpelmann et al., 1996). In an interesting cost analysis, Smythe et al. (1994) reported that PCA with pethidine accounted for $24.63 per day, whereas well-controlled intramuscular therapy by the nursing staff needed only $2.92 (Smythe et al., 1994). Although PCA was judged slightly better in this study, the question remains: Is PCA still justified in a majority of patients? Obviously, intravenous application is not the only solution. Prophylactic intramuscular or subcutaneous pain management in combination with pain measurements at regular intervals and dose adjustment according to individual needs has been shown to be equally effective (Rawal and Beggren, 1994). Interestingly, PCA was found to provide better pain relief than IM injections, but it also led to greater fatigue and less vigor (Passchier et al., 1993). Some studies have demonstrated that PCA improved recovery (i.e., there were fewer postoperative pulmonary or thromboembolic complications and shorter hospital stays) (Boulanger et al., 1993; Searle et al., 1994); others, however, have indicated that all effective pain management strategies are equivalent in this respect (Beattie et al., 1993; Christopherson et al., 1993).

Wherever the basics are not yet established (and I assume this holds for most hospitals), their introduction will cost money. If people believe PCA is the best solution, PCA devices have to be paid for. If others think the job can be done with adequate training of doctors and nurses, they have to allocate their funds to this end. I suggest,

Table 14.6. *Postoperative Fentanyl Consumption Following Various Types of Surgery*

	n	Male/Female	µg/kg/hour	RPS
Orthopaedics	20	(5/15)	0.53 ± 0.39	0.89 ± 0.55
Abdominal Surgery	45	(29/16)	0.63 ± 0.29	1.44 ± 1.17
Hysterectomies	92	(0/92)	0.65 ± 0.35	2.16 ± 1.28
Thoracotomies	19	(13/ 6)	0.68 ± 0.39	0.84 ± 0.83

Note: Demand dose 34.5 µg, infusion rate 4 µg/hour, lockout time 1 minute, hourly maximum dose 0.25 mg/hour; results as arithmetic mean ± SD (Lehmann, 1995).

however, that PCA be used to change the staff mindset; thereafter the staff must be trained according to a more conventional regimen.

Uses of PCA for Research

As soon as PCA was accepted as a clinical method for the treatment of pain, a number of studies were undertaken to use PCA designs for research purposes (see references in Lehmann, 1993, 1994a, 1995). Supposing that postoperative analgesic consumption reflects pain intensities after surgical operations, a rank order of painfulness could be established on that basis. It has been shown, however, that physicians' prescribing practices and nursing staff's application of physicians' orders are greatly influenced by tradition and fears of side effects rather than by individual patient needs. Thus, retrospective analyses of analgesic dosages are more likely to indicate what patients received than what they needed. For this reason only complete independence from normal drug administration procedures would justify the assumptions just given. Table 14.6 demonstrates our own results. Although all patients had virtually free access to the fentanyl dosage, drug intake as well as retrospective pain judgment varied significantly. Thus, it must be concluded that even under PCA, drug consumption alone does not allow a valid comparison of the degree of pain associated with various surgical operations. Additional classical pain measurements must be performed. It has been the author's impression with hysterectomy patients that the meaning of the operation to the patient (e.g., loss of an aspect of womanhood) was of utmost importance in the judgment of postoperative well-being, which is certainly reflected in the retrospective pain classification and possibly in analgesic consumption (Schonecke et al., 1993; Schonecke et al., 1994). It should always be kept in mind that interpretation of PCA results is complicated by considerable individual variations, which render statistical comparisons difficult.

So far, only a few studies have compared the effect of premedication or anesthetic

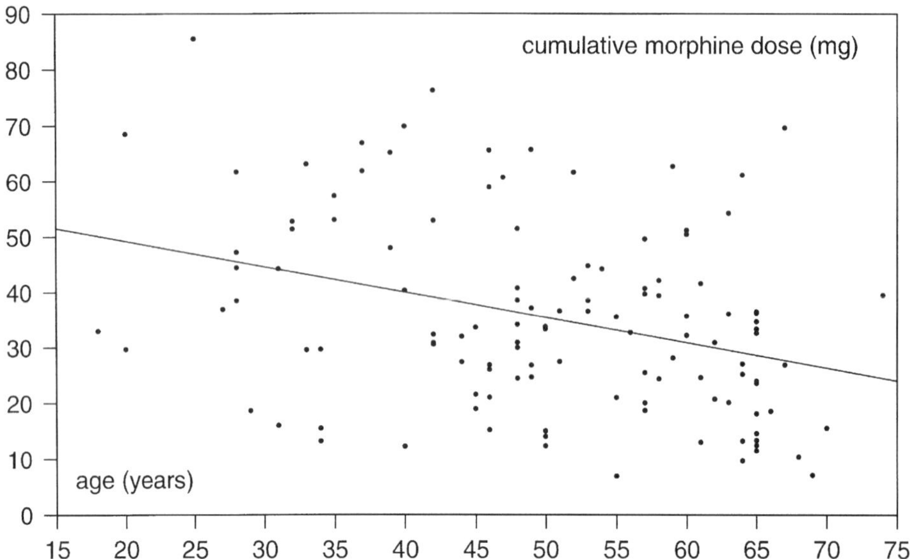

Figure 14.2. Self-administered morphine doses during the first 24 hours after major abdominal or orthopedic surgery, plotted against age.

technique on postoperative pain. Personality (Jamison et al., 1993; Perry et al., 1994), age (Figure 14.2), gender, drug history, and so on, are additional factors that presumably predict postoperative pain. Conclusive PCA studies are still rare (Gil et al., 1990; Chapman, 1992; Thomas et al., 1995; Taylor et al., 1996). Results are often conflicting, but most investigations have failed to find statistically significant differences. Interestingly, some trials have found a correlation between postoperative analgesic consumption and preoperative neurotransmitter concentrations (endorphins, substance P) in CSF (Sjöstrom et al., 1988).

Many investigations have used PCA to assess the efficacy of non-PCA pain treatment – for example, systemic, transdermal, intra-articular, and spinal opioids or clonidine, spasmolytic agents, local anaesthetics, cryoanalgesia, and transcutaneous electrical nerve stimulation or acupuncture. Similar studies were performed to demonstrate drug interactions between opioids and calcium channel blockers, cholecystokinin antagonists, antiemetics, tricyclic antidepressants, respiratory analeptics, and opiate antagonists. Recently, the number of similar trials has considerably increased, but usually with conflicting results. Particularly interesting is that whereas some investigators believed that PCA data confirmed the importance of pre-emptive analgesia, the majority of studies contradicted this conclusion.

Equipotency of Analgesic Drugs

Estimation of relative potency should be possible when analgesic consumption using PCA is analyzed in comparable groups of patients. Particularly interesting, however,

Table 14.7. *Minimum Effective Concentrations (MEC) during Postoperative PCA*

Analgesic	Median	Minimum	Maximum	Variability (%)	
	(ng/ml)			Intrasubject	Intersubject
Sufentanil	0.04	0.01	0.56	80.0	81.0
Buprenorphine	0.38	0.01	6.56	67.9	107.3
Fentanyl	1.16	0.18	8.01	27.2	63.9
Alfentanil	14.87	0.57	99.20	37.0	62.5
Tramadol	287.7	20.20	936.30	38.2	59.1

Sources: Lehmann, 1993, 1994.

is that comparative studies have often revealed differences in overall therapeutic outcome, depending on the analgesic studied, despite the fact that maximum doses were virtually unlimited. Again, it does not seem justified to merely examine drug consumption without taking into account drug efficacy. For this reason, in the author's studies the product of mean analgesic consumption and mean retrospective pain score was calculated (Tables 14.2 and 14.3). The resulting figures take into account both the intensity and the duration of drug effect. It should be stressed that this attempt must be preliminary as long as nonoptimum demand doses are used, that simply multiplying the variables may be questionable, and that the approach is possibly not valid for agonist-antagonists, for which analgesic ceiling effects limit an increase of efficacy with increasing doses. Further controlled investigations on this subject are highly desirable.

"Analgesic" Plasma Concentrations

Plasma concentrations alone are of only minor value unless the correlation between concentration and pharmacodynamic effects is also known. Comprehensive studies have now been done for most analgesics. Unfortunately, their value for clinical practice is controversial because the concentration-effect relationship is extremely variable. Most studies reported a close correlation only if individual pharmacokinetic parameters derived from intraoperative analysis were used for comparison with postoperative data from the same patient; intersubject variability, however, was very high for all analgesics studied. Much time was spent in the author's own experiments to determine analgesic "threshold" concentrations (minimum effective concentrations, MEC) for some opiates. For this reason, venous blood samples were taken immediately before a patient demand, that is, at a point in time at which the patient was just becoming dissatisfied with analgesia. Figure 14.3 displays tramadol results. It is evident that a generizable threshold concentration does not exist. There are always

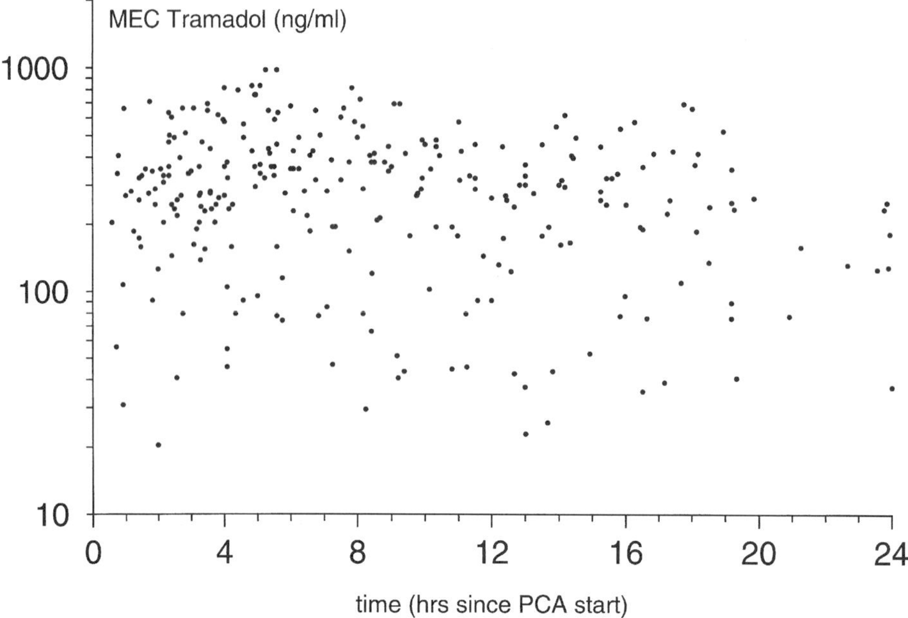

Figure 14.3. Minimum effective tramadol plasma concentrations during postoperative PCA (40 patients recovering from major gynecologic surgery, 278 samples), plotted against duration of treatment.

some patients who have intraindividually stable MEC, who are different from other subjects, whereas other patients show remarkable intraindividual variation. MECs are usually log normally distributed, and the range is very broad. In general, intraindividual variability in MEC is consistently lower than interindividual variability (Table 14.7); individual regression analyses never give an indication of accumulation. In view of the available data, it seems wise to use the term *therapeutic window* instead of *threshold,* and it should be kept in mind that the window is rather wide. When one looks at Figures 14.1 and 14.2, which illustrate the tremendous variability in drug consumption among patients, one cannot be surprised by the conclusion that the corresponding plasma concentrations vary as well.

Summary

As far as we know today, it is impossible to predict accurately how much pain a patient will experience after an operation or what analgesic dosage will be required to provide adequate pain relief. PCA has opened new possibilities for the management of pain and analgesics studies. Since patients have virtually free access to the dose, different agents or strategies can be compared more or less objectively. Patients usually control their analgesic demand within the limits available to them, and they seem to strike a balance between the desirable analgesic effect of the drug and the undesirable effects such as nausea, sedation, and dysphoria. In other words, demand rates are determined not only by the drug's analgesic properties but also by the drug's overall acceptability. A drug's acceptability includes the idea, although still not very well understood, that some patients are prepared to tolerate a certain amount of pain whereas others are not. The influence of psychological variables on pain behavior during PCA must not be neglected. PCA researchers also have the strong impression that most patients seem to use PCA to become comfortable rather than pain free.

On the whole, results available so far suggest that PCA is not only efficacious and well accepted by patients but that it can also improve conventional techniques. Objective documentation of individual variability in analgesic demand, which is often much higher than anticipated from clinical "experience," must consequently lead to a greater confidence in patients' opinions.

What do patients expect from adequate postoperative pain management? Owen et al. (1990) suggested that the most important goal is immediate action as soon as an individual's pain-tolerance threshold is exceeded. The insight that thresholds are unpredictable in individual patients, both subjective thresholds and "objective" parameters such as plasma drug concentrations (Lehmann, 1991), is one of the greatest merits of PCA. Any technique based on this knowledge and commited to immediate reaction (the PCA principle) can in theory be considered equivalent. One might even argue that different PCA modes (by any route or device) are not superior to nurse-controlled techniques. Although self-control may offer some subjective advantages to some patients, PCA expenses are usually costly enough that suitable devices are not available to all patients, and low-cost techniques based on the PCA principle have been shown to be highly effective.

Are specialized PCA devices still needed? In my opinion, PCA was of utmost importance until the PCA principle was discovered. Who would have believed the huge opioid doses that were sometimes needed for effective analgesia? Who would have imagined how much was wrong in the management of simple postoperative pain? Would the concept of an Acute Pain Service, and the newer international recommendations for adequate pain management, have emerged without PCA experience? I doubt it. PCA is still one of the best ways to achieve patient satisfaction and recuperation in the postoperative period. But even those who have no (or not enough) PCA devices available can apply the PCA principle. To do so involves trusting the patient, providing adequate monitoring and appropriate documentation, and, of course, raising the educational level of the staff on the surgical ward.

The name of the game is individual variability. Although not described in detail, this opinion was already in the air at the first PCA workshop in 1984. To deal with individual variability, we first needed our eyes opened by patients, who showed us the variability that exists. Now, we need well-educated and well-organized staff to implement this lesson.

REFERENCES

Alexander, R., Lovell, A.T., and Seingry, D. (1995). Comparison of ondansetron and droperidol in reducing postoperative nausea and vomiting associated with patient-controlled analgesia. *Anaesthesia.* **50,** 1086–1088.

Ashburn, M.A., Lind, G.H., Gillie, M.H., de Boer, A.J.F., Pace, N.L., and Stanley T.H. (1993). Oral transmucosal fentanyl citrate (OTFC) for the treatment of postoperative pain. *Anesth. Analg.* **76,** 377–381.

Ashburn, M.A., Love, G., and Pace, N.L. (1994). Respiratory-related critical events with intravenous patient-controlled analgesia. *Clin. J. Pain.* **10,** 52–56.

Ashburn, M.A., Stephen, R.L., Ackerman, E., Petelenz, T.J., Hare, B., Pace, N.L., and Hofman, A.A. (1992). Iontophoretic delivery of morphine for postoperative analgesia. *J. Pain Symptom Management.* **7,** 27–33.

Atchison, N.E., Osgood, P.F., Carr, D.B., and Szyfelbein, S.K. (1991). Pain during burn dressing change in children: Relationship to burn area, depth and analgesic regimens. *Pain.* **47,** 41–45.

Ballantyne, J.C., Carr, D.B., Chalmers, T.C., Dear, K.B.G., Angelillo, I.F., and Mosteller, F. (1993). Postoperative patient-controlled analgesia: Meta-analysis of initial randomized control trials. *J. Clin. Anesth.* **5,** 182–193.

Beattie, W.S., Buckley, D.N., and Forrest, J.B. (1993). Epidural morphine reduces the risk of postoperative myocardial ischaemia in patients with cardiac risk factors. *Can. J. Anaesth.* **40,** 532–541.

Bernard, J.M., Faintreny, A., Lienhart, A., and Souron, R. (1996). Patient-controlled premedication by iv midazolam for ambulatory surgery. *Acta Anaesthesiol. Scand.* **40,** 331–337.

Black, A.M.S., Goodman, N.W., Bullingham, R.E.S., and Lloyd, J. (1990). Intramuscular ketorolac and morphine during patient-controlled analgesia (PCA) after hysterectomy: Does PCA lock-out time reveal an efficacy limitation of ketorolac? *Eur. J. Anaesthesiol.* **7,** 9–17.

Boulanger, A., Choinière, M., Roy, D., Bouré, B., Chartrand, D., Choquette, R., and Rousseau, P. (1993). Comparison between patient-controlled analgesia and intramuscular meperidine after thoracotomy. *Can. J. Anaesth.* **40,** 409–415.

Brown, D.V., and McCarthy, R.J. (1995). Epidural and spinal opioids. *Curr. Opin. Anaesth.* **8,** 337–341.

Bruera, E., MacMillan, K., Hanson, J., and MacDonald, R.N. (1991). The Edmonton injector: A simple device for patient-controlled subcutaneous analgesia. *Pain.* **44,** 167–169.

Bruera, E., Brenneis, C., Michaud, M., MacMillan, K., Hanson, J., and MacDonald, N. (1988). Patient-controlled subcutaneous hydromorphone versus subcutaneous infusion for the treatment of cancer pain. *J. Natl. Cancer. Inst.* **88,** 1152–1154.

Carl, P., Crawford, M.E., Madsen, N.B.B., Ravlo, O., Bach, V., and Larsen, A.I. (1987). Pain relief after major abdominal surgery: A double-blind controlled comparison of sublingual buprenorphine, intramuscular buprenorphine, and intramuscular meperidine. *Anesth. Analg.* **66,** 142–146.

Caudle, C.L., Freid, E.B., Bailey, A.G., Valley, R.D., Lish, M.C., and Azizkhan, R.G. (1993). Epidural fentanyl infusion with patient-controlled epidural analgesia for postoperative analgesia in children. *J. Pediatr. Surg.* **28,** 554–559.

Chan, V.W., Chung, F., McQuestion, M., and Gomez, N. (1995). Impact of patient-controlled analgesia on required nursing time and duration of postoperative recovery. *Reg. Anesth.* **20,** 506–514.

Chapman, C.R. (1992). Psychological aspects of postoperative pain control. *Acta Anaesthesiol. Belg.* **43,** 41–52.

Chauvin, M., Hongnat, J.M., Mourgeon, E., Lebrault, C., Bellenfant, F., and Alfonsi P. (1993). Equivalence of postoperative analgesia with patient-controlled intravenous or epidural alfentanil. *Anesth. Analg.* **76,** 1251–1258.

Chraemmer Jorgensen, B., Schmidt, F.J., Hertel, S., Banning, A.M., and Risbo, A. (1988). Patient-controlled analgesic therapy by sublingual buprenorphine. *Clin. J. Pain.* **4,** 75–79.

Christopherson, R., Beattie, C., Frank, S.M., Norris, E.J., Meinert, C.L., Gottlieb, S.O., Yates, H., Rock, P., Parker, S.D., Perler, B.A., and Williams, G.M. (1993). Perioperative morbidity in patients randomized to epidural or general anesthesia for lower extremity vascular surgery. *Anesthesiology.* **79,** 422–434.

Cohen, S., Amar, D., Pantuck, C.B., Pantuck, E.J., Goodman, E.J., Widroff, J.S., Kanas, R.J., and Brady, J.A. (1993). Postcesarean delivery epidural patient-controlled analgesia. Fentanyl or sufentanil? *Anesthesiology.* **78,** 486–491.

Cohen, S., Amar, D., Pantuck, E.J., Singer, N., and Divon, M. (1994). Decreased incidence of headache after accidental dural puncture in caesarean delivery patients receiving continuous postoperative intrathecal analgesia. *Acta Anaesthesiol. Scand.* **38,** 716–718.

Cohen, S.E., Subak, L.L., Brose, W.G., and Halpern, J. (1991). Analgesia after cesarean delivery: Patient evaluation and costs of five opioid techniques. *Reg. Anesth.* **16,** 141–149.

Cook, L.B., Lockwood, G.G., Moore, C.M., and Whitwam, J.G. (1993). True patient-controlled sedation. *Anaesthesia.* **48,** 1039–1044.

Cork, R.C., Heaton, J.F., Campbell, C.E., and Kihlstrom, J.F. (1996). Is there implicit memory after propofol sedation? *Br. J. Anaesth.* **76,** 492–498.

Curry, P.D., Pascoo, C., and Heap, D.G. (1994). Patient-controlled epidural analgesia in obstetric anaesthetic practice. *Pain.* **57,** 125–128.

Dahlström, B., Tamsen, A., Paalzow, L., and Hartvig, P. (1982). Patient-controlled analgesic therapy, part IV: Pharmacokinetics and analgesic plasma concentrations of morphine. *Clin. Pharmacokinet.* **7,** 266–279.

Dell. R. (1996). A review of patient-controlled sedation. *Eur. J. Anaesthesiol.* **13,** 547–552.

Demartini, L., Coven, G., Cimino, F., Zizzi, S., Noli, S., Bettaglio, R., and Bonezzi, C. (1995). Postoperative PCA with morphine in abdominal surgery. Influence of the loading dose in pain control. *Eur. J. Pain.* **16,** 49–51.

Dickert, T., Hoffmann, H., Zucker, T.P., Hagemann, U., and Hopf, H.B. (1993). Niedrig dosiertes Midazolam reduziert den Alfentanilverbrauch bei alten, nicht aber bei jungen Patienten während extrakorporaler Stoβwellenlithotrypsie. *Anaesthesiol. Intensivmed. Notfallmed. Schmerzther.* **28,** 13–17.

Domsky, M., and Tarantino, D. (1992). Patient-controlled spinal analgesia for postoperative pain control. *Anesth. Analg.* **75,** 453–455.

Doyle, E., Byers, G., McNicol, L.R., and Morton, N.S. (1994). Prevention of postoperative nausea and vomiting with transdermal hyoscine in children using patient-controlled analgesia. *Br. J. Anaesth.* **72,** 72–76.

Doyle, E., Harper, I., and Morton, N.S. (1993). Patient-controlled analgesia with low dose background infusion after lower abdominal surgery in children. *Br. J. Anaesth.* **71,** 718–722.

Doyle, E., Mottard, K.J., Marshall,C., and Morton, N.S. (1994). Comparison of different bolus doses of morphine for patient-controlled analgesia in children. *Br. J. Anaesth.* **72,** 160–163.

Doyle, E., Morton, N.S., and McNicol, L.R. (1994). Comparison of patient-controlled analgesia in children by i.v. and s.c. routes of administration. *Br. J. Anaesth.* **72,** 533–536.

Doyle, E., Robinson, D., and Morton, N.S. (1993). Comparison of patient-controlled analgesia with and without a background infusion after lower abdominal surgery in children. *Br. J. Anaesth.* **71,** 670–673.

Dunbar, P.J., Buckley, P., Gavrin, J.R., Sanders, J.E., and Chapman, C.R. (1995). Use of patient-controlled analgesia for pain control for children receiving bone marrow transplantation. *J. Pain Symptom Management.* **10,** 604–611.

Egan, K.J., and Ready, L.B. (1994). Patient satisfaction with intravenous PCA or epidural morphine. *Can. J. Anaesth.* **41,** 6–11.

Egbert, A.M., Parks, L.H., Short, L.M., and Burnett, M.L. (1990). Randomized trial of postoperative patient-controlled analgesia vs. intramuscular narcotics in frail elderly men. *Arch. Intern. Med.* **150,** 1897–1903.

Etches, R.C. (1994). Respiratory depression associated with patient-controlled analgesia: A review of eight cases. *Can. J. Anaesth.* **41,** 125–132.

Ferrante, F.M., Barber, M.J., Segal, M., Hughes, N.J., and Datta, S. (1995). 0.0625% bupivacaine with 0.0002% fentanyl via patient-controlled epidural analgesia for pain of labor and delivery. *Clin. J. Pain.* **11,** 121–126.

Ferrante, F.M., Ostheimer, G.W., and Covino, B.G. (eds). (1990). *Patient-controlled analgesia.* Boston: Blackwell Scientific Publications.

Ferrante, M.F., Lu, L., Jamison, S.B., and Datta, S. (1991). Patient-controlled epidural analgesia: Demand dosing. *Anesth. Analg.* **73,** 547–552.

Ferrell, B.R., Nash, C.C., and Warfield, C. (1992). The role of patient-controlled analgesia in the management of cancer pain. *J. Pain Symptom Management.* **7,** 149–154.

Fine, P.G., Marcus, M., De Boer, A.J., and Van der Oord, B. (1991). An open label study of oral transmucosal fentanyl citrate (OTFC) for the treatment of breakthrough cancer pain. *Pain.* **45,** 149–153.

Fleming, B.M., and Coombs, D.W. (1992). A survey of complications documented in a quality-control analysis of patient-controlled analgesia in the postoperative patient. *J. Pain Symptom Management.* **7,** 463–469.

Fredman, B., Olsfanger, D., Flor, P., and Jedeikin, R. (1996). Ketorolac does not decrease postoperative pain in elderly men after transvesical prostatectomy. *Can. J. Anaesth.* **43,** 438–441.

Gambling, D.R., McMorland, G.H., Yu, P, and Lazlo, C. (1990). Comparison of patient-controlled epidural analgesia and conventional intermittent "top-up" injections during labor. *Anesth. Analg.* **70,** 256–261.

Gambling, D.R., Huber, C.J., Howell, P., Swenerton, J.E., Ross, P.L.E., Chrochetière, C.T., and Pavy, T.J.G. (1993). Patient-controlled epidural analgesia in labour: Varying bolus dose and lockout interval. *Can. J. Anaesth.* **40,** 211–217.

Gan, T.J., Alexander, R., Fennelly, M., and Rubin, A.P. (1995). Comparison of different methods of administering droperidol in patient-controlled analgesia in the prevention of postoperative nausea and vomiting. *Anesth. Analg.* **80,** 81–85.

Geller, R.J. (1993). Meperidine in patient-controlled analgesia: A near-fatal mishap. *Anesth. Analg.* **76,** 655–657.

Gil, K.M., Ginsberg, B., Muir, M., Sykes, D., and Williams, D.A. (1990). Patient-controlled analgesia in postoperative pain: The relation of psychological factors to pain and analgesic use. *Clin. J. Pain.* **6,** 137–142.

Ginsberg, B., Gil, K.M., Muir, M., Sullivan, F., Williams, D.A., and Glass, P.S.A. (1995). The influence of lockout intervals and drug selection on patient-controlled analgesia following gynecological surgery. *Pain.* **62,** 95–100.

Gonzalez, E.R., Bahal, N., Hansen, L.A., Ware, D., Bull, D.S., Ornato, J.P., and Lehman, M.E. (1991). Intermittent injections vs. patient-controlled analgesia for sickle cell crisis pain. Comparison in patients in the emergency department. *Arch. Intern. Med.* **151,** 1373–1376.

Gouverneur, J.M., and Singelyn, F. (1992). PCA and peripheral nerve blocks. *Acta Anaesthesiol. Belg.* **43,** 63–65.

Grass, J.A., Zuckerman, R.L., Sakima, N.T., and Harris, A.P. (1994). Patient-controlled analgesia after cesarean delivery. Epidural sufentanil versus intravenous morphine. *Reg. Anesth.* **19,** 90–97.

Grond, S., Meuser, T., Zech, D., Hennig, U., and Lehmann, K.A. (1995). Analgesic efficacy and safety of tramadol enantiomers in comparison with the racemate: A randomized, double-blind study with gynecological patients using intravenous patient-controlled analgesia. *Pain.* **62,** 313–320.

Grover, E.R., and Heath, M.L. (1992). Patient-controlled analgesia. A serious incident. *Anaesthesia.* **47,** 402–404.

Hamid, S.K., Wong, P.K., Carmichael, F., White, K., and Ashbury, A.J. (1996). A novel device for patient-controlled sedation: Laboratory and clinical evaluation of the Baxter Intermate LV250 infusor and patient-control-module. *Anaesthesia.* **51,** 145–150.

Harmer, M., Rosen, M., and Vickers, M.D. (eds.). (1985). *Patient-controlled analgesia.* Oxford: Blackwell Scientific Publications.

Harmer, M., Slattery, P.J., Rosen, M., and Vickers, M.D. (1983). Intramuscular on demand analgesia: Double blind controlled trial of pethidine, buprenorphine, morphine, and meptazinol. *Br. Med. J.* **286,** 680–682.

Hecker, B.R., and Albert, L. (1980). Patient-controlled analgesia: A randomized, prospective comparison between two commercially available PCA pumps and conventional analgesic therapy for postoperative analgesia. *Pain.* **35,** 115–120.

Herrick, I.A., Ganapathy, S., Komar, W., Kirkby, J., Moote, R.A., Dobkowski, W., and Eliasziw, M. (1996). Postoperative cognitive impairment in the elderly. Choice of patient-controlled analgesia opioid. *Anaesthesia.* **51,** 356–360.

Herrick, I.A., Gelb, A.W., Nichols, B., and Kirkby, J. (1996). Patient-controlled sedation for elderly patients: Safety and patient attitude toward control. *Can. J. Anaesth.* **43,** 1014–1018.

Hill, H.F., Coda, B.A., Mackie, A.M., and Iverson, K. (1992). Patient-controlled analgesic infusions: Alfentanil versus morphine. *Pain.* **49,** 301–310.

Hill, H.F., and Mather, L.E. (1993). Patient-controlled analgesia. Pharmacokinetic and therapeutic considerations. *Clin. Pharmacokinet.* **24,** 124–140.

Irwin, M., Gillespie, J.A., and Morton, N.S. (1992). Evaluation of a disposable patient-controlled analgesia device in children. *Br. J. Anaesth.* **68,** 411–413.

Irwin, M.G., Campbell, R.C.H., Lun, T.S., and Yang, J.C.S. (1996). Patient maintained target-controlled infusion for analgesia during extracorporeal shock wave lithotripsy. *Can. J. Anaesth.* **43,** 919–924.

Jadad, A.R., Carrol, D., Glynn, C.J., Moore, R.A., and McQuay, H.J. (1992). Morphine responsiveness of chronic pain: Double-blind randomized crossover study with patient-controlled analgesia. *Lancet* **339,** 1367–1371.

Jamison, R.N., Taft, K., O'Hara, J.P., and Ferrante, F.M. (1993). Psychosocial and pharmacologic predictors of satisfaction with intravenous patient-controlled analgesia. *Anesth. Analg.* **77,** 121–125.

Johnson, T., and Daugherty, M. (1992). Oversedation with patient-controlled analgesia. *Anaesthesia.* **47,** 81–82.

Juhl, I.U., Christensen, V., Bülow, H.H., Wilbek, H., Dreijer, N.C., and Egelund, B. (1993). Postoperative pain relief, from the patients' and the nurses' point of view. *Acta Anaesthesiol. Scand.* **37,** 404–409.

Kalso, E., Heiskanen, T., Rantio, M., Rosenberg, P.H., and Vainio, A. (1996). Epidural and subcutaneous morphine in the management of cancer pain: A double-blind cross-over study. *Pain.* **67,** 443–449.

Kluger, M.T., and Owen, H. (1990). Patients' expectations of patient-controlled analgesia. *Anaesthesia.* **45,** 1072–1074.

Kluger, M.T., and Owen, H. (1991). Patient-controlled analgesia: Can it be made safer? *Anaesth. Intensive Care.* **19,** 412–420.

Koh, P., and Thomas, V.J. (1994). Patient-controlled analgesia (PCA): Does time saved by PCA improve patient satisfaction with nursing care? *J. Adv. Nurs.* **20,** 61–70.

Kreitzer, J.M., Kirschenbaum, L.P., and Eisenkraft, J.B. (1989). Safety of PCA devices. *Anesthesiology.* **70,** 881.

Lam, F.Y. (1993). Patient-controlled analgesia by proxy. *Br. J. Anaesth.* **70,** 113.

Lehmann, K.A., Abu-Shibika, M., and Horrichs-Haermeyer, G. (1990). Postoperative Schmerztherapie mit l-Methadon und Metamizol. Eine randomisierte Untersuchung im Rahmen der intravenösen On-Demand Analgesie. *Anaesth. Intensivther. Notfallmed.* **25,** 152–159.

Lehmann, K.A., Brand-Stavroulaki, A., and Dworzak, H. (1986). The influence of demand- and loading dose on the efficacy of postoperative patient-controlled analgesia with tramadol. A randomized double-blind study. *Schmerz-Pain-Douleur* **7,** 146–152.

Lehmann, K.A. (1991). Patient-controlled intravenous analgesia for postoperative pain relief. *Adv. Pain. Res. Ther.* **18,** 481–506.

Lehmann, K.A. (1993). Intravenous patient-controlled analgesia for post-operative pain management and research. In *Anesthésie-Réanimation/Pitié-Salpêtrière. Analgésie périopératoire,* ed. Balagn E. et al. Paris: Arnette.

Lehmann, K.A. (1994a). Patientenkontrollierte Analgesie. In *Der postoperative Schmerz,* 2nd ed., ed. K.A. Lehmann. Berlin: Springer-Verlag.

Lehmann, K.A. (1994b). Tramadol for the management of acute pain. *Drugs.* **47** (Suppl 1), 19–32.

Lehmann, K.A. (1995). New developments in patient-controlled postoperative analgesia. *Ann. Med.* **27,** 271–282.

Lehmann, K.A., Asoklis, S., and Grond, S. (1993). Kontinuierliches Monitoring der Spontanatmung in der postoperativen Phase. Teil 4. Auswirkungen der postoperativen Schmerztherapie auf kutane Sauerstoff- und Kohlendioxidpartialdrücke nach gynäkologischen Eingriffen unter Neuroleptanalgesie. *Anaesthesist.* **42,** 441–447.

Lehmann, K.A., and Klaschik, E. (eds.). (1991). *On-demand-analgesie.* Wiesbaden: Wissenschaftliche Verlagsabteilung, Abbott.

Lehmann, K.A., Mehler, O., and Grond, S. (1992). Klinischer Vergleich verschiedener Infusionsregime im Rahmen der postoperativen On-demand-Analgesie mit Fentanyl. *Anaesth. Intensivmed. Notfallmed. Schmerzther.* **27,** 346–353.

Lehmann, K.A., and Zech, D. (1993). Morphine-6-glucuronide, a pharmacologically active morphine metabolite. A review of the literature. *Eur. J. Pain.* **14,** 28–35.

Litman, R.S., and Shapiro, B.S. (1992). Oral patient-controlled analgesia in adolescents. *J. Pain Symptom Management.* **4,** 78–81.

Looi-Lyons, L.C., Chung, F.F., Cahn, V.W., and McQuestion, M. (1996). Respiratory depression: An adverse outcome during patient-controlled analgesia. *J. Clin. Anesth.* **8,** 151–156.

Lubenow, T.R., Tanck, E.N., Hopkins, E.M., McCarthy, R.J., and Ivankovich, A.D. (1994). Comparison of patient-assisted epidural analgesia with continuous-infusion epidural analgesia for postoperative patients. *Reg. Anesth.* **19,** 206–211.

Macintyre, P.E., and Jarvis, D.A. (1996). Age is the best predictor of postoperative morphine requirements. *Pain.* **64,** 357–364.

McCormack, J.P., Li, R., Zarowny, D., and Singer, J. (1993). Inadequate treatment of pain in ambulatory HIV patients. *Clin. J. Pain.* **9,** 279–283.

McCoy, E.P., Furness, G., and Wright, P.M.C. (1993). Patient-controlled analgesia with and without background infusion. Analgesia assessed using the demand:delivery ratio. *Anaesthesia.* **48,** 256–265.

McKenzie, R., Tantisira, B., Jackson, D., Bach, T., and Riley, T. (1995). Antiemetic efficacy of a droperidol-morphine combination in patient-controlled analgesia. *J. Clin. Anesth.* **7,** 141–147.

Meyer, G.S., and Eagle, K.A. (1992). Patient-controlled analgesia masking pulmonary embolus in a postoperative patient. *Crit. Care. Med.* **20,** 1619–1621.

Mies, R.H.M., van der Aa, Dixon, C.L., Kaltenbach, M., Derendorf, H., and Gravenstein, N. (1994). Computer-modulated patient-controlled analgesia. Preliminary evaluation of a prototype. *Reg. Anesth.* **19,** 270–276.

Murphy, D.F., and Opie, N.J. (1991). Nurse-controlled intravenous analgesia. Effective pain control after thoracotomy. *Anaesthesia.* **46,** 772–774.

Nimmo, W.S. (1992). Novel delivery systems: Electrotransport. *J. Pain Symptom Management.* **7,** 160–162.

Nitschke, L.F., Schlösser, C.T., Berg, R.L., Selthafner, J.V., Wengert, T.J., and Acevilla, C.S. (1996). Does patient-controlled analgesia achieve better control of pain and fewer adverse effects than intramuscular analgesia? A prospective randomized trial. *Arch. Surg.* **131,** 417–423.

Oates, J.D.L., Snowdon, S.L., and Jayson, D.W.H. (1994). Failure of pain relief after surgery. Attitudes of ward staff and patients to postoperative analgesia. *Anaesthesia.* **49,** 755–758.

Osborne, G.A., Rudkin, G.E., Jarvis, D.A., Young, I.G. Barlow, J., and Leppard, P.I. (1994). Intra-operative patient-controlled sedation and patient attitude to control. A crossover comparison of patient preference from patient-controlled propofol and propofol by continuous infusion. *Anaesthesia.* **49,** 287–292.

Owen, H., McMillan, V., and Rogowski, D. (1990). Postoperative pain therapy: A survey of patients' expectations and their experiences. *Pain.* **41,** 303–307.

Owen, H., Plummer, J.L., Armstrong, I., Mather, L.E., and Cousins, J. (1989). Variables of patient-controlled analgesia. 1. Bolus size. *Anaesthesia.* **44,** 7–18.

Owen, H., Plummer, L., Ilsley A., Hawkins, R., Arfeen, Z., and Tordoff, K. (1995). Variable-dose patient controlled analgesia. A preliminary report. *Anaesthesia.* **58,** 855–857.

Owen, H., Szekely, S.M., Plummer, J.L., Cushnie, J.M., and Mather, L.E. (1989). Variables of patient-controlled analgesia. 2. Concurrent infusion. *Anaesthesia.* **44,** 11–13.

Paech, M.J. (1992). Patient-controlled epidural analgesia in labour – is a continuous infusion of benefit? *Anaesth. Intensive Care.* **20,** 15–20.

Paech, M.J., Moore, J.S., and Evans, S.F. (1994). Meperidine for patient-controlled analgesia after cesarean section. *Anesthesiology.* **80,** 1268–1276.

Parker, R.K., Holtmann, B., and White, P.F. (1992). Effect of nighttime opioid infusion with

PCA therapy on patient comfort and analgesic requirements after abdominal hysterectomy. *Anesthesiology.* **76,** 362–367.

Passchier, J., Rupreht, J., Koenders, E.F., Orlee, M., Luitwieler, R.L., and Bonke, B. (1993). Patient-controlled analgesia (PCA) leads to more postoperative pain relief, but also to more fatigue and less vigour. *Acta Anaesthesiol. Scand.* **37,** 659–663.

Perry, F., Parker, R.K., White, P.F., and Clifford, P.A. (1994). Role of psychological factors in postoperative pain control and recovery with patient-controlled analgesia. *Clin. J. Pain.* **10,** 57–63.

Petros, J.G., Realica, R., Ahmad, S., Rimm, E.B., and Robillard, R.J. (1995). Patient-controlled analgesia and prolonged ileus after uncomplicated colectomy. *Am. J. Surg.* **170,** 371–374.

Purdie J., Reid, J., Thorburn, J., and Asbury, A.J. (1992). Continuous extradural analgesia: Comparison of midwife top-ups, continuous infusions and patient controlled administration. *Br. J. Anaesth.* **68,** 580–584.

Rawal, N., and Beggren, L. (1994). Organizing of acute pain services: A low cost model. *Pain.* **57,** 117–123.

Roberts, C.J., Millar, J.M., and Goat, V.A. (1995). The antiemetic effectiveness of droperidol during morphine patient-controlled analgesia. *Anaesthesia.* **50,** 559–562.

Rodrigo, M.R.C., and Tong, C.K.A. (1994). A comparison of patient and anaesthetist controlled midazolam sedation for dental surgery. *Anaesthesia.* **49,** 241–244.

Russel, D., Duncan, L.A., Frame, W.T., Higgins, P.J., Asbury, A.J., and Millar, K. (1996). Patient-controlled analgesia with morphine and droperidol following caesarean section under spinal anaesthesia. *Acta Anaesthesiol. Scand.* **40,** 600–605.

Säwe, J., Hansen, J., Ginman, C., Hartivg, P., Jakobsson, P.A., Nilsson, N.I., Rane, A., and Änggard, E. (1981). Patient-controlled dose regimen of methadone for chronic cancer pain. *Br. Med. J.* **282,** 771–773.

Schelling, G., Mendl, G., Weber, W., Pauletzki, J., Sackmann, M., Pöppel, E., and Peter, K. (1992). Patient controlled analgesia for extracorporeal shock wave lithotripsy of gallstones. *Pain.* **48,** 355–359.

Schonecke, O.W., Muck-Weich, C., and Lehmann, K.A. (1993). Schmerzverhalten während der postoperativen "Patientenkontrollierten Analgesie" (PCA). I. Schmerzverhalten und Schmerzerleben. *Z. Med. Psychol.* **2,** 62–71.

Schonecke, O.W., Muck-Weich, C., and Lehmann, K.A. (1994). Schmerzverhalten während der postoperativen "Patienten-kontrollierten Analgesie" (PCA). II. Prädiktoren von Schmerzverhalten und Schmerzerleben. *Z. Med. Psychol.* **3,** 28–38.

Schug, S.A., and Large, R.G. (1993). Economic considerations in pain management. *PharmacoEconomics.* **3,** 260–267.

Schug, S.A., and Fry, RA. (1994). Continuous regional analgesia in comparison with intravenous opioid administration for routine postoperative pain control. *Anaesthesia.* **49,** 528–532.

Schug, S.A., and Torrie, J.J. (1993). Safety assessment of postoperative pain management by an acute pain service. *Pain.* **55,** 387–391.

Searle, N.R., Roy, M., Bergeron, G., Perrault, J., Roof, J., Heermans, C., Courtemanche, M., Demers, C., and Cartier, R. (1994). Hydromorphone patient-controlled analgesia (PCA) after coronary artery bypass surgery. *Can. J. Anaesth.* **41,** 198–205.

Shapiro, B.S., Cohen, D.E., and Howe, C.J. (1993). Patient-controlled analgesia for sickle-cell-related pain. *J. Pain Symptom Management.* **8,** 22–28.

Sittl, R., Tillig, J., Huber, H., Braun, G., and Katalinic, A. (1995). Schmerztherapie bei

Kindern und Erwachsenen nach Trichterbrustkorrektur. Eine retrospektive Analyse der Analgetikamedikation nach Bedarf und mittels PCA. *Schmerz.* **9,** 179–184.

Sjöström, S., Tamsen, A., Hartvig, P., Folkesson, R., and Terenius, L. (1988). Cerebrospinal fluid concentrations of substance P and (Met)enkephalin-Arg6-Phe7 during surgery and patient-controlled analgesia. *Anesth. Analg.* **67,** 976–981.

Smith, C.V., Rayburn, W.F., Karaisakis, P.T., Morton, R.D., and Novell, M.J. (1991). Comparison of patient-controlled analgesia and epidural morphine for postcesarean pain and recovery. *J. Reprod. Med.* **36,** 430–434.

Smythe, N., Loughlin, K., Schad, R.F., and Lucarroti, R.L. (1994). Patient-controlled analgesia versus intramuscular analgesic therapy. *Am. J. Hosp. Pharm.* **51,** 1433–1440.

Stehr-Zirngibl, S., Zirngibl, H., Angster, R., and Taeger K. (1995). Patientenkontrollierte Analgesie (PCA) auf Allgemeinstationen: Ein Erfahrungsbericht. *Anästh. Intensivmed.* **36,** 128–134.

Stevens, P.E., Dibble, S.L., and Miaskowski, C. (1995). Prevalence, characteristics, and impact of postmastectomy pain syndrome: An investigation of women's experiences. *Pain.* **61,** 61–68.

Stone, P.A., Macintyre, P.E., and Jarvis, D.A. (1993). Norpethidine toxicity and patient-controlled analgesia. *Br. J. Anaesth.* **71,** 738–740.

Stratton Hill, C. (1993). The barriers to adequate pain management with opioid analgesics. *Sem. Oncol.* **20** (Suppl. 1), 1–5.

Striebel, H.W., Ölmann, T., Spies, C., and Brummer, G. (1995). Patient-controlled intranasal analgesia (PCINA) for the management of postoperative pain – a pilot study. *J. Clin. Anesth.* **8,** 4–8.

Sümpelmann, R., Schröder, D., Krohn, S., Strauß, K.M., and Hausdörfer, J. (1996). Patientenkontrollierte Analgesie bei Kindern. *Anästh. Intensivmed.* **37,** 19–26.

Swenson, J.D., Hullander, R.M., Bready, R.J., and Leivers, D. (1994). A comparison of patient controlled epidural analgesia with sufentanil by the lumbar versus thoracic route after thoracotomy. *Anesth. Analg.* **78,** 215–218.

Taylor, N.M., Hall, G.N., and Salmon, P. (1996). Patients' experiences of patient-controlled analgesia. *Anaesthesia.* **51,** 525–528.

Thomas, V., Heath, M., Rose, D., and Flory, P. (1995). Psychological characteristics and the effectiveness of patient-controlled analgesia. *Br. J. Anaesth.* **74,** 271–276.

VanDerCar, D.H., Martinez, A.P., and de Lisser, E.A. (1991). Sleep apnea syndromes: A potential contraindication for patient-controlled analgesia. *Anesthesiology.* **74,** 623–624.

Vercauteren, M.P. (1992). PCA by epidural route (PCEA). *Acta Anaesthesiol. Belg.* **43,** 33–39.

Viscomi, C., and Eisenach, J.C. (1991). Patient-controlled epidural analgesia during labor. *Obstet. Gynecol.* **77,** 348–351.

Wakerlin, G., and Larson, C.P. (1990). Spouse-controlled analgesia. *Anesth. Analg.* **70,** 119.

Walder, A.D., and Aitkenhead, A.R. (1995). A comparison of droperidol and cyclizine in the prevention of postoperative nausea and vomiting associated with patient-controlled analgesia. *Anaesthesia.* **50,** 654–656.

Weldon, B.C., Connor, M., and White, P.F. (1993). Pediatric PCA: The role of concurrent opioid infusions and nurse-controlled analgesia. *Clin. J. Pain.* **9,** 26–33.

Wheatley, R.G., Shepherd, D., Jackson, I.J.B., Madej, T.H., and Hunter, D. (1992). Hypoxaemia and pain relief after upper abdominal surgery: Comparison of i.m. and patient-controlled analgesia. *Br. J. Anaesth.* **69,** 558–561.

Whipple, J.K., Lewis, K.S., Quebbeman, E.J., Esser, M.J., Gottlieb, M.S., McKindley, D.S.,

Hess, M., Boucher, B.A., Jancik, L.C., Erstad, B., and Ausman, R.K. (1995). Current patterns of prescribing and administering morphine in trauma patients. *Pharmacotherapy.* **15,** 210–215.

White, P.F. (1990). Subcutaneous-PCA: An alternative to IV-PCA for postoperative pain management. *Clin. J. Pain.* **6,** 297–300.

Witjes, W.P.J., Crul, B.J.P., Vollhaard, E.J., Joosten, H.J.M., and Egmond, J. (1992). Application of sublingual buprenorphine in combination with naproxen or paracetamol for postoperative pain relief in cholecystectomy patients in a double-blind study. *Acta Anaesthesiol. Scand.* **36,** 323–327.

Woodhouse, A., Hobbes, A.F.T., Mather, L.E., and Gibson, M. (1996). A comparison of morphine, pethidine and fentanyl in the postsurgical patient-controlled environment. *Pain.* **64,** 115–121.

Wrench, I.J., Ward, E.J.H., Walder, A.D., and Hobbs, G.J. (1996). The prevention of postoperative nausea and vomiting using a combination of ondansetron and droperidol. *Anaesthesia.* **51,** 776–778.

Yu, P.Y.H., and Gambling, D.R. (1993). A comparative study of patient-controlled epidural fentanyl and single dose epidural morphine for post-caesarean analgesia. *Can. J. Anaesth.* **40,** 416–420.

Zech, D., Grond, S., and Lynch, J. (1993). Subcutaneous and transdermal administration of opioids in cancer pain. A review. *Eur. J. Pain.* **14,** 69–78.

Zech, D.F.J., Grond, S.U.A., Lynch, J., Dauer, H.G., Stollenwerk, B., and Lehmann, K.A. (1992). Transdermal fentanyl and initial dose-finding with patient-controlled analgesia in cancer pain. A pilot study with 20 terminally ill cancer patients. *Pain.* **50,** 293–301.

CHAPTER 15

Opioids in Chronic Nonmalignant Pain

DWIGHT E. MOULIN

Introduction

Chronic pain, usually considered to be continuous or episodic pain of at least six months duration, is a common cause of major disability. A recent survey of randomly selected adult Americans estimated that almost one individual in five, or 30 million people, suffers from chronic pain (Jorensen and Lietman, 1994). Given the magnitude of the problem, every approach of potential therapeutic value deserves to be studied in a rigorous manner. Although the place of opioid analgesics in the management of cancer pain is beyond question (Levy, 1996), a systematic approach to the role of opioid analgesics in chronic nonmalignant pain has been hindered by perceived risks of serious adverse events. The traditional view has been that, despite reports of partial pain relief, opioid use will lead to impaired cognition and drug-seeking behavior that will ultimately impair quality of life. This view has been reinforced by leading journals, which continue to stigmatize the use of opioid analgesics in the management of chronic nonmalignant pain. For instance, a recent review article in the *New England Journal of Medicine* on the management of the complications of diabetes mellitus states that, in reference to the treatment of painful neuropathy, "narcotic agents should be avoided because of their high potential for abuse" (Clark and Lee, 1995). Given this mindset, reluctance to use long-term opioid therapy in patients with chronic nonmalignant pain is understandable. However, there is emerging evidence that this view is very much distorted and that in selected patients chronic opioid treatment is appropriate and justified.

Published Reports of Opioid Use

Extensive survey data on opioid use in chronic nonmalignant pain has accumulated over the past 15 years. Representative studies are listed in Table 15.1. Some surveys report significant pain relief in response to long-term opioid therapy (Taub, 1982; Portenoy and Foley, 1986; Tennant et al., 1988; Bouckoms et al., 1992); others describe the additional benefit of improvement in performance status (Tennant and Uelman, 1983; France et al., 1984). A relatively recent study (Zenz et al., 1992) is

Christoph Stein, ed., *Opioids in Pain Control: Basic and Clinical Aspects*. Printed in the United States of

Table 15.1. *Representative Published Surveys and Randomized Controlled Trials* of Opioids for Chronic Nonmalignant Pain*

Author	n	Diagnosis	Daily Dose Equivalent	Duration	Outcome
Maruta and Swanson (1981)	42	Musculoskeletal	Low-dose (30 mg) and high-dose (>30 mg) oxycodone	1 month	Significantly lower treatment success rate than 158 nonusers of opioids
Taub (1982)	313	Somatic and neuropathic	Mean 10–20 mg oral methadone	Up to 6 years	Generalized benefit; abuse in 13 patients (8 had prior history drug abuse)
Turner et al. (1982)	92	Musculoskeletal	Not stated; roughly half on opioids and half on opioids and sedatives	Not stated	Greater physical impairment and higher hypochondriasis and hysteria scores than in 39 nonusers
Portenoy and Foley (1986)	38	Mixed	Median 10–20 mg parenteral	Median 3–4 years	Adequate or partial relief in 24 patients; little functional improvement; abuse in 2
Tennant et al. (1988)	52	Mixed	Range 10–240 mg oral methadone	Average >12 years	Adequate or partial relief in all patients; constipation in 20, edema in 12
Zenz et al. (1992)	100	Mixed	Oral morphine range 20–2,000 mg	Mean 224 days	Good or partial pain relief in 79 patients; overall improvement in performance status; no abuse
Arkinstall et al. (1995)*	30	Musculoskeletal	Mean oral codeine 273 mg	7 days in cross-over study	Significant pain relief and improvement in function
Moulin et al. (1996)*	46	Musculoskeletal	Mean oral morphine 83.5 mg	9 weeks in cross-over study	Significant pain relief; no improvement in function or psychological status; no abuse

typical of those surveys suggesting overall benefit. One hundred patients with predominantly neuropathic pain and back pain were followed for a mean of 224 days. They were treated with dihydrocodeine, buprenorphine, or morphine in a dose range of 20–2,000 mg of oral morphine equivalents daily. Greater than 50% pain relief was obtained by 51 patients, and 25–50% pain relief was reported by 28 patients. Pain reduction was associated with a significant increase in performance status. There were no cases of respiratory depression or addiction to opioids. In contrast, studies originating in multidisciplinary pain-management programs suggest that chronic opioid therapy leads to greater psychological distress, impaired cognition, and poor outcome (Maruta et al., 1979; Maruta and Swanson, 1981; Turner et al., 1982; McNairy et al., 1984). All of these studies likely suffer from lack of adequate controls and inherent biases. Surveys declaring benefit from opioid analgesics are subject to extraneous factors that might be responsible for improvement. Patients are seen regularly for prescription refills, and the treatment team has usually communicated that pain management is a high priority. A quality assurance study of 248 patients with chronic nonmalignant pain revealed that there was little correlation between pain severity and satisfaction with the treatment (Ward and Gordon, 1994). Satisfaction was, however, related to communication by the health-care team that treatment of pain was considered very important. Patients may therefore report benefit because of the attitude of the caregivers rather than as a function of the analgesics prescribed. Negative reports from multidisciplinary pain clinics may reflect selection bias. Patients admitted to these treatment programs who are already on opioid analgesics may be preselected to have poor outcomes by virtue of their greater physical impairment and psychological distress (Maruta and Swanson, 1981; Turner et al., 1982).

Only two randomized controlled trials address the issue of efficacy of oral opioid analgesics in chronic nonmalignant pain. One group reported on 30 patients with predominantly musculoskeletal pain who were treated for one week with sustained-release codeine or placebo in a cross-over study (Arkinstall et al., 1995). With a mean daily codeine dose of 273 mg, there was an overall reduction in pain intensity of 29% and a reduction in the Pain Disability Index of an identical 29%. However, virtually all of these patients had previously been treated with codeine, and the mean duration of opioid use prior to the study was 6 years. It is therefore not surprising that three-quarters of the patients declared a blinded treatment preference for codeine, and over 90% requested long-term open-label treatment with sustained-release codeine. Another group conducted a double blind cross-over trial in which 46 patients with chronic musculoskeletal pain who had not responded to codeine, anti-inflammatory agents, or antidepressants were randomized to sustained-release morphine or active placebo (benztropine) for 9 weeks (Moulin et al., 1996). The mean daily dose of morphine was 83.5 mg. The morphine group showed a significant reduction in pain intensity relative to placebo, but the benefit was modest. Of the 40% of patients who declared a blinded treatment preference for morphine, the mean pain intensity (visual analog scale 0–10 cm) dropped from 8.2 to 7.1 – a 13% reduction. There were no significant differences in psychological features, functional status, or cognition between morphine and placebo, and there was no evidence of psychological dependence or addiction.

Opioid Responsiveness

Pain can generally be classified as nociceptive, neuropathic, or idiopathic in nature (Payne, 1990) and can be further classified as acute or chronic. Opioid responsiveness, defined as the balance between analgesia and dose-limiting toxicity during dose titration (Portenoy et al., 1990), varies tremendously among these types of pain. Nociceptive pain that is acute (e.g., postoperative pain) or related to progressive tissue injury (e.g., tumor infiltration) usually responds exceedingly well to opioid analgesics (Bonica, 1989; Foley and Inturrisi, 1989) – reflecting a favorable balance between analgesia and side effects. Chronic nociceptive pain of myofascial or musculoskeletal origin does not respond nearly as well. As previously discussed, two randomized controlled trials involving chronic pain of musculoskeletal origin showed only modest benefit from opioid analgesics, with reductions in pain intensity in the 15–30% range (Arkinstall et al., 1995; Moulin et al., 1996). The morphine trial is especially striking because the mean daily dose of 83.5 mg was at least four times more potent than the pretrial analgesic, and this was reflected in the side effect profiles and cardiovascular responses (Moulin et al., 1996). This relative lack of opioid responsiveness may be explained in part by the mechanism of action of opioids on the central nervous system to relieve pain. Opioids act directly on the spinal cord and indirectly through descending inhibitory projections from the brainstem to depress nociceptor transmission through the dorsal horn (Dickenson, 1994; Gogas et al., 1996). Chronic pain involves affective, behavioral, and social dimensions that may not respond to opioid analgesics (Turk, 1994).

Opioid responsiveness to chronic neuropathic pain remains controversial. Two placebo-controlled studies were particularly influential in asserting the notion that neuropathic pain responds poorly to opioids (Arner and Meyerson, 1988; Kupers et al., 1991). The latter study suggested that morphine reduced the affective but not the sensory dimension of neuropathic pain. Reported clinical experience with neuropathic cancer pain also suggests diminished opioid responsiveness (Bruera et al., 1989a; Moulin and Foley, 1990). However, a randomized controlled trial involving patients with postherpetic neuralgia showed significant pain relief with morphine (Rowbatham et al., 1991), and a combined analysis of several controlled single-dose studies in cancer patients demonstrated that neuropathic pain responds to standard opioid doses, although the response was less than that to nociceptive pain (Cherny et al., 1994). Two studies involving patient-controlled analgesic systems suggest that a favorable balance between analgesia and side effects is less likely to occur among persons with neuropathic pain than nociceptive pain (McQuay et al., 1992; Jadad et al., 1992). Overall, the extant literature indicates that neuropathic pain does respond to opioids in a classic dose-dependent fashion, but this involves a shift to the right in the dose-response curve, which may increase the risk of side effects and therefore compromise quality of life (Portenoy et al., 1990).

Two placebo-controlled trials suggest that idiopathic pain is not opioid responsive (Arner and Meyerson, 1988; Kupers et al., 1991). This finding may in part explain the reluctance of most clinicians to use opioids for idiopathic pain as compared to pain with a clear-cut etiology. Although this conclusion has to be interpreted cautiously, chronic pain that has no identifiable initiating event or cause or that is determined primarily by psychological factors is less likely to respond to any pharmacologic intervention.

Potential Complications of Chronic Opioid Use

Organ Toxicity

Although there have been no systematic longitudinal studies of opioid use to assess organ damage, extensive clinical experience in the cancer population and in methadone programs to treat opioid addiction indicate that the risk of major organ toxicity must be exceedingly low (Portenoy, 1994). Opioids have the potential to release histamine from mast cells, and the result can be itching and urticaria (Jaffe and Martin, 1985). However, major complications such as laryngeal edema and airway obstruction are extremely unlikely. Pulmonary edema has been reported, but in patients dying from advanced cancer who were given very high opioid doses (Bruera and Miller, 1989). Animal studies have suggested that opioid exposure can alter cell-mediated immunity (Molitor et al., 1991). Although there is no clinical confirmation of this observation, further evaluation is required in otherwise well patients who receive long-term treatment for chronic nonmalignant pain.

Side Effects, Including Cognitive Impairment

Opioids produce several clinically significant effects other than analgesia. Nausea, vomiting, and sedation can produce serious morbidity, but in the cancer population tolerance to these adverse effects frequently develops, or patients can be switched from one opioid analgesic to another with a more favorable side effect profile (Foley, 1991). Constipation, a persistent problem, usually responds to an aggressive bowel regimen involving stimulants and stool softeners (Levy, 1996). In the methadone maintenance population approximately 10–25% of patients complain of persistent constipation, sweating, insomnia, and decreased sexual function (Kreek, 1978). In a morphine trial over 9 weeks for chronic nonmalignant pain, nausea, vomiting, poor appetite, dizziness, and constipation occurred in at least a third of patients and usually required specific treatment (Moulin et al., 1996). However, this study may have overestimated the risk of side effects because the structured protocol did not allow for individualized dose titration, which would be available in the clinical setting.

The issue of cognitive impairment is particularly important in the management of chronic nonmalignant pain because mental clouding due to opioids could compromise a rehabilitation program. Cognitive impairment has been reported in surveys of patients referred to multidisciplinary pain-management programs (Maruta, 1978; McNairy et al., 1984). It has also been reported in some surveys of methadone maintenance programs (Gritz et al., 1975; Rounsaville et al., 1981) but not in others (Appel and Gordon, 1976; Lombardo et al., 1976). More recent studies strongly suggest that persistent sedation is uncommon in the patient without other predisposing causes of encephalopathy. A survey of patients with advanced cancer noted significant cognitive impairment when opioid doses increased by 30% or more in the previous two days but not when doses were stable (Bruera et al., 1989a). A randomized controlled trial of oral morphine 15 mg in healthy subjects did not show significant cognitive or psychomotor dysfunction (Hanks et al., 1995). Oral morphine titration to a mean dose of 83.5 mg daily over 3 weeks and then maintained for 6 weeks in patients with chronic nonmalignant pain did not reveal cognitive impairment using a sensitive cognitive screen (Moulin et al., 1996). A controlled trial of driving skills in cancer patients on oral morphine at a mean dose of 209 mg daily did not show any significant psychomotor dysfunction (Vainio et al., 1995). These findings strongly suggest that tolerance usually develops to the cognitive effects of opioid drugs.

Analgesic Tolerance

Tolerance occurs when exposure to a drug results in the lessening of its effect or the need for higher doses to maintain it (Foley, 1991). As previously discussed, the development of tolerance to the adverse pharmacologic effects of opioid analgesics is common. What about tolerance to analgesic effects? Although tolerance to the antinociceptive effects of opioid drugs can be easily demonstrated in animal models (Louie and Way, 1991), pharmacodynamic tolerance as the result of drug exposure per se appears uncommon in the clinical setting. Numerous longitudinal studies in both cancer and noncancer populations show that opioid doses typically stabilize for extended periods of time (Portenoy and Foley, 1986; Hill et al., 1990; Plummer et al., 1991; Schug et al., 1992). When cancer patients undergo dose escalation to maintain analgesic effects, there is usually evidence of disease progression or increased psychological distress to explain it (Gonzales et al., 1991; Schug et al., 1992). These observations suggest that tolerance attributable to drug exposure is unlikely to complicate the management of chronic pain patients.

Risk of Psychological Dependence or Addiction

It is crucial to differentiate between physical and psychological dependence to assess the risk of addiction when opioid analgesics are used in the management of chronic pain. Physical dependence is a physiologic phenomenon, characterized by the development of withdrawal symptoms following abrupt discontinuation of treatment, substantial dose reduction, or antagonistic drug administration (Jaffe, 1985). The potential for an abstinence syndrome exists whenever repeated doses of analgesic have been administered for more than a few days. However, abstinence symptoms are usually self-limiting and can be avoided by 50% dose reductions every two to three days. Yet, psychological dependence or addiction can be defined as compulsive drug use despite harm, an overwhelming preoccupation with the securing of the drug, and the tendency to relapse after withdrawal (Jaffe, 1985). Addiction reflects a behavioral pattern of drug use when medication is taken for its psychic effects rather than for its analgesic properties. Aberrant drug-related behavior indicative of addiction includes selling prescription drugs, forging prescriptions, multiple episodes of prescription loss, and deterioration in performance that appears related to drug use (Portenoy, 1994). The term *pseudoaddiction* was introduced to describe behavior related to the threat of drug withdrawal when specific benefits such as pain relief have already been realized (Weissman and Haddox, 1989). Pseudoaddiction has been observed in the cancer pain population when undertreatment of pain is met with aberrant behavior in an attempt to secure more drug. When the pain is relieved, the behavior ceases. Pseudoaddictive behavior includes aggressive complaining about the need for more drug, drug hoarding during periods of reduced symptoms, and attempts to acquire the same or similar analgesics from other physicians (Portenoy, 1994). Such behavior is less predictive of true psychological dependence or addiction.

Two older studies were particularly influential in supporting the notion that chronic opioid therapy leads to addiction (Kolb, 1925; Rayport, 1954). In particular, the latter study reported that opioids prescribed for painful medical disorders were responsible for iatrogenic addiction in 27% of an addicted population. Although this was a retrospective study that relied on the ability of addicts to remember accurately their medical and social history, it had a tremendous negative impact on opioid use for both acute and chronic pain. This view was reinforced by the irrational link between physical and psychological dependence and by reports of aberrant drug-related behavior in patients attending multidisciplinary pain clinics (Maruta et al., 1979; Turner and Romano, 1984; Buckley et al., 1986). However, experience with opioid use in more heterogeneous populations does not support this view. Only four of 11,882 patients without a history of substance abuse who were treated with opioids in hospital developed evidence of addiction (Porter and Jick, 1980). A national survey of burn units did not reveal a single case of iatrogenic addiction in over 10,000 patients treated for burn pain (Perry and Heidrich, 1982), and a survey of 2,269 patients attending a headache clinic uncovered only three cases of opioid abuse (Medina and Diamond, 1977). Patients allowed to self-administer an opioid for the treatment of mucositis-related pain following bone marrow transplantation did not develop aberrant drug-related behavior (Chapman and Hill, 1989). Cancer patients who have been successfully weaned from an opioid drug because of the availability of other treatment modalities rarely evidence addictive behavior (Moulin and Foley, 1990). These studies indicate that the inherent reinforcing properties of a drug are not sufficient to produce addiction. Other factors include genetic predisposition and the situational and psychological milieu of the patient (Jaffe, 1985). The importance of situational factors is highlighted by the observation that war veterans who became addicted while serving in Vietnam had far lower recedivism rates following detoxification and return to the United States than other addict populations (Robins et al., 1974). The extant literature strongly suggests that the overall risk of addiction associated with the long-term administration of opioid analgesics to patients with chronic nonmalignant pain is quite low if there is no prior history of substance abuse and no evidence of a major personality disorder or social disruption. Obviously, the older patient with an established track record of licit drug use and emotional stability is least likely to develop iatrogenic addiction.

Impact of Government Regulations

Unfortunately, regulatory and law-enforcement agencies remain notoriously naive regarding the risk of psychological dependence or addiction in patients given opioid drugs for chronic pain. According to a survey of U.S. state medical legislators, only 12% thought that the administration of opioids to patients with chronic nonmalignant pain and no history of substance abuse was lawful and acceptable medical practice, and almost none could accurately distinguish between physical dependence, psychological dependence, and tolerance (Joranson et al., 1992). Perceived government interference leads to underutilization of opioid analgesics in patients who clearly need analgesics for pain relief. The implementation of triplicate prescription programs has been consistently followed by a greater than 50% reduction in the prescribing of controlled drugs in the United States (Portenoy, 1994). Regulatory bodies have a responsibility to prevent the inappropriate use of medication, such as the selling of controlled drugs, but they should also support the legitimate use of opioids when the primary goal is pain relief.

Goals of Treatment

The traditional view of chronic pain management is that opioid analgesics provide the mainstay of treatment for cancer pain whereas nonpharmacologic multidisciplinary pain-management programs are the accepted approach to chronic pain of nonmalignant origin. The latter approach is based on the primary goal of functional restoration with the hope that psychological and rehabilitative treatments will also provide some degree of pain relief. However, most patients and primary caregivers are oriented more to the conventional medical model of making a specific diagnosis and then eliminating the pain. This goal is frequently untenable – the specific diagnosis is often elusive (Deyo et al., 1990), and complete pain relief is unrealistic. Given these inadequacies, what priority should be assigned to pain relief relative to functional restoration in the management of chronic nonmalignant pain? (Fig. 15.1). Large and Schug (1995) have posited that the suffering associated with chronic pain leads to loss of control and autonomy and that reliance on medication might lead to

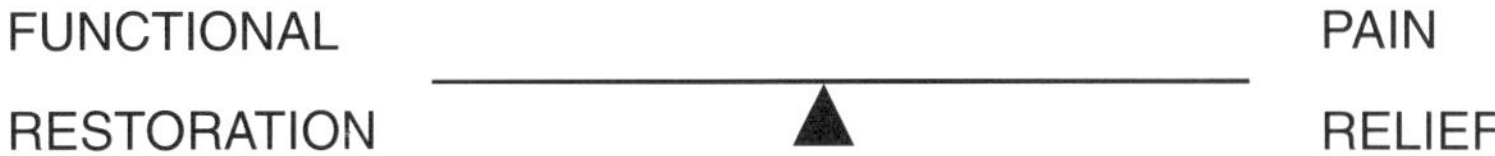

Figure 15.1. The balance between functional restoration and pain relief in the management of chronic nonmalignant pain: the use of opioid analgesics may seem counterproductive rather than complementary.

further loss of autonomy – the locus of control is externalized so that patients no longer feel in control of their management. Somerville (1995) has countered that if opioid treatment is reasonably safe, according to the doctrine of informed consent, it should be offered to the patient and that to deny access to opioids actually reduces autonomy. Clinical experience suggests that a treatment program which focuses on analgesics without incorporating psychosocial and behavioral approaches can reinforce pain-related behavior and undermine a rehabilitative program targeted to function restoration (Fordyce, 1992; Turk and Meichenbaum, 1994). Yet, numerous reviews of multidisciplinary pain-treatment programs show significant improvements in physical and psychological function and reduced medication use but limited pain relief (Large and Peters, 1991; Flor et al., 1992; Williams et al., 1996).

How do we come to a common ground regarding the dual goals of pain relief and functional restoration in the treatment of chronic nonmalignant pain? Extensive survey data and limited controlled trials provide some guidance regarding the long-term administration of opioid drugs. First, there is a low risk of psychological dependence or addiction in the absence of a history of substance abuse. Second, cognitive impairment is unlikely to compromise the treatment program, and other side effects are usually controllable with individualized dose titration and pharmacologic measures such as antiemetics and bowel stimulants. Third, opioid treatment probably provides modest but significant pain relief in selected patients and may in fact facilitate rehabilitative goals. If one accepts these tenets, compatibility between opioid therapy and multidisciplinary pain-management programs could be facilitated by making analgesic use purely time contingent and not pain contingent after initial dose titration. This compromise (i.e., the avoidance of analgesics for breakthrough pain) might allow the patient to focus on "well behavior" rather than on pain behavior (Fordyce, 1978) – especially if sustained-release opioid preparations are used. An exception to this model would be the elderly or very disabled patient in which the primary goal is clearly pain relief and not functional restoration.

Guidelines for Opioid Therapy in Chronic Nonmalignant Pain

Guidelines for opioid maintenance therapy in patients with chronic nonmalignant pain are provided in Table 15.2. These guidelines are similar to those that have appeared in previous publications (Merry et al., 1992; Portenoy, 1994; Hagen et al., 1995), but they include modifications based on the information in this chapter. They are also based on the premise that functional restoration is at least as important a goal as pain relief.

Table 15.2. *Guidelines for Opioid Therapy in Chronic Nonmalignant Pain*

- Consider after other reasonable therapies have failed.
- Perform a complete pain and psychosocial history and a physical examination. A history of isolated tension-type headaches, substance abuse, major personality disorder, or social disruption are relative contraindications to opioid therapy.
- A single physician who sets up a contract with the patient should be responsible for opioid prescriptions. The agreement should specify the drug regimen, the goals of treatment, possible side effects, the functional restoration program, and violations that will result in the abrupt termination of opioid therapy.
- The opioid analgesic of choice (preferably a sustained-release preparation) should be administered around the clock with an initial titration phase of 3–6 weeks to minimize side effects. Dosing should generally be time contingent rather than pain contingent except during the titration phase where rescue doses for breakthrough pain should be used to help determine the maintenance dose.
- Incremental dosing during the titration phase should result in a graded analgesic response or at least partial pain relief. Failure to realize at least partial analgesia at initial doses may mean that the pain syndrome is unresponsive to opioid treatment.
- The patient should be seen monthly for the first six months and every two months thereafter. At each visit the patient should be assessed for analgesia, opioid-related side effects, compliance with functional goals, and the presence of aberrant drug-related behavior. All of this information should be documented in the medical record.
- The patient should be reminded that the goal of opioid therapy is to make the pain tolerable and perhaps to improve function as part of a comprehensive treatment program.

A complete history and physical examination are essential. The psychosocial history is especially pertinent because the patient's psychiatric and psychological profile can be a major determinant of pain behavior and disability. Chronic pain that appears idiopathic (i.e., has no identifiable antecedent event or cause) or is determined primarily by psychogenic factors is less likely to respond to pharmacologic measures. With rare exceptions, isolated tension-type headaches should not be treated with opioid drugs because the risk of inducing chronic daily headaches from analgesic rebound is significant (Rapaport, 1988).

An agreement should be established between the prescribing physician and the patient that discusses the drug regimen and possible side effects. Functional goals, including a graduated exercise program, should also be agreed upon. The contract should clearly state that there is to be no unsanctioned dose escalation and no procurement of opioids from any other physician. It should be made clear that violation of this agreement will result in the termination of opioid treatment. The agreement can take the form of a consent discussion that addresses these issues with documentation in the medical record or can take the form of a formal written consent.

Careful monitoring is required during the titration phase to assess pain relief and side effects. Failure of a graded analgesic response to incremental doses may mean that opioid therapy is ineffective, and consideration should be given to terminating treatment. Patients should be seen monthly for the first six months and every two months thereafter. At each visit, patients should be assessed for analgesia, opioid-related side effects, compliance with functional goals, and presence of aberrant drug-related behavior.

The goal of chronic opioid therapy is to make the pain tolerable and perhaps improve function. For some patients even modest pain relief can make the difference between bearable and unbearable pain. Science and good clinical judgment should replace myth and fear of recrimination in the use of opioid analgesics for chronic nonmalignant pain (Melzack, 1990).

REFERENCES

Appel, P.W., and Gordon, N.B. (1976). Digit-symbol performance in methadone-treated ex-heroin addicts. *Am. J. Psychiatry.* **133,** 1337–1340.

Arkinstall, W., Sandler, A., Goughnour, B., et al. (1995). Efficacy of controlled-release codeine in chronic nonmalignant pain: A randomized, placebo-controlled clinical trial. *Pain.* **62,** 169–178.

Arner, S., and Meyerson, B.A. (1988). Lack of analgesic effect of opioids on neuropathic and idiopathic forms of pain. *Pain.* **33,** 11–23.

Bonica, J.J. (1989). Post-operative pain. In Bonica, J.J., Loeser, J.D., Chapman, C.R., and Fordyce, W.E. (eds)., *The management of pain,* Vol. 1, 2nd ed. Philadelphia: Lea and Febiger, 461–480.

Bouckoms, A.J., Masand, P., Murray, G.B., Cassem, E.H., Stern, T.A., and Tesar, G.E. (1992). Chronic nonmalignant pain treated with long-term oral narcotic analgesics. *Ann. Clin. Psychiatry.* **4,** 185–192.

Bruera, E., MacMillan, D., Hanson, J., and MacDonald, R.N. (1989a). The Edmonton staging system for cancer pain: Preliminary report. *Pain.* **37,** 203–210.

Bruera, E., MacMillan, K., Hanson, J., and MacDonald, R.N. (1989b). The cognitive effects of the administration of narcotic analgesics in patients with cancer pain. *Pain.* **39,** 13–16.

Bruera, E., and Miller, M.J. (1989). Non-carcinogenic pulmonary edema after narcotic treatment for cancer pain. *Pain.* **39,** 297–300.

Buckley, F.P, Sizemore, W.A., and Charlton, J.E. (1986). Medication management in patients with chronic nonmalignant pain. A review of the use of a drug withdrawal protocol. *Pain.* **26,** 153–166.

Chapman, C.R., and Hill, H.F. (1989). Prolonged morphine self-administration and addiction liability: Evaluation of two theories in a bone marrow transplant unit. *Cancer.* **63,** 1636–1644.

Cherny, N.I., Thaler, H.T., Friedlander-Klar, H., et al. (1994). Opioid responsiveness of cancer pain syndromes caused by neuropathic or nociceptive mechanisms: A combined analysis of controlled single-dose studies. *Neurology.* **44,** 857–861.

Clark, C.M., and Lee, D.A. (1995). Prevention and treatment of the complications of diabetes mellitus. *N. Engl. J. Med.* **332,** 1210–1217.

Deyo, R.A., Walsh, N.E., Martin, D.C., Schoenfeld, L.S., and Ramamurthy, S. (1990). Controlled trial of transcutaneous electrical nerve stimulation (TENS) and exercise for chronic low back pain. *N. Engl. J. Med.* **23,** 1627–1634.

Dickenson, A.H. (1994). Where and how do opioids act? In Gebhart, G.S., Hammond, D.L., and Jensen, T.S. (eds.), *Progress in pain research and management,* Vol. 2. Seattle: IASP Press, 525–552.

Flor, H., Fydrich, T., and Turk, D.C. (1992). Efficacy of multidisciplinary pain treatment centers: A meta-analytic review. *Pain.* **49,** 221–230.

Foley, K.M. (1991). Clinical tolerance to opioids. In Basbaum, A.I., and Besson, J.-M. (eds.), *Towards a new pharmacotherapy of pain.* Chichester: John Wiley, 181–203.

Foley, K.M., and Inturrisi, C.E. (1989). Pharmacological approaches to cancer pain. In Foley, M.K., and Payne, R. (eds.), *Current therapy of pain.* Toronto: B.C. Decker, 303–331.

Fordyce, W.E. (1978). Learning process in pain. In Sternback, R.A. (ed.)., *The psychology of pain.* New York: Raven Press, 2–19.

Fordyce, W.E. (1992). Opioids, pain and behavioural outcomes. *APS Journal.* **1,** 282–284.

France, R.D., Urban, B.J., and Keefe, F.J. (1984). Long-term use of narcotic analgesics in chronic pain. *Soc. Sci. Med.* **19,** 1379–1382.

Gogas, K.R., Cho, H.J., Botchkina, G.I., Levine, J.D., and Basbaum, A.I. (1996). Inhibition of noxious stimulus-evoked pain behaviours and neuronal fos-like immunoreactivity in the spinal cord of the rat by supraspinal morphine. *Pain.* **65,** 9–15.

Gonzales, G.R., Elliott K.J., Portenoy, R.K., and Foley, K.M. (1991). The impact of a comprehensive evaluation in the management of cancer pain. *Pain.* **47,** 141–144.

Gritz, E.R., Shiffman, S.M., Jarvik, M.E., Haber, J., Dymond, A.M., Coger, R., Charuvastra, V., and Schlesinger, J. (1975). Physiological and psychological effects of methadone in man. *Arch. Gen. Psychiatry.* **32,** 237–242.

Hagen, N., Flynne, P., Hays, H., and MacDonald, N. (1995). Guidelines for managing chronic non-malignant pain: Opioids and other agents. *Can. Fam. Physician.* **41,** 49–53.

Hanks, G.W., O'Neill, W.M., Simpson, P., and Wesnek, K. (1995). The cognitive and psychomotor effects of opioid analgesics. II. A randomized controlled trial of single doses of morphine, lorazepam and placebo in healthy subjects. *Eur. J. Clin. Pharmacol.* **48**(6), 455–460.

Hill, H.F., Chapman, C.R., Kornell, J.A., Sullivan, K.M., Saeger, L.C., and Benedetti, C. (1990). Self-administration of morphine in bone marrow transplant patients reduces drug requirement. *Pain.* **40,** 121–129.

Jadad, A.R., Carroll, D., Glynn, C.J., Moore, R.A., and McQuay, H.J. (1992). Morphine responsiveness of chronic pain: Double blind randomized crossover study with patient-controlled analgesia. *Lancet.* **339,** 1367–1371.

Jaffe, J.H. (1985). Drug addiction and drug abuse. In Gilman, A.G., Goodman, L.S., Rall, T.W., and Murad, F. (eds.), *The pharmacological basis of therapeutics,* 7th ed. New York: Macmillan, 532–581.

Jaffe, J.H., and Martin, W.R. (1985). Opioid analgesics and antagonists. In Gilman, A.G., Goodman, L.S., Rall, T.W., and Murad, F. (eds.), *The pharmacological basis of therapeutics,* 7th ed. New York: Macmillan, 491–531.

Joranson, D.E., Cleeland, C.S., Weissman, D.E., et al. (1992). Opioids for chronic cancer and noncancer pain: A survey of state medical board members. *J. Med. Licen. Discipl.* **79,** 15–49.

Joranson, D.E., and Lietman, R. (1994). *The McNeil National Pain Study.* New York: Louis Harris and Associates.

Kolb, L. (1925). Types and characteristics of drug addicts. *Men. Hyg.* **9,** 300–313.

Kreek, M.J. (1978). Medical complications in methadone patients. *Ann. NY Acad. Sci.* **311,** 110–134.

Kupers, R.C., Konings, H., Adriansen, H., and Gybels, J.M. (1991). Morphine differentially affects the sensory and affective pain rating in neurogenic and idiopathic forms of pain. *Pain.* **47,** 5–12.

Large, R., and Peters, J. (1991). A critical appraisal of outcome of multidisciplinary pain clinic treatments. In Bond, M.R., Charlton, J.E., and Woolf., C.J. (eds.), *Proceedings of the VIth World Congress on Pain.* Elsevier Science Publishers BV, 417–427.

Large, R.G., and Schug, S.A. (1995). Opioids for chronic pain of non-malignant origin – caring or crippling? *Health Care Analysis.* **3,** 5–11.

Levy, M.H. (1996). Pharmacologic treatment of cancer pain. *N. Engl. J. Med.* **335,** 1124–1132.

Lombardo, W.K., Lombardo, B., and Goldstein, A. (1976). Cognitive functioning under moderate and low dose methadone maintenance. *Int. J. Addict.* **11,** 389–401.

Louie, A.K., and Way, E.L. (1991). Overview of opiate tolerance and physical dependence. In Almeida, O.F., and Shippenberg, T.S. (eds.), *Neurobiology of opioids.* New York: Springer-Verlag.

Maruta, T. (1978). Prescription drug-induced organic brain syndrome. *Amer. J. Psychiatry* **135,** 376–377.

Maruta, T., and Swanson, D.W. (1981). Problems with the use of oxycodone compound in patients with chronic pain. *Pain.* **11,** 389–396.

Maruta, T., Swanson, D.W., and Finlayson, R.E. (1979). Drug abuse and dependency in patients with chronic pain. *Mayo Clin. Proc.* **54,** 241–244.

McNairy, S.L., Maruta, T., Ivnik, R.J., Swanson, D.W., and Ilstrup, D.M. (1984). Prescription medication dependence and neuropsychologic function. *Pain.* **18,** 169–177.

McQuay, H.J., Jadad, A.R., Carroll, D., Faura, C., Glynn, C.J., Moore, R.A., and Liu, Y. (1992). Opioid sensitivity of chronic pain: A patient-controlled analgesia method. *Anaesthesia.* **47,** 757–767.

Medina, J.L., and Diamond, S. (1977). Drug dependency in patients with chronic headache. *Headache.* **17,** 12–14.

Melzack, R. (1990). The tragedy of needless pain. *Sci. Am.* **262,** 27–33.

Merry, A.F., Schug, S.A., Richards, E.G., and Large, R.G. (1992). Opioids in chronic pain of nonmalignant origin: State of the debate in New Zealand. *Eur. J. Pain.* **13,** 39–43.

Molitor, T.W., Morilla, A., Risdahl, J.M., Murtaugh, M.P., Chao, C.C., and Peterson, P.K. (1991). Chronic morphine administration impairs cell-mediated immune responses in swine. *J. Pharmacol. Exp. Ther.* **260,** 581–586.

Moulin, D.E., and Foley, K.M. (1990). Review of a hospital-based pain service. In Foley, K.M., Bonica, J.J., and Ventafridda, V. (eds.), *Advances in pain research and therapy,* Vol. 16. Second International Congress on Cancer Pain. New York: Raven Press, 413–427.

Moulin, D.E., Iezzi, A., Amireh, R., Sharpe, W.K.J., Boyd, D., and Merskey, H. (1996). Randomised trial of oral morphine for chronic non-cancer pain. *Lancet.* **347,** 143–147.

Payne, R. (1990). Pathophysiology of cancer pain. *Adv. Pain. Res. Therapy.* **16,** 13–26.

Perry, S., and Heidrich, G. (1982). Management of pain during debridement: A survey of U.S. burn units. *Pain.* **13,** 267–280.

Plummer, J.L., Cherry, D.A., Cousins, M.J., Gourlay, G.K., Onley, M.M., and Evans, K.H.A. (1991). Long-term spinal administration of morphine in cancer and non-cancer pain: A retrospective study. *Pain.* **44,** 215–220.

Portenoy, R.K. (1994). Opioid therapy for chronic nonmalignant pain: Current status. In Fields, H.L., and Liebeskind, J.C. (eds.), *Progress in pain research and management,* Vol. 1. Seattle: IASP Press, 247–287.

Portenoy, R.K., and Foley, K.M. (1986). Chronic use of opioid analgesics in non-malignant pain. Report of 38 cases. *Pain.* **25,** 171–186.

Portenoy, R.K., Foley, K.M., and Inturrisi, C.E. (1990). The nature of opioid responsiveness and its implications for neuropathic pain: New hypotheses derived from studies of opioid infusions. *Pain.* **43,** 273–286.

Porter, J., and Jick, H. (1980). Addiction rare in patients treated with narcotics. *N. Engl. J. Med.* **302,** 123.

Rapaport, A.M. (1988). Analgesic rebound headache. *Headache.* **28,** 662–665.

Rayport, M. (1954). Experience in the management of patients medically addicted to narcotics. *J.A.M.A.* **156,** 684–691.

Robins, L.N., Davis, D.H., and Nurco, D.N. (1974). How permanent was Vietnam drug addiction? *Amer. J. Publ. Health.* **64,** 38–43.

Rounsaville, B.H., Novelly, R.A., Kleber, H.D., and Jones, C. (1981). Neuropsychological impairment in opiate addicts: Risk factors. *N.Y. Acad. Sci.* **362,** 79–90.

Rowbatham, M.C., Reisner-Keller, L.A., and Fields, H.L. (1991). Both intravenous lidocaine and morphine reduce the pain of postherpetic neuralgia. *Neurology.* **41,** 1024–1028.

Schug, S.A., Zech, D. Grond, S., Jung, H., Meurser, T., and Stobbe, B. (1992). A long-term survey of morphine in cancer pain patients. *J. Pain Symptom Management.* **7,** 259–266.

Somerville, M.A. (1995). Opioids for chronic pain of non-malignant origin – coercion or consent? *Health Care Analysis.* **3,** 12–14.

Taub, A. (1982). Opioid analgesics in the treatment of chronic intractable pain of non-neoplastic origin. In Kitahata, L.M., and Collins, D. (eds.), *Narcotic analgesics in anaesthesiology.* Baltimore, MD: Williams and Wilkins, 199–208.

Tennant, F.S., Robinson, D., Sagherian, A., and Seecof, R. (1988). Chronic opioid treatment of intractable non-malignant pain. *Pain Management.* Jan.–Feb., 18–36.

Tennant, F.S., and Uelman, G.F. (1983). Narcotic maintenance for chronic pain: Medical and legal guidelines. *Postgrad. Med.* **73,** 81–94.

Turk, D.C., and Meichenbaum, D. (1994). A cognitive-behavioural approach to pain management. In Wall, P.D., and Melzack, E. (eds.), *Textbook of pain,* 3rd ed. Edinburgh: Churchill Livingstone, 1337–1348.

Turner, J.A., Calsyn, D.A., Fordyce, W.E., and Ready, L.B. (1982). Drug utilization pattern in chronic pain patients. *Pain.* **12,** 357–363.

Turner, J.A., and Romano, J.M. (1984). Evaluation psychologic interventions for chronic pain: Issues and recent developments. In Benedetti, C., Chapman, C.R., and Moricca, G. (eds.), *Advances in pain research and therapy,* Vol. 7. Management of Pain. New York: Raven Press, 257–296.

Vainio, A., Ollila, J., Matikainen, E., Rosenberg, P., and Kalso, E. (1995). Driving ability in cancer patients receiving long-term morphine analgesia. *Lancet.* **346,** 667–670.

Ward, S.E., and Gordon, D. (1994). Application of the American Pain Society quality assurance standards. *Pain.* **56,** 299–306.

Weissman, D.E., and Haddox, K.D. (1989). Opioid pseudo addiction – an iatrogenic syndrome. *Pain.* **36,** 363–366.

Williams, A.C.de C., Richardson, P.H., Nicholas, M.K., Pither, C.E., Harding, V.R., Ridout, K.L., Ralphs, J.A., Richardson, I.H., Justins, D.M., and Chamberlain, J.H. (1996). Inpatient vs. outpatient pain management: Results of a randomised controlled trial. *Pain.* **66,** 13–22.

Zenz, M., Strumpf, M., and Tryba, M. (1992). Long-term oral opioid therapy in patients with chronic nonmalignant pain. *J. Pain Symptom Management.* **7,** 69–77.

CHAPTER SIXTEEN

Opioids in Cancer Pain

EDUARDO BRUERA, PAUL WALKER, AND PETER LAWLOR

Introduction

Opioids are the most effective treatment in patients with cancer pain (Health and Welfare, Canada, 1984; Foley, 1985). The general principles of pharmacology that are described elsewhere apply also to cancer patients. However, pain syndromes in cancer are unique in intensity and duration, so that opioids must be used at the highest doses in clinical medicine. In addition, cancer patients present with a number of devastating symptoms that require specific treatment, including nausea, delirium, asthenia, and dyspnea. These symptoms and the drugs used in their treatment influence the pattern of opioid use.

This chapter discusses some of the unique characteristics of pain syndromes and clinical situations of cancer patients and their implications for opioid management of cancer pain.

Characteristics of Patients with Cancer Pain

Approximately 80% of cancer patients develop pain before death (Health and Welfare, Canada, 1984; Foley, 1985). Pain occurs more frequently in patients with locally advanced or metastatic cancer, and in approximately 80% of cases the pain is due to the presence of the tumor (Foley, 1985). However, almost one in five advanced cancer patients experience pain as a function of the treatment (radiotherapy or surgical fibrosis, chemotherapy-induced neuropathies), general weakness (tendon retraction, pressure ulcers), or unrelated conditions. Therefore, it is crucial to establish the cause of the pain even in patients with documented disseminated cancer.

In addition to pain, advanced cancer patients have a number of clinical syndromes and are frequently receiving drugs that may influence opioid treatment. For example, anorexia, chronic nausea, and constipation are frequently present in these patients, and these conditions may be aggravated by opioids (Dunlop, 1996; Vigano, 1996). Emesis may decrease the bioavalibility of opioids or result in dehydration due to decreased oral intake. Dehydration or renal failure can result in decreased renal excre-

Christoph Stein, ed., *Opioids in Pain Control: Basic and Clinical Aspects*. Printed in the United States of America.

Table 16.1. *Frequent Myths About Opioids in Cancer Pain*

- Opioids cause addiction.
- Physical dependence equals addiction.
- Tolerance equals addiction.
- Opioids decrease survival.
- Opioids cause frequent respiratory depression.
- Oral opioids are ineffective.

tion of active opioid metabolites with resulting neurotoxicity (see later in this chapter). Cancer patients often experience clinical and subclinical delirium that can be aggravated by opioid treatment (Bruera, 1992). Anitiemetics with central effect such as prochlorperazine, chlorpromazine, dimenhydrinate, tricyclic antidepressants, and benzodiazepines can all result in increased sedation or confusion in these patients. Finally, cancer patients and their families frequently fear the effects of opioids. Among the most frequent myths are that opioids can reduce survival, cause addiction, or induce chronic cognitive failure or that if opioids are used fully now, there may be intractable pain in the future (Health and Welfare, Canada, 1984; Foley, 1985).

The Use of Opioids

Patterns of Use

Opioids have been consistently underused in the treatment of cancer pain (World Health Organization, 1986; Bruera, 1987; Sjernsward et al., 1995). Physicians, nurses, and pharmacists share many of the myths previously described for patients and families (some of these myths are listed in Table 16.1).

In developed countries, the main reasons for the undertreatment of cancer pain are inadequate physician education, poor assessment of the patient's condition, and patient and family reluctance to espouse opioids (Von Roenn et al., 1993; Cleeland et al., 1994). In developing countries the main barriers are poverty and legal and regulatory obstacles to opioid prescription (World Health Organization, 1986; Bruera, 1993; Sjernward et al., 1995).

The World Health Organization and a number of researchers have documented the main obstacles and proposed strategies for an improvement in cancer pain treatment (Health and Welfare, Canada, 1984; Foley, 1985; World Health Organization, 1986; Cleeland et al., 1994; Sjernsward et al., 1995). As a result of these initiatives, the use of opioid analgesics has increased dramatically in both developed and developing countries (World Health Organization, 1990; DeLima and Bruera, 1996). However, even today the majority of cancer patients in the world die of their disease without ever having received a single dose of a strong opioid for the management of their pain.

Current Recommendations

The guidelines of the Agency for Health Care Policy and Research in the United States, the Canadian Ministry of Health, and the World Health Organization, as well as a number of authoritative reviews (Health and Welfare, Canada, 1985; World Health Organization, 1986; U.S. Depart. Health, 1994; Levy, 1996) suggest that patients receive regular opioids, either as intermittent doses or as continuous infusions. However, selected patients can also achieve good analgesia using patient-controlled analgesia, both orally and subcutaneously (Bruera, Brenneis et al., 1988; Bruera and Schoeller, 1992).

Opioid receptor agonists such as codeine, oxycodone, hydromorphone, morphine, and fentanyl are effective analgesics (Foley, 1985; Levy, 1996). Meperidine offers short-acting analgesia and significant neurotoxicity because of the accumulation of active metabolites such as normepridine and should not be used for cancer pain (Health and Welfare, Canada, 1985; U.S. Depart. Health, 1994; World Health Organization, 1986; Levy, 1996). Pentazocine has a high incidence of psychotomimetic effects and, as in the case of all other agonist/antagonists opioids, there is the potential for triggering a withdrawal reaction in dependent patients (Health and Welfare, Canada, 1984; U.S. Depart. Health, 1994; Levy, 1996). Methadone has recently emerged as an alternative in patients with rapid tolerance or neurotoxicity and will be discussed later in this chapter.

Patients should undergo careful titration using a single opioid until good analgesia or dose-limiting toxicity occurs (most frequently nausea or sedation). At this point a trial of an alternative opioid or the addition of adjuvant drugs should be considered (Bruera, 1993; Portenoy, 1993).

The oral route is safe, inexpensive, and effective in the great majority of patients. Slow-release preparations allow for the administration every 12 hours of drugs such as morphine, hydromorphone, codeine, and oxycodone (U.S. Depart. Health and Human Services, 1994; Levy, 1996). Novel preparations of morphine also allow for the administration every 24 hours (Sweet et al., 1996). Two important considerations for slow release opioids are:

1. Patients should always be titrated with a rapid-release opioid until good pain control is achieved. If patients develop severe pain aggravation on a slow-release opioid, they should be retitrated on a rapid-release opioid before the slow-release opioid is restarted at the new equivalent dose. This approach will prevent both delays in achieving pain control and toxicity due to excessive dosing.
2. All patients on slow-release opioids should be provided with rescue doses of rapid-release opioids for extra pain. Most groups provide doses of approximately 10% of the daily opioid dose (U.S. Depart. Health, 1994; Cherny and Foley, 1996; Levy, 1996).

Table 16.2. *Difficult Cancer Pain Syndromes*

- Neuropathic pain
- Incidental pain
- History of alcoholism/drug abuse
- Somatization
- Rapid tolerance

Patients and families should be routinely educated about the importance of regular administration as well the different side effects and be provided with laxatives and antiemetics. Education should also take place routinely about the most common opioid myths (Table 16.1). Special effort should be made to discuss addiction and life shortening, stressing the fact that patients on opioids should be able to function physically and cognitively better than patients in pain.

Difficult Pain Syndromes

Pain can be effectively controlled in most cancer patients with minimal toxicity until death. However, during recent years it has become apparent that some patient characteristics are associated with more difficult treatment. These patients often require multimodal treatment by specialized multidisciplinary groups. The early recognition of these cases will ensure rapid referral and prevent unnecessary pain and opioid-related toxicity (Bruera et al., 1989, 1995).

Table 16.2 summarizes clinical conditions in which opioid treatment may be particularly difficult.

Neuropathic Pain

There has been significant controversy about the role of opioids in neuropathic pain (Aner and Meyerson, 1988; Portenoy et al., 1990; Dubner, 1991). Neuropathic pain has been found to be a poor independent prognostic factor for pain control in cancer patients (Bruera et al., 1989; Bruera, Schoeller et al., 1995). However, most patients with neuropathic cancer pain do improve on opioid analgesics (Bruera et al., 1989; Portenoy et al., 1990; Bruera, Schoeller et al., 1995). Patients with neuropathic cancer pain require significantly higher doses than those with non-neuropathic syndromes (Bruera, Schoeller et al., 1995; Vigano et al., 1996). However, a recent prospective open study suggests that more than two-thirds of patients with neuropathic cancer pain achieve good analgesia with opioids alone (Bruera et al., 1996). Since the effectiveness of adjuvant drugs, including tricyclic antidepressants, anticonvulsants, mexilitine, and baclofen, has rarely been reported to exceed 30% (Bruera and Ripamonti, 1993; Portenoy, 1993), opioids remain the first line of treatment in these patients. Adjuvant drugs should be added when patients reach dose-limiting toxicity (Bruera, 1993; Portenoy, 1993).

Incidental Pain

These patients have no pain or mild pain when resting, but the pain intensity becomes severe when performing certain maneuvres such as sitting, walking, swallowing, or having a bowel movement (Portenoy and Hagen, 1990). The opioid dose capable of controlling pain when resting is ineffective during the incidental episode. The dose that might control pain during the incidental episode would cause unacceptable sedation or cognitive failure at rest.

Most of these patients have bone metastases, and they may benefit from local radiation therapy, orthopedic procedures, or bisphosphonate infusions for pain (Bruera, 1992; Ernst et al., 1992). Neurosurgical procedures such as percutaneous cordotomy (Sanders and Zuurmond, 1995) and spinal opioids (Samlelsson, 1995) can be useful alternatives in these patients.

Systemic opioid treatment should be titrated until dose-limiting toxicity is observed. At that point adjuvant analgesics can be added. When the dose-limiting toxicity is sedation, some patients may be able to receive a higher opioid dose if metholphenidate is started in order to antagonize opioid-induced sedation (Bruera et al., 1992).

Alcoholism and Drug Addiction

A history of alcoholism or drug addiction is a poor prognostic factor for analgesic response in patients with cancer pain (Bruera et al., 1989; Bruera, Schoeller et al., 1995).

Recent research suggests that the mechanism of reward associated with alcohol intake is at least partially mediated by endorphins (O'Brien and McLellan, 1996). Treatments including naltrexone have succeeded in increasing abstinence by blocking such a reward mechanism (O'Brien and McLellan, 1996).

Although most patients with cancer pain and history of alcoholism are not actively consuming alcohol, they are more likely to cope chemically with the distress associated with their illness. This results in increased pain expression with consequent increased opioid dose and risk of toxicity (Bruera, Moyano et al., 1995). Unfortunately, the majority of alcoholic patients are not diagnosed by family physicians and specialists (Moore et al., 1989). Approximately 28% of 200 patients with cancer pain retrospectively screened for alcoholism in a palliative care unit were found to screen positively for alcoholism according to the CAGE Questionnaire (Bruera, Moyano et al., 1995). Only 33% of these outpatients who screened positively on the CAGE questionnaire had been previously diagnosed (Bruera, Moyano et al., 1995). When alcoholic patients and their families received careful opioid titration and counseling on coping chemically, together with ongoing support, both pain intensity and opioid dose were not significantly different from those in nonalcoholic patients (Bruera, Moyano et al., 1995). These findings suggest that patients in whom alcoholism is not detected and treated will achieve worse pain control and use higher doses than nonalcoholic patients (Bruera et al., 1989; Bruera, Schoeller et al., 1995). However, with adequate counseling their outcome can be as good as that of nonalcoholics (Bruera, Moyano et al., 1995). Simple screening tools such as the CAGE questionnaire can be administered in minutes by staff with minimal training and should be used in the routine management of cancer pain (Moore et al., 1989; Bruera, Moyano et al., 1995). Because of the greater complexity of these patients it is likely that a significant proportion of patients with a history of severe alcoholism or drug addiction will need to be referred to specialized cancer pain or palliative care groups upon detection.

Somatization

The expression of psychosocial distress as somatic symptoms such as pain or nausea has been associated mostly with affective disorders such as depression or anxiety. Somatization is a poor independent prognostic factor for response to opioid analgesics (Bruera et al., 1989; Bruera, Schoeller et al., 1995). Patients with a previous history of somatization following major stressors are at higher risk of somatization. A combination of counseling, distraction, and pharmacologic management of affective disorders may be required in order to decrease the intensity of pain expression.

Tolerance

Approximately 20% of patients consume more than 70% of the opioids in some hospitals (Coyle et al., 1990; Fainsinger, 1991). The need for frequent and massive dose increase may lead to severe side effects (Bruera, 1996). Opioid rotation may decrease the level of dose escalation (see later). Methadone appears to be particularly effective in decreasing tolerance (Bruera, Watanabe et al., 1995). This may be due to partial cross tolerance with other opioids such as morphine or hydromorphone or to a suggested role of methadone as an NMDA antagonist (Ebert et al., 1995). Since excitatory amino acids such as NMDA have been associated with both neurotoxicity of opioids and tolerance development in animals (Shimoyama et al., 1996), there is great interest in trying some of the antagonists of excitatory amino acids for the prevention of opioid tolerance. Animal studies strongly suggest that agents such as dextrometorphan, ketamine, and new synthetic competitive and noncompetitive blockers delay and reverse opioid tolerance (Bruera, 1996; Shimoyama et al., 1996).

Traditional and Emerging Toxicities

Table 16.3 summarizes some of the traditionally recognized side effects of opioid analgesics in cancer pain patients. During recent years, probably due to treatment of patients with increasing doses of opioids for prolonged periods of time (Bruera et al.,

Table 16.3. *Traditional Toxicities of Opioids in Cancer Pain*

- Sedation
- Nausea
- Constipation
- Sweating
- Pruritus

Table 16.4. *Emerging Opioid Toxicities*

- Myoclonus – grand mal seizures
- Delirium – hallucinations
- Hyperalgesia
- Noncardiogenic pulmonary edema

1987, 1990; World Health Organization, 1990) and also due to increased vigilance about neuropsychiatric toxicity (Bruera et al., 1992, 1996), a series of emerging toxicities have been described (see Table 16.4). These emerging toxicities have been described overwhelmingly in patients exposed to a high opioid dose for a prolonged period of time or in association with renal failure, dehydration, delirium, or psychoactive drugs.

Noncardiogenic Pulmonary Edema

A frequent complication of acute overdose in opioid addicts is noncardiogenic pulmonary edema (Bogartz and Miller, 1971). However, it can also occur in cancer patients who are undergoing rapid opioid titration (Bruera and Miller, 1989). Because of the terminal nature of the illness in many of these patients, aggressive measures for resuscitation, including mechanical ventilation, are not appropriate. Therefore, this complication will be better managed with a reduction in opioid dose accompanied by oxygen and other respiratory support measures.

Excitatory Symptoms

During recent years a large number of authors have described cases of excitatory toxicity, including generalized myoclonus, grand mal seizures, hallucinations, hyperactive delirium, and hyperalgesia in patients with advanced cancer receiving high doses of opioid analgesics (DeConno et al., 1991; Morley et al., 1992; MacDonald et al., 1993; Sjogren et al., 1993; Sjogren et al., 1994; Bruera, Franco et al., 1995; deStoutz et al., 1995; Lawlor et al., 1997).

Table 16.5. *Management of Neuropsychiatric Toxicity*

• Opioid rotation
• Dose reduction
• Hydration
• Drugs (midazolam, barbiturates, baclofen)

In animal models, both opioid analgesics and their active metabolites are capable of causing excitatory symptoms such as those observed in cancer patients (Crain and Shen, 1990; Chen and Huang, 1991; Huang, 1992).

Lately, it has been recognized that opioid agonists, including morphine, hydromorphone, oxycodone, codeine, and meperidine have active metabolites. Some of these metabolites, such as morphine-6-glucuronide and oxymorphone, are capable of binding to the opioid receptors and have analgesic and sedative effects. Other metabolites, such as normeperidine, normorphine, and morphine-3-glucuronide, do not have analgesic properties. These metabolites are possibly capable of causing central irritability by nonopioid mechanisms (Kaiko et al., 1983; Glare et al., 1990; Smith and Watt, 1990; Bruera, 1996).

In patients in whom active metabolites of the opioid-stimulating nature accumulate, opioid toxicity will resemble the traditional "opioid intoxication" syndrome: sedation, miosis, cognitive failure, hypotension, respiratory depression. Yet, patients in whom the accumulation of the nonopioid active metabolite occurs, may present with the "excitatory" toxicities: myoclonus/seizures, hyperalgesia, hyperactive delirium/hallucinations. Since most patients produce a combination of both types of metabolites, most patients with severe opioid toxicity present with mixed syndromes, combining features of the opioid and excitatory side effects. Table 16.5 summarizes a number of strategies proposed for the management of opioid neuropsychiatric toxicity.

A number of authors have reported significant improvement or complete disappearance of opioid neurotoxicity with both opioid rotation and dose reduction (DeConno et al., 1991; Eisele et al., 1992; MacDonald et al., 1993; Caraceni et al., 1994; Sjogren et al., 1994; Bruera, Franco et al., 1995; deStoutz et al., 1995). The principle behind this strategy is that the change in the type of opioid agonist will result in rapid decrease in the circulating levels of the active metabolites and/or parent compound responsible for the neurotoxicity. Most authors have changed from one opioid agonist to another using generally accepted equianalgesic tables (Health and Welfare, Canada, 1984; Foley, 1985; U.S. Dept. Health, 1994; Levy, 1996).

The main exception to this observation has been methadone. This synthetic opioid agonist has the advantage of its extremely low cost, excellent oral bioavailability, and lack of demonstrated active opioid metabolites (Fainsinger et al., 1993). Its main drawback is its long and unpredictable half-life. It has recently become apparent that

Table 16.6. *Alternate Routes of Opioid Administration*

Regular Use
- Subcutaneous
- Rectal
- Transdermal
- Intravenous

Experimental
- Sublingual
- Buccal
- Inhalatory

in patients receiving a regular opioid for cancer pain, the equianalgesic dose ratio between methadone and opioid agonists such as morphine and hydromorphone is approximately 10 times more potent than previously reported (Bruera, Watanabe et al., 1995; Bruera et al., 1996). In addition, a unique characteristic of methadone is that the equianalgesic dose ratio increases in patients exposed to higher doses of opioids. This is different from other opioid agonists in which the equianalgesic ratio appears to be independent of the opioid exposure. These findings suggest that there is only partial cross tolerance between other opioid agonists and methadone. A recent finding that methadone could have NMDA antagonist properties (Ebert et al., 1995) suggests that this drug might be particularly useful for patients who develop neuropsychiatric toxicity due to massive opioid dose. However, randomized clinical trials of blind dose titration are required in order to appropriately establish the efficacy and safety of methadone as a second-line opioid. In the meantime, opioid rotations to methadone should be performed with extreme caution, particularly in patients previously exposed to high doses of other opioid agonists.

Anecdotal reports suggest that a number of psychoactive drugs, including midazolam, barbiturates, and baclofen, can be used for the management of opioid neuropsychiatric toxicity (Bruera, 1996). However, these drugs are likely to further increase sedation and cognitive failure and should probably be tried only after unsuccessful opioid rotation or dose reduction.

Alternate Routes of Administration

Approximately 70% of cancer patients will require alternate routes for opioid delivery before death for periods ranging from hours to months (Coyle et al., 1986; Bruera, 1990). Table 16.6 summarizes the most frequently used routes for systemic delivery of opioids in cancer patients. Because of limited information on both pharmacokinetics and pharmacodynamics, the sublingual, buccal, and inhalational routes are considered experimental. More research is needed in order to clarify the role of these routes.

Subcutaneous Route

This route has become the most commonly used alternate route to oral opioid administration (Bruera, Chadwick et al., 1988; Bruera and Ripamonti, 1993). Most opioid agonists, including morphine, hydromorphone, fentanyl, oxycodone, diamorphine, and meperidine, can be safely administered subcutaneously. Methadone can cause serious local irritation and should not be delivered by this route (Bruera et al., 1991). Opioids can be used subcutaneously as continuous infusions or intermittent injections or as patient-controlled analgesia (Bruera, Brenneis et al., 1988; Bruera, Chadwick et al., 1988; Bruera and Ripamonti, 1993). The subcutaneous site of injection lasts for approximately 5 to 7 days (Bruera, 1990). In patients in whom local irritation develops, a siolotic needle is significantly more expensive but results in the longer duration of the site of infusion (McMillan et al., 1994).

Patients receiving subcutaneous opioids at home have access to a number of portable devices, ranging from expensive electronic devices (Bruera and Ripamonti, 1993) to extremely low-cost injection systems that can be used in rural areas or developing countries (Bruera et al., 1993).

Rectal Route

The rectal route allows for the effective absorption of a number of opioid agonists administered as both suppositories and liquid solutions (Bruera and Ripamonti, 1993; DeConno et al., 1995). Major limitations of this route are the insufficient strength of commercially available preparations and the need for frequent administration of suppositories of rapid-release formulations. During recent years slow-release suppositories of morphine have been found to be equivalent in both pharmacokinetics and pharmacodynamics to subcutaneous morphine (Bruera, Fainsinger et al., 1995a, 1995b). Custom-made suppositories of methadone are a very low-cost and simple technique for the administration of a wide range of doses of methadone (Bruera, Watanabe et al., 1995). The excellent absorption of parenteral solutions with the rectal route suggests that this route can also be used for breakthrough pain in patients receiving regular slow-release rectal opioids (DeConno et al., 1995).

Transdermal Route

Transdermal fentanyl is well absorbed and can be a useful treatment in patients with stable cancer pain (Bruera and Ripamonti, 1993). The transdermal route is particularly effective in patients who are receiving relatively low opioid doses and are in excellent pain control. Transdermal fentanyl can be considered an alternative to slow-release oral or rectal opioids. The main limitation of this route is the considerable length of time required to achieve steady state in blood and the slow elimination of this drug. Therefore, similar to slow-release oral and rectal opioids, patients should be in stable pain control receiving a known dose of a previous opioid before transdermal fentanyl is started. If patients experience sudden deterioration in pain control, they should be retitrated using a rapid-release opioid before being restarted on transdermal fentanyl at the new effective equivalent analgesic dose.

Intravenous Route

In patients who require an intravenous route for other reasons, opioids can be safely and effectively administered intravenously. However, if the only reason for starting an intravenous is the administration of parenteral opioids, this will result in more discomfort, less ability to use the limbs freely, and higher cost than subcutaneous opioid delivery.

Choice of Alternative Route

The success of the alternate route will depend on matching the ideal route, opioid type and dose, and the patient and family's choice. Some patients will prefer the rectal route to carrying needles and injection devices.

Patients with diarrhea, rectal pain or hemorrhoids, or colostomies would not qualify for rectal opioids. Yet, patients with severe edema or coagulation disorders may be inappropriate candidates for subcutaneous opioids.

It is crucial before discharge to educate the patient and family on alternative routes in order to ensure compliance and early identification of potential problems with the delivery system.

Summary

Opioids remain the most effective treatment of cancer pain. Cancer patients have unique problems that require special consideration in the use of opioids, including chronic nausea, polypharmacy, multiple other symptoms, and a high incidence of delirium. Current guidelines recommend the use of regular doses of oral opioid agonists with titration according to analgesia and side effects such as nausea and sedation. Some specific situations are more difficult to treat, including neuropathic pain, incidental pain, alcoholism or drug addiction, tolerance, and somatization. These patients often require multiple modes of treatment by specialized multidisciplinary teams. Because of the increased use of opioids in higher dosages, during recent years a number of neuropsychiatric side effects have been described, including delirium, myoclonus, grand mal seizures, and hyperalgesia. A change in the type of opioid and/or other drugs may be required in these cases. Most patients require alternative routes of opioid delivery before death. The subcutaneous and rectal routes are simple, effective, safe, and low cost in this case, particularly for patients at home.

REFERENCES

Aner, S., and Meyerson, B.A. (1988). Lack of analgesic effects of opioids on neuropathic and idiopathic forms of pain. *Pain.* **33,** 11–23.

Bogartz, L., and Miller, W. (1971). Pulmonary edema associated with propoxyphene intoxication. *J.A.M.A.* **215,** 259–262.

Bruera, E. (1990). Subcutaneous administration of opioids in the management of cancer pain. In Foley, K., and Ventafridda, V. (eds.), *Advances in pain research and therapy.* New York: Raven Press, 203–218.

Bruera, E. (1992). Bone pain due to cancer. "Why Do We Care?" Pain and Symptom Control, Psychiatric Issues and Ethical Dilemmas in the Care of Patients with Cancer. Syllabus of the Postgraduate Course. New York: Memorial Sloan-Kettering Cancer Center, 279–284.

Bruera, E. (1993). Palliative care in Latin America. *J. Pain Symptom Management.* **8**(6), 365–368.

Bruera, E. (in press). New insights into opioids. Paper presented at the 8th World Congress on Pain, Vancouver, Canada, August 17–22, 1996. Seattle: IASP Press.

Bruera, E., and Miller, M.J. (1989). Non-cardiogenic pulmonary edema after narcotic treatment for cancer pain. *Pain.* **39,** 297–300.

Bruera, E., and Ripamonti, C. (1993). Adjuvants to opioid analgesics. In Patt, R. (ed.), *Cancer pain.* Philadelphia: J.B. Lippincott, 143–159.

Bruera, E., and Ripamonti, C. (1993). Alternate routes of administration of opioids for the management of cancer pain. In Patt, R. (ed.), *Cancer pain.* Philadelphia: J.B. Lippincott, 161–184.

Bruera, E., and Schoeller, T. (1992). Patient controlled analgesia in cancer pain. *Principles Practice Oncol.* **6**(4), 1–7.

Bruera, E., Brenneis, C., Michaud, M., Macmillan, K., Hanson, J., and MacDonald, N. (1988). Patient-controlled subcutaneous hydromorphone vs. continuous subcutaneous infusion for the treatment of cancer pain. *J. Nat. Cancer Inst.* **80**(14), 1152–1154.

Bruera, E., Chadwick, S., Brenneis, C., Michaud, M., Bacovsky, R., Emeno, A., and MacDonald, R.N. (1988). Use of the subcutaneous route for the administration of narcotics in patients with cancer pain. *Cancer.* **62**(2), 407–411.

Bruera, E., Fainsinger, R., MacEachern, T., and Hanson, J. (1992). The use of methylphenidate in patients with incident cancer pain receiving regular opiates. A preliminary report. *Pain.* **50,** 75–77.

Bruera, E., Fainsinger, R., Moore, M., Thibault, R., Spoldi, E., and Ventafridda, V. (1991). Clinical note: Local toxicity with subcutaneous methadone. Experience of two centers. *Pain.* **45,** 141–143.

Bruera, E., Fainsinger, R., Spachynski, K., Babul, N., Harsanyi, Z., and Darke, A.C. (1995). Clinical efficacy and safety of a novel controlled release morphine suppository and subcutaneous morphine in cancer pain: A randomized evaluation. *J. Clin. Oncol.* **13**(6), 1520–1527.

Bruera, E., Fainsinger, R.L., Spachynski, K., Babul, N., Harsanyi, Z., and Darke, A.C. (1995). Steady-state pharmacokinetic evaluation of a novel, controlled release morphine suppository and subcutaneous morphine in cancer pain. *J. Clin. Pharmacol.* **35**(7), 666–672.

Bruera, E., Fox, R., Chadwick, S., Brenneis, C., and MacDonald, R.N. (1987). Changing pattern in the treatment of pain and other symptoms in advanced cancer patients. *J. Pain Symptom Management.* **2**(3), 139–145.

Bruera, E., Franco, J.J., Maltoni, M., Watanabe, S., and Suarez-Almazor, M. (1995). Changing pattern of agitated impaired mental status in patients with advanced cancer: Association with cognitive monitoring, hydration and opiate rotation. *J. Pain Symptom Management.* **10**(4), 287–291.

Bruera, E., Macmillan, K., Hanson, J., and MacDonald, R.N. (1989). The Edmonton staging system for cancer pain: Preliminary report. *Pain.* **37,** 203–209.

Bruera, E., Macmillan, K., Hanson, J., and MacDonald, R.N. (1990). Palliative care in a cancer center: Results in 1984 vs. 1987. *J. Pain Symptom Management.* **5**(1), 1–5.

Bruera, E., Miller, L., McCallion, J., Macmillan, K., Krefting, L., and Hanson, J. (1992). Cognitive failure in patients with terminal cancer: A prospective study. *J. Pain Symptom Management.* **7**(4), 192–195.

Bruera, E., Moyano, J., Seifert, L., Fainsinger, R.L., Hanson, J., and Suarez-Almazor, M. (1995). The frequency of alcoholism among patients with pain due to terminal cancer. *J. Pain Symptom Management.* **10**(8), 599–603.

Bruera, E., Pereira, J., Watanabe, S., Belzile, M., Kuehn, N., and Hanson, J. (1996). Opioid rotation in patients with cancer pain. A retrospective comparison of dose ratios between methadone, hydromorphone and morphine. *Cancer.* **78**(4), 852–857.

Bruera, E., Schoeller, T., Wenk, R., MacEachern, T., Marcelino, S., Suarez-Almazor, M., and Hanson, J. (1995). A prospective multi-center assessment of the Edmonton Staging System for cancer pain. *J. Pain Symptom Management.* **10**(5), 348–355.

Bruera, E., Velasco, A., Fainsinger, R., Watanabe, S., and Hanson, J. (1996). A prospective study of neuropathic (N) pain (P) in cancer patients (PTS). **217,** 175. Seattle: IASP Press.

Bruera, E., Velasco-Leiva, A., Spachynski, K., Fainsinger, R., Miller, M.J., and MacEachern, T. (1993). The use of the Edmonton Injector (EI) for parenteral opioid management of cancer pain: A study of 100 consecutive patients. *J. Pain Symptom Management.* **8**(8), 525–528.

Bruera, E., Watanabe, S., Fainsinger, R., Spachynski, K., Suarez-Almazor, M., and Inturrisi, C. (1995). Custom-made capsules and suppositories of methadone for patients on high dose opioids for cancer pain. *Pain.* **62,** 141–146.

Caraceni, A., Martini, C., De Conno, F., et al. (1994). Organic brain syndromes and opioid administration for cancer pain. *J. Pain Symptom Management.* **9,** 527–533.

Chen, L., and Huang, L.Y. (1991). Sustained potentiation of NMDA receptor mediated glutamate responses through activation of protein kinase C by a MU opioid. *Neuron.* **7,** 319–326.

Cherny, N.I., and Foley, K.M. (1996). Non-opioid and opioid analgesic pharmacotherapy of cancer pain. *Haematol./Oncol. Clin. N. Am.* **10**(1), 79–102.

Cleeland, C.S., Gonin, R., Hatfield, A.K., Edmonson, J.H., et al. (1994). Pain and its treatment in outpatients with metastatic cancer. *N. Engl. J. Med.* **331**(22), 1528.

Coyle, N., Adelhardt, J., Foley, K., and Portenoy, R.K. (1990). Character of terminal illness in the advanced cancer patient: Pain and other symptoms during the last four weeks of life. *J. Pain Symptom Management.* **5,** 93.

Coyle, N., Manuskop, A., Maggard, J., and Foley, K. (1986). Continuous subcutaneous infusions of opioids in cancer patients with pain. *Oncol. Nursing Forum.* **12,** 52–57.

Crain, S.M., and Shen, K.F. (1990). Opioids can evoke direct receptor mediated excitatory effects in sensory neurons. *Trends Pharmacol. Sci.* **11,** 77–81.

De Conno, F., Caraceni, A., Martini, C., Spoldi, E., Salvetti, M., and Ventafridda, V. (1991). Hyperalgesia and myoclonus with intrathecal infusion of high-dose morphine. *Pain.* **47,** 337–339.

De Conno, F., Ripamonti, C., Saita, L., MacEachern, T., Hanson, J., and Bruera, E. (1995). The role of the rectal route in treating cancer pain: A randomized crossover clinical trial of oral vs. rectal morphine administration of opioid-naive cancer patients with pain. *J. Clin. Oncol.* **13**(4), 1004–1008.

De Lima, L., and Bruera, E. (1996). From Florianopolis (1994) to Santo Domingo (1996): A progress report on opioid availabiltiy. *Cancer Pain Release.* **9**(1), 4.

de Stoutz, N.D., Bruera, E., and Suarez-Almazor, M. (1995). Opioid rotation (OR) for toxicity reduction in terminal cancer patients. *J. Pain Symptom Management.* **10**(5), 378–384.

Dubner, R. (1991). A call for more science, not more rhetoric, regarding opioids and neuropathic pain. *Pain.* **47,** 1–2.

Dunlop, R. (1996). Clinical epidemiology of cancer cachexia. In Bruera, E., and Higginson, I. (eds.), *Cachexia-anorexia in cancer patients.* Oxford: Oxford University Press, **5,** 76–82.

Ebert, B., Andersen, S., and Krogsgaard-Larsen, P. (1995). Ketobemidone, methadone and pethidine are non-competitive N-Methyl-D-Aspartate (NMDA) antagonists in the rat cortex and spinal cord. *Neurosci. Lett.* **187,** 165–168.

Eisele, J.H., Grigsby, E.J., and Dea, G. (1992). Clonazepam treatment of myoclonic contractions associated with high-dose opioids: Case report. *Pain.* **49,** 231–232.

Ernst, D.S., MacDonald, R.N., Paterson, A.H.G., Jensen, J., Brasher, P., and Bruera, E. (1992). A double-blind crossover trial of intravenous clodronate in metastatic bone pain. *J. Pain Symptom Management.* **7**(1), 4–11.

Fainsinger, R., Bruera, E., Miller, M.J., Hanson, J., and MacEachern, T. (1991). Symptom control during the last week of life on a palliative care unit. *J. Palliat. Care.* **7**(1), 5–11.

Fainsinger, R., Schoeller, T., and Bruera, E. (1993). Methadone in the management of cancer pain: A review. *Pain.* **52, 137–147.**

Foley, K. (1985). The treatment of cancer pain. *N. Engl. J. Med.* **313,** 84–95.

Glare, P.A., Walsh, T.D., and Pippenger, C.E. (1990). Normorphine, a neurotoxic metabolite. *Lancet.* **335**(8691), 725–726.

Health & Welfare, Canada. (1984). *Cancer pain: a monograph on the management of cancer pain.* Minister of Supply and Services Canada, Ottawa H42–2/5 1984E.

Huang, L.Y. (1992). The excitatory effects of opioids. *Neurochem. Int.* **29,** 463–468.

Kaiko, R.F., Foley, K., and Grabinski, P.Y. (1983). Central nervous system excitatory effects of meperidine in cancer patients. *Ann. Neurol.* **13,** 150–185.

Lawlor, P., Walker, P., Bruera, E., and Mitchell, S. (in press). Severe opioid toxicity and somatization of psychosocial distress in a cancer patient with a background of chemical dependence. *J. Pain Symptom Management.*

Levy, M.H. (1996). Pharmacologic treatment of cancer pain. *N. Engl. J. Med.* **335**(15), 1124–1132.

MacDonald, R.N., Der, L., Allen, S., and Champion, F. (1993). Opioid hyperexcitability: The application of an alternate opioid therapy. *Pain.* **53,** 353–355.

Macmillan, K., Bruera, E., Kuehn, N., Selmser, P., and Macmillan, A. (1994). A prospective comparison study between a butterfly needle and a Teflon cannula for subcutaneous (SC) narcotic administration. *J. Pain Symptom Management.* **9**(2), 82–84.

Moore, R., Bone, L., Geller, G., et al. (1989). Prevalence, detection and treatment of alcoholism in hospitalized patients. *J.A.M.A.* **261,** 403–407.

Morley, J.S., Miles, J.B., and Bowsher, D. (1992). Paradoxical pain. *Lancet.* **340,** 1045.

O'Brien, C.P., and McLellan, A.T. (1996). Myths about the treatment of addiction. *Lancet.* **347**(8996), 237–241.

Portenoy, R., Foley, K.M., and Inturrisi, C.E. (1990). The nature of opioid responsiveness and its implications for neuropathic pain: New hypothesis derived from studies of opioid infusions. *Pain.* **43,** 273–286.

Portenoy, R.K. (1993). Adjuvant analgesics in pain management. In Doyle, D., Hanks, G., and MacDonald, N. (eds.), *Oxford textbook of palliative medicine.* London: Oxford Medical Publications, 187–203.

Portenoy, R.K., and Hagen, N.A. (1990). Breakthrough pain definition, prevalence and characteristics. *Pain.* **41,** 273–281.

Samlelsson, H., Malmberg, F., Eriksson, M., and Hedner, T. (1995). Outcomes of epidural morphine treatment in cancer pain: Nine years of clinical experience. *J. Pain Symptom Management.* **10**(2), 105–112.

Sanders, M., and Zuurmond, W. (1995). Safety of unilateral and bilateral percutaneous cervical cordotomy in 80 terminally ill cancer patients. *J. Clin. Oncol.* **13,** 1509–1512.

Shimoyama, N., Shimoyama, M., Intrurrisi, C.E., and Elliott, K. (in press). Ketamine attenuates and reverses analgesic tolerance to morphine. Paper presented at the 8th World Congress on Pain, Vancouver, Canada, August 17–22, 1996. Seattle: IASP Press.

Sjernsward, J., Joranson, D., Montejo, G., Castillo, G., Pazos, M., Pruvost, M., Mendez, E., and Olalla, J. (1995). Opioid availability in Latin America: The Declaration of Florianopolis. *J. Pain Symptom Management.* **10**(3), 233–236.

Sjogren, P., Jensen, N.H., and Jensen, T.S. (1994). Disappearance of morphine-induced hyperalgesia after discontinuing or substituting morphine with other opioid agonists. *Pain.* **59,** 313–316.

Sjogren, P., Jonsson, T., Jensen, N.H., Drenck, N.E., and Jensen, T.S. (1993). Hyperalgesia and myoclonus in terminal cancer patients treated with continuous intravenous morphine. *Pain.* **55,** 93–97.

Smith, M.T., and Watt, J.A. (1990). Morphine-3-glucoronide – a potent antagonist of morphine analgesia. *Life Sciences.* **47,** 579–585.

Sweet, P., Miah, Y., Barklam, B., Larsen, V., Hanna, M., and Peat, S. (1996). Morphine once daily versus twice daily: A double-blind cross over study comparing an oral 24 hour release morphine preparation with MST continus. Paper presented at the 8th World Congress on Pain, August 17–22, Vancouver, Canada. Seattle: IASP Press.

U.S. Department of Health and Human Services. (March 1994). *Management of cancer pain. Clinical practice guidelines.* Rockville, MD: AHCPR Publications, No. 94–0592.

Vigano, A., and Bruera, E. (1996). Enteral and parenteral nutrition in cancer patients. In Bruera, E., and Higginson, I., (eds.), *Cachexia-anorexia in cancer patients.* Oxford: Oxford University Press, **8,** 110–127.

Vigano, A., Suarez-Almazor, M., Fan, D., Hanson, J., DeConno, F., Ripamonti, C., and Bruera, E. (1996). Age, pain intensity and opioid dose in advanced cancer patients, **45,** 16. Seattle: IASP Press.

Von Roenn, J.H., Cleeland, C.S., Gonin, R., Hatfield, A.K., and Pandya, K.J. (1993). Physi-

cian attitudes and practice in cancer pain management. A survey from the Eastern Cooperative Oncology Group. *Ann. Intern. Med.* **119**(2), 121–126.
World Health Organization. (1986). *Cancer pain relief.* Geneva, 19.
World Health Organization. (1990). *Cancer pain relief and palliative care.* Report of a WHO Expert Committee. Geneva.

CHAPTER SEVENTEEN

Opioids in Visceral Pain

G. F. GEBHART, JYOTIRINDRA N. SEGUPTA, AND XIN SU

Introduction

When given systemically, the prototypical opioid analgesic morphine attenuates pain arising from the viscera. Indeed, malignancies and obstructions of the viscera caused by tumors are routinely treated with opioids such as morphine. Although it has long been held that opioids produce analgesia principally by actions in the central nervous system, it is now widely appreciated that opioids also have direct effects in the periphery, particularly in the presence of tissue injury (as detailed in Chapter 5 of this volume). Because of an interest in mechanisms of visceral pain, we undertook development of an appropriate model (colorectal distension in the rat) and then carried out studies to examine the efficacy and potency of opioids in the modulation of responses to colonic distension. That colorectal distension is both an appropriate and useful model for the study of visceral pain in humans and nonhuman animals has been documented (Ness and Gebhart, 1988; Ness et al., 1990; Gebhart and Sengupta, 1995). Balloon distension of the gut produces sensations similar in intensity, quality, and localization to those experienced in functional bowel disorders. In unanesthetized rats, responses to colorectal distension include supraspinally organized visceromotor and pressor responses. Both the visceromotor and pressor responses to distension are attenuated by morphine, whether given systemically or directly into the intrathecal space where afferent fibers innervating the colon terminate (Ness and Gebhart, 1988; Danzebrink et al., 1995; Harada et al., 1995).

In examination of opioid actions in the model of colorectal distension, the effects of δ- and κ-opioid receptor agonists were also studied, and it was noted that although morphine (and other μ-opioid receptor agonists) and δ-opioid receptor agonists were effective when given into the intrathecal space, the κ-opioid receptor agonist U-50,488 was not effective (Danzebrink et al., 1995; Harada et al., 1995). When given systemically, however, U-50,488 did significantly attenuate responses to noxious colorectal distension (Danzebrink et al., 1995; Harada et al., 1995). This observation suggested that κ-opioid receptor agonists might have useful peripheral or/and supraspinal antinociceptive effects in visceral pain, particularly in treatment of the functional bowel disorders. Discomfort and pain are common features of functional

Christoph Stein, ed., *Opioids in Pain Control: Basic and Clinical Aspects*. Printed in the United States of America.

bowel disorders such as irritable bowel syndrome and nonulcer dyspepsia, and current treatment has been largely unsuccessful. Accordingly, we began to examine systematically the actions of opioids on primary afferent sensory fibers innervating the pelvic viscera of the rat. The novel outcome of these electrophysiologic studies, which examined responses of decentralized pelvic nerve afferent fibers innervating the urinary bladder or colon in the rat, is that κ- but not either μ- or δ-opioid receptor agonists dose dependently attenuate such responses.

Location of Opioid Receptors

The distribution of opioid receptors in peripheral tissues has been investigated. In spinal dorsal root ganglion cells in the rat, the presence of μ-, δ-, and κ-opioid receptors (or their messenger RNAs) has been documented (Schafer et al., 1994; Ji et al., 1995; Minami et al., 1995). Opioid receptors are preferentially localized to small-diameter dorsal root ganglion cells, those typically associated with unmyelinated or thinly myelinated axons generally assumed to play roles in nociception (see Willis and Coggeshall, 1991). These small-diameter sensory neuron cell bodies are those that generally contain substance P and/or calcitonin gene-related peptide; many also contain the excitatory amino acid transmitters glutamate or aspartate (Battaglia and Rustioni, 1988). Mu-opioid receptors are reported to be present on about 21% of lumbar dorsal root ganglion cells in the rat; 14% of the cells have δ-opioid receptors, and 9% of the cells have κ-opioid receptors. Ji et al. (1995) reported that the percentage of δ- and κ-opioid receptors decreases in the ipsilateral dorsal root ganglia one and three days after experimental hindpaw inflammation, whereas the percentage of μ-opioid receptors increases significantly. In support, Stein et al. (1988) reported that experimental hindpaw inflammation increases the potency of μ- and κ-opioid receptor agonists in the periphery; they later reported that the κ-opioid receptor-preferring ligand dynorphin was present in the periphery on nerve fibers and immunocytes during inflammation (Hassan et al., 1992). It is now clear from various studies that the tissue content of both opioid receptors and endogenous opioid peptides increases in consequence of tissue injury.

It has long been appreciated that opioid receptors are present in the gut (Pert and Snyder, 1973). Subsequent pharmacologic and electrophysiologic investigations provided early evidence for opioid effects localized to the gastrointestinal tract; binding studies subsequently documented the presence of opioid receptors on nerve and smooth muscle in the gastrointestinal tract (Miller and Kirning, 1989; Daniel and Fox-Threlkeld, 1992; Kuemmerle et al., 1992; Bagnol et al., 1995). The most recent study, using antibodies raised to the cloned μ- and κ-opioid receptors, found that smooth muscle cells in the rat colon contained neither μ- nor κ-opioid receptors (Bagnol et al., 1995, 1997). Both μ- and κ-opioid receptors, however, were reported to be present on myenteric and submucosal plexus neurons, as well as on interstitial cells. Localization of these opioid receptors in the rat colon suggests possible roles related to absorption, secretion, motility, and visceral sensation.

Opioid Effects on Sensory Afferent Fibers

Relatively few studies have examined the effects of opioids on primary afferent fibers. Russell et al. (1987) examined the effects of μ- and κ-opioid receptor agonists on the spontaneous discharges of afferent fibers innervating the inflamed knee joint of the cat. Morphine reduced the spontaneous activity of three fibers and had no effect on six other fibers. The peptide μ-opioid receptor agonist DAMGO reduced the spontaneous activity of five of ten fibers tested. The authors noted that κ-opioid receptor agonists appeared to be more effective: κ-opioid receptor agonists U-50,488 reduced spontaneous activity in six of seven fibers studied, and ethylketocyclazocine reduced spontaneous activity in nine of fourteen fibers studied. More recently, Andreev and co-workers (Andreev et al., 1994) examined the effects of opioids on cutaneous polymodal nociceptors contained in the saphenous nerve innervating the hindpaw of the rat. After ultraviolet irradiation to produce an inflammation, these polymodal nociceptors became spontaneously active (i.e., were sensitized), and both morphine and the κ-opioid receptor selective agonist U-69,593 produced concentration-dependent suppression of spontaneous activity. Interestingly, the peptide δ-opioid receptor agonist DPDPE was without effect.

In studies in which tissue has not been inflamed, opioids that were tested were found not to affect spontaneous discharges of C-polymodal nociceptors in normal skin or the responses of these nociceptors to noxious stimuli. Neither morphine nor fentanyl, when applied directly to the radial nerve, or fentanyl, when given intravenously, affected heat-evoked responses of polymodal nociceptors recorded in the cat (Senami et al., 1986). Shakhanbeh and Lynn (1993) observed that morphine reduced the spontaneous activity of C-polymodal nociceptors innervating rat skin only after carrageenan-produced inflammation.

Three studies have examined the effects of opioids on visceral afferent fibers, and all have reported that the fibers were activated. Kumazawa and co-workers (Kumazawa et al., 1989) reported that morphine, a δ-opioid receptor agonist (DADLE) and the κ-opioid receptor agonist dynorphin all increased the discharges of polymodal nociceptors in a dog testis-spermatic nerve in vitro preparation. Curiously, the excitatory effects of morphine were typically produced only on initial bath application of the drug; considerable tachyphylaxis appeared to develop upon subsequent testing. In a study of visceral mechanoreceptors with low thresholds for response, Balkowiec and co-workers (Balkowiec et al., 1994) reported that morphine applied to the thoracic visceral receptive field activated 19 of 21 vagal or splanchnic nerve afferent fibers tested after induction of an experimental pericarditis in cats. Recently, Eastwood and Grundy (1995) reported that morphine, DAMGO and DADLE (but not U-50,488), activated both vagal and nonvagal intestinal afferent fibers in the rat. That morphine activates vagal afferent fibers has been interpreted as contributing to the analgesia produced when morphine is given systemically (see Randich et al., 1991, for discussion). It is difficult, however, to understand how activation of visceral afferent fibers in other nerves (e.g., splanchnic or spermatic) relate to the principal action of opioids, namely, to attenuate visceral pain.

Kappa-Opioid Receptor Agonists

Several years ago, we began systematically to evaluate the effects of μ-, δ-, and κ-opioid receptor agonists on responses of pelvic nerve afferent fibers innervating the descending colon or urinary bladder of the rat (Sengupta et al., 1996; Su et al., 1997a, 1997b). These studies focused on mechanosensitive pelvic nerve afferent fibers that responded to noxious intensities of either colorectal distension or urinary bladder distension. We recorded from the decentralized S1 (colon) or decentralized L6 (urinary bladder) dorsal root in anesthetized rats. Because the afferent input was decentralized, effects observed in such experiments were restricted to the periphery: at receptors in the tissue, along the sensory axons, or on dorsal root ganglion cell bodies. Unexpectedly, neither morphine nor fentanyl, which has greater intrinsic efficacy than morphine, affected responses to colorectal distension after cumulative doses of 16 mg/kg morphine or 300 μg/kg fentanyl (Sengupta et al., 1996) (Fig. 17.1, for example). Similarly, δ-opioid receptor agonists (the peptide agonist DPDPE and the nonpeptide agonist SNC-80) were also without effect on responses of mechanosensitive pelvic nerve afferent fibers to noxious colorectal distension. Cumulative doses of κ-opioid receptor agonists, however, produced dose-dependent attenuation of responses to colorectal distension (Fig. 17.1). In a subsequent study (Su et al., 1997a), μ- and δ-opioid receptor agonists were found to be without effect on responses of pelvic nerve afferent fibers innervating the urinary bladder. The κ-opioid receptor agonists U-50,488, U-69,593, and U-62066, however, all dose dependently inhibited the responses of pelvic nerve mechanosensitive afferent fibers to noxious intensities of urinary bladder distension. In both studies (Sengupta et al., 1996; Su et al., 1997a), the colon or the urinary bladder was inflamed acutely, and the effects of drugs were examined 60–120 minutes following acute inflammation of the tissue. We found that the inflammation sensitized the afferent fibers (i.e., response magnitude increased and response threshold decreased), but found no changes in drug potency. We had expected that perhaps the μ-opioid receptor agonists that were ineffective in the absence of inflammation might attenuate responses to organ distension when the viscus was inflamed. We also did not note a leftward shift in the dose-response function to the κ-opioid receptor agonists in the presence of inflammation, contrary to other reports examining peripheral (cutaneous) inflammation (e.g., Joris et al., 1987; Stein et al., 1988, 1989). Although there is abundant evidence to suggest that inflammation leads to an up-regulation of opioid receptors in the periphery (e.g., see Hassan et al., 1993), we believe that the failure to see changes in potency of the opioid receptor agonists tested is due to an inadequate time for de novo receptor synthesis following urinary bladder or colonic inflammation. Alternatively, such changes as established in cutaneous models of inflammation do not occur in the viscera.

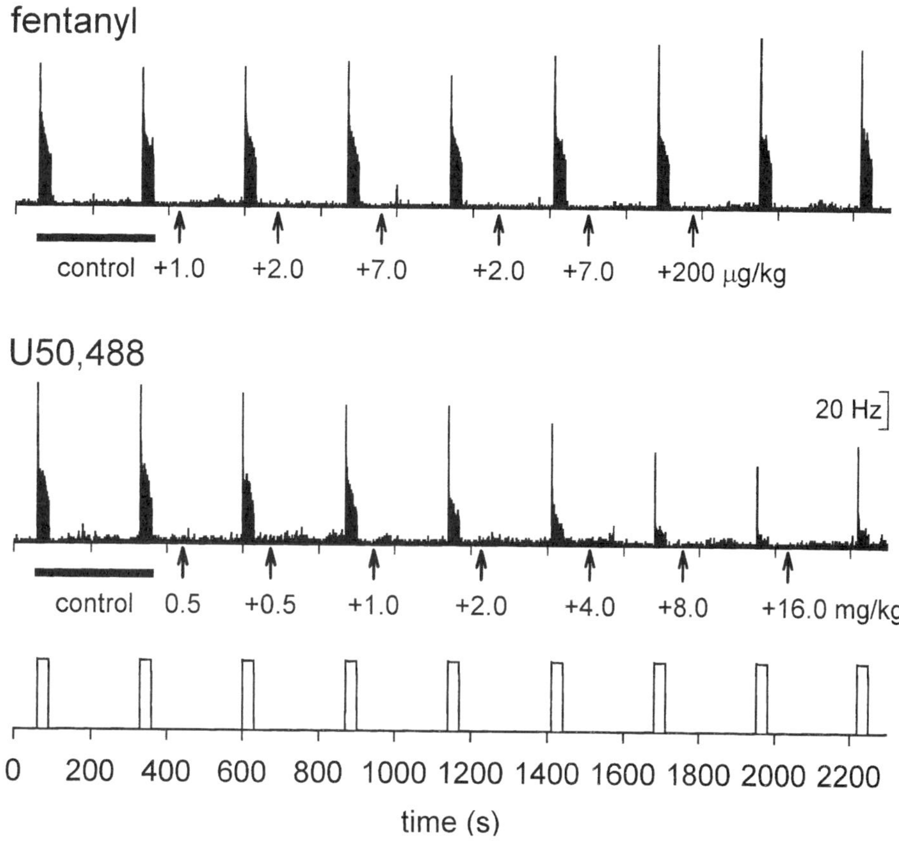

Figure 17.1. Examples of the effects of fentanyl and U-50,488 on responses of pelvic nerve afferent fibers to colorectal distension (80 mmHg, 30 seconds every 4 minutes; shown bottommost). Drugs were injected intraarterially in cumulative doses as indicated (↑).

Because the effects of the κ-opioid receptor agonists just described were antagonized by naloxone, we believe that the effects are produced at opioid receptors in the periphery. Specifically, μ-opioid receptor selective doses of naloxone did not block the effects of κ-opioid receptor agonists on responses to urinary bladder or colonic distension; greater, nonreceptor-selective doses of naloxone did reliably antagonize the effects of the κ-opioid receptor agonists tested. Interestingly, putative κ-opioid receptor-selective antagonists nor-BNI and DIPPA were ineffective in preventing or reversing the effects of any of the κ-opioid receptor agonists tested. In a subsequent study (Su et al., 1997b), we examined κ-opioid receptor agonists selective for putative κ_1, κ_2, and κ_3 opioid receptors. Again, we found dose-dependent inhibition of responses of pelvic nerve afferent fibers to noxious intensities of colorectal distension. The effects were antagonized by appropriate doses of naloxone (i.e., non–μ-opioid receptor-selective doses), but not by κ-opioid receptor-selective antagonists (nor-BNI, DIPPA). Interestingly, when the dose-response functions for all of the

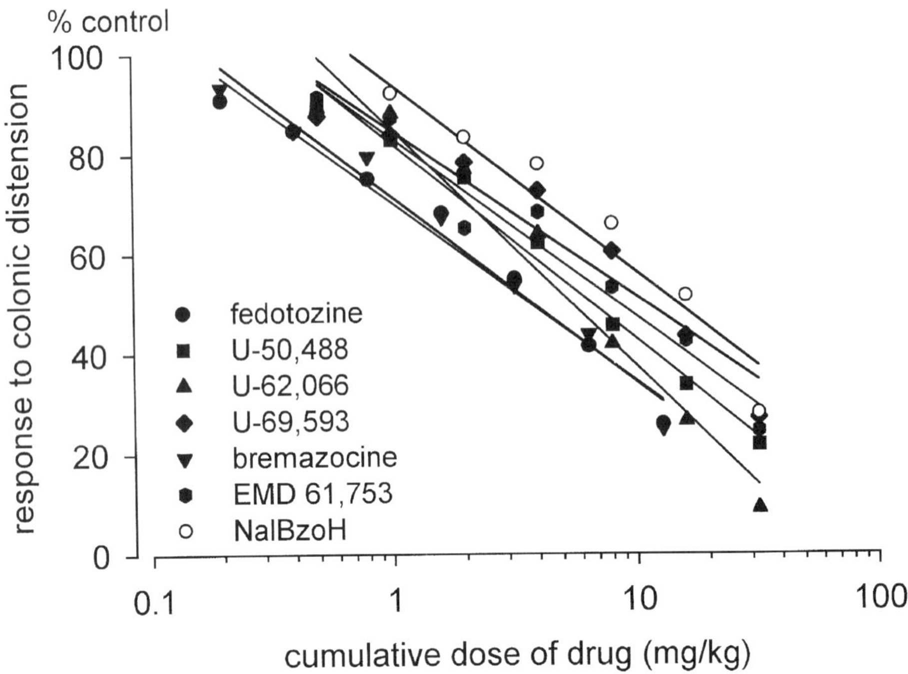

Figure 17.2. Dose-dependent inhibition by κ-opioid receptor agonists on responses of pelvic nerve afferent fibers to noxious colorectal distension (80 mmHg, 30 seconds).

κ-opioid receptor agonists tested are plotted together, one notes that the dose-response functions are parallel and tightly grouped (Fig. 17.2). Indeed, the effective dose-50s range between approximately 5 and 15 mg/kg, which is clearly at odds with the more than 100-fold range of effective antinociceptive doses reported in the literature for these same κ-opioid receptor agonists in other models. We speculated, on the basis of these results, that κ-opioid receptor agonists produced their effects at a κ-like opioid receptor different from that which has been cloned from the central nervous system.

Most recently, we have reinvestigated the potency of opioid receptor agonists in the presence of chronic colonic inflammation (Snider et al., 1997). In these experiments we used TNBS (trinitrobenzine sulfonic acid) to inflame the colon and tested rats 3–4 days after intracolonic instillation of TNBS. Neither morphine nor the non-peptide δ-receptor agonist SNC-80 attenuated responses of pelvic nerve afferent fibers to colonic distension in these inflamed rats. The peripherally restricted κ-opioid receptor agonist EMD 61,753, however, exhibited greater potency in the presence of chronic inflammation (Fig. 17.3). Whereas the effective dose 50 of EMD 61,753 was the same in untreated and acutely inflamed rats (about 8 mg/kg), the effective dose 50 was reduced to about 3.5 mg/kg in rats with TNBS-inflamed colons. Accordingly, the receptor at which the κ-opioid receptor agonists act to attenuate responses from the pelvic viscera studied up-regulates in the presence of chronic inflammation.

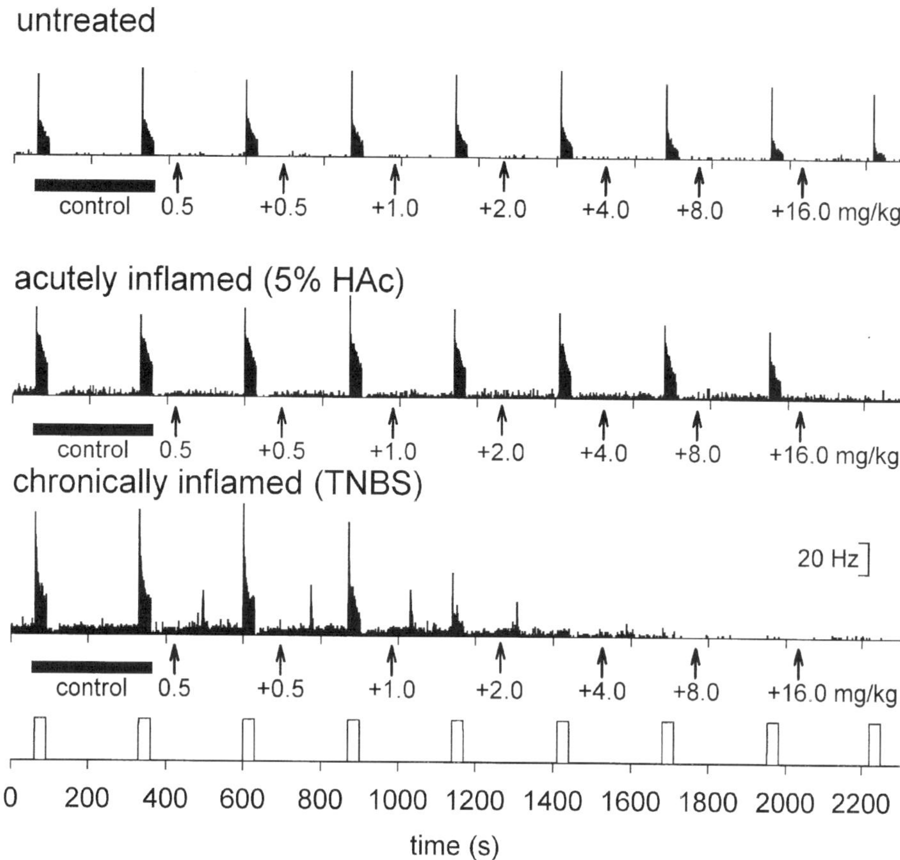

Figure 17.3. Examples of the effects of EMD 61,753 on responses of pelvic nerve afferent fibers to colorectal distension (80 mmHg, 30 seconds every 4 minutes; shown bottom-most). EMD 61,753 was tested on afferent fibers from untreated colons, from acute acetic acid (HAc)-inflamed colons, and from TNBS-inflamed colons.

Finally, we have recently documented that κ-opioid receptor agonists administered intracolonically can significantly attenuate responses of pelvic nerve afferent fibers to noxious colorectal distension (Su et al., 1998), providing additional evidence for direct and potent actions of this class of opioid agonists.

Summary

The results briefly reviewed here confirm that opioid effects studied in cutaneous and mononeuropathic models of pain do not necessarily extend to the viscera. That is, while μ-opioid receptors have been shown to up-regulate in some of these models, and their potency increases in the presence of inflammation, this does not occur in pelvic viscera. Our observations lead to several conclusions and speculations.

- The well-documented efficacy and utility of morphine and other opioids in the treatment of visceral pain arising from the colon or bladder involves sites of action restricted to the central nervous system.
- Peripherally restricted κ-opioid receptor agonists may be particularly useful in the treatment of pelvic visceral pain associated, for example, with functional bowel disorders such as irritable bowel syndrome. This speculation may extend to other visceral disorders (e.g., nonulcer dyspepsia). In unpublished work (Ozaki, Sengupta, and Gebhart), the κ-opioid receptor agonist EMD 61,753 has been observed to attenuate responses of mechanosensitive vagal afferent fibers innervating the stomach of the rat. Interestingly, in these same studies, low doses of morphine increase the spontaneous activity of about one-half of the vagal afferent fibers studied to date.
- The receptor in the viscera at which the κ-opioid receptor agonists act is likely different than the κ-opioid receptor agonists cloned from the central nervous system.

ACKNOWLEDGMENTS: The authors thank Susan Birely for secretarial assistance and Michael Burcham for preparation of the figures. The authors are supported by National Institutes of Health awards DA 02879, NS 19912 and NS35790.

REFERENCES

Andreev, M., Urban, L., and Dray, A. (1994). Opioids suppress spontaneous activity of polymodal nociceptors in the rat paw skin induced by ultraviolet irradiation. *Neurosci.* **58,** 793–798.

Bagnol, D., Mansour, A., Akil, H., and Watson, S.J. (1995). Localization of mu and kappa opioid receptors in rat colon by antibodies to the cloned opioid receptors. *Analgesia.* **1,** 4–6.

Bagnol, D., Mansour, A., Akil, H., and Watson, S.J. (1997). Cellular localization and distribution of the cloned mu and kappa receptors in rat gastrointestinal tract. *Neuroscience.* **81,** 579–591.

Balkowiec, A., Kukula, K., and Szulczyk, P. (1994). Influence of morphine on the activity of low-threshold visceral mechanoreceptors in cats with acute pericarditis. *Pain.* **59,** 251–259.

Battaglia, G., and Rustioni, A. (1988). Coexistence of glutamate and substance P in dorsal root ganglion neurons of the rat and monkey. *J. Comp. Neurol.* **277,** 302–312.

Daniel, E.E., and Fox-Threlkeld, J.E.T. (1992). Role of opioid receptor subtypes in control of the gastrointestinal tract. In Holle, G.H., and Wood, J.D. (eds.), *Advances in the innervation of the gastrointestinal tract.* Amsterdam: Elsevier, 329–340.

Danzebrink, R.M., Green, S.H., and Gebhart, G.F. (1995). Spinal mu and delta but not kappa opioid receptor agonists attenuate responses to noxious colorectal distension in the rat. *Pain.* **63,** 39–47.

Eastwood, C., and Grundy, D. (1995). Morphine stimulates intestinal afferent discharge via μ- and δ- but not κ-opioid receptors. *Gastroenterol.* **108,** A594.

Gebhart, G.F., and Sengupta, J.N. (1995). Evaluation of visceral pain. In Gaginella, T. (ed.),

Handbook of methods in gastrointestinal pharmacology. Boca Raton, FL: CRC Press, 359–373.

Harada, Y., Nishioka, K., Kitahata, L.M., Nakatani, K., and Collins, J.G. (1995). Contrasting actions of intrathecal U-50,488H on visceromotor responses to colorectal distension as compared to intrathecal morphine and DPDPE or intravenous U-50,488H in the rat. *Anesthesiology.* **83,** 336–343.

Hassan, A.H.S., Pzewlocki, R., Herz, A., and Stein, C. (1992). Dynorphin, a preferential ligand for the κ-opioid receptors, is present in nerve fibers and immune cells within inflamed tissue of the rat. *Neurosci. Lett.* **140,** 85–88.

Hassan, A.H.S., Ableitner, A., Stein, C., and Herz, A. (1993). Inflammation of the rat paw enhances axonal transport of opioid receptors in sciatic nerve and increases their density in the inflamed tissue. *Neuroscience.* **55,** 185–195.

Ji, R.-R., Zhang, Q., Law, P.Y., Low, H.H., Elde, R., and Hokfelt, T. (1995). Expression of μ-, δ-, and κ-opioid receptor-like immunoreactivities in rat dorsal root ganglion after carrageenan-induced inflammation. *J. Neurosci.* **15,** 8156–8166.

Joris, J.L., Dubner, R., and Hargreaves, K.M. (1987). Opioid analgesia at peripheral sites: A target for opioids released during stress and inflammation. *Anesth. Analg.* **66,** 1277–1281.

Kuemmerle, J.F., Grider, J.R., Murthy, K.S., Souquet, J.-C., Hellstrom, P., Martin, D.C., and Makhlouf, G.M. (1992). Characterization of receptors for neuropeptides on muscle cells of the gut. In Holle, G.H., and Wood, J.D. (eds.), *Advances in the innervation of the gastrointestinal tract.* Amsterdam: Elsevier, 341–356.

Kumazawa, T., Mizumura, K., Satoh, J., and Minagawa, M. (1989). Facilitatory effects of opioid on the discharges of visceral nociceptors. *Brain Res.* **497,** 231–238.

Miller, R.J., and Kirning, L.D. (1989). Opioid peptides of the gut. In Schultz, S.T., Makhlouf, G.N., and Rauner, B.B. (eds.), *Handbook of physiology, the gastrointestinal tract,* vol. 2. Bethesda, MD: American Physiological Society, 631–660.

Minami, M., Maekawa, K., Yabuuchi, K., and Satoh, M. (1995). Double *in situ* hybridization study on coexistence of μ-, δ-, and κ-opioid receptor mRNAs with preprotachykinin A mRNA in the rat dorsal root ganglia. *Molec. Brain Res.* **30,** 203–210.

Ness, T.J., and Gebhart, G.F. (1988). Colorectal distension as a noxious visceral stimulus: Physiologic and pharmacologic characterization of pseudoaffective reflexes in the rat. *Brain Res.* **450,** 153–169.

Ness, T.J., Metcalf., A.M., and Gebhart, G.F. (1990). A psychophysiological study in humans using phasic colonic distension as a noxious visceral stimulus. *Pain.* **43,** 377–386.

Pert, C.B., and Snyder, S.H. (1973). Opiate receptors: Demonstration in nervous tissue. *Science.* **179,** 1011–1014.

Randich, A., Thurston, C.L., Ludwig, P.S., Timmerman, M.R., and Gebhart, G.F. (1991). Antinociception and cardiovascular responses produced by intravenous morphine: The role of vagal afferents. *Brain Res.* **543,** 256–270.

Russell, N.J.W., Schaible, H.-G., and Schmidt, R. (1987). Opiates inhibit the discharges of fine afferent units from inflamed knee joint of the cat. *Neurosci. Lett.* **76,** 107–112.

Schafer, M.K.-H., Bette, M., Romero, H., Schwaeble, W., and Weihe, E. (1994). Localization of κ-opioid receptor mRNA in neuronal subpopulations of rat sensory ganglia and spinal cord. *Neurosci. Lett.* **167,** 137–140.

Senami, M., Aoki, M., Kitahata, L.M., Collins, J.G., Kumeta, Y., and Murata, K. (1986). Lack of opiate effects on cat C polymodal nociceptive fibers. *Pain.* **27,** 81–90.

Sengupta, J.N., Su, X., and Gebhart, G.F. (1996). κ, but not μ or δ, opioids attenuate responses to distension of afferent fibers innervating the rat colon. *Gastroenterol.* **111,** 968–980.

Shakhanbeh, J., and Lynn, B. (1993). Morphine inhibits antidromic vasodilation without affecting the excitability of C-polymodal nociceptors in the skin of the rat. *Brain Res.* **607,** 314–318.

Snider, A.A., Sengupta, J.N., and Gebhart, G.F. (1997). Effects of morphine and a peripherally-acting kappa-opioid receptor agonist on the visceromotor response to colonic distension in the rat. *Gastroenterol.* **112,** A828.

Stein, C., Millan, M.J., Yassoudris, A., and Herz, A. (1988). Antinociceptive effects of μ- and κ-agonists in inflammation are enhanced by a peripheral opioid receptor-specific mechanism. *Europ. J. Pharmacol.* **155,** 255–264.

Stein, C., Millan, M.J., Shippenberg, T.S., Peter, K., and Herz, A. (1989). Peripheral opioid receptors mediating antinociception in inflammation: Evidence for involvement of mu, delta and kappa receptors. *J. Pharmacol. Exp. Therap.* **248,** 1269–1275.

Su, X., Julia, V., and Gebhart, G.F. (in press). Modulation of mechanosensitive pelvic nerve afferents by intracolonic κ-opioid agonists. *Soc. Neurosci. Abstracts.*

Su, X., Sengupta, J.N., and Gebhart, G.F. (1997a). Effects of opioids on mechanosensitive pelvic nerve afferent fibers innervating the urinary bladder of the rat. *J. Neurophysiol.* **77,** 1566–1580.

Su, X., Sengupta, J.N., and Gebhart, G.F. (1997b). Effects of kappa opioid receptor-selective agonists on responses of pelvic nerve afferents to noxious colorectal distension. *J. Neurophysiol.* **78,** 1003–1012.

Willis, W.D., and Coggeshall, R.E. (1991). *Sensory mechanisms of the spinal cord,* 2nd ed. New York: Plenum.

CHAPTER EIGHTEEN

Opioids in Obstetrics

MARCO M. E. MARCUS, WIEBKE GOGARTEN,
AND HUGO VAN AKEN

Introduction

The use of pain-relieving drugs during labor is now common, but expectant mothers are still concerned about the effects of anesthetics on their unborn babies. However, mothers-to-be should be told that excessive pain or anxiety during labor may harm the fetus more than the judicious use of analgesic drugs. Psychological stress is difficult to quantify, but in the primate mother it can cause hypoxia and acidosis in the fetus, probably because of a reduction in uterine blood flow (Moore, 1993). The body reacts to stress by releasing endogenous opioids. The administration of exogenous opioids is another way to modulate the stress response. The modern use of synthetic opioid narcotics for analgesia during labor started with the use of meperidine in 1939. However, despite the widespread popularity of meperidine, the perinatal pharmacokinetics of meperidine remained long unknown and the pharmacodynamics of the drug not understood (Moore, 1993). Although a wide variety of narcotics are now available, only a few are used currently in obstetrics; these include morphine, meperidine, fentanyl, and sufentanil. These narcotics cause a variety of side effects in the mother, including respiratory depression, orthostatic hypotension, nausea, vomiting, and delay of gastric motility. All narcotics are rapidly transferred across the placenta and are capable of producing neonatal respiratory depression and changes in the neurobehavior of the child. To diminish the usual side effects observed with systematically and intramuscularly administered opioids, alternative ways of administration have been sought. Spinal and epidural delivery of opiates was introduced in 1979, and the practice has been widely accepted in obstetric analgesia, although this mode of opiate delivery has some disadvantages. This chapter discusses the advantages and disadvantages associated with the use of opioids in obstetrics, administered both systemically and by epidural and spinal routes.

Endogenous Opioids

Regardless of the method of delivery, exogenous opioids engage an endogenous system composed of opiate receptors and opiatelike substances. Understanding this

Christoph Stein, ed., *Opioids in Pain Control: Basic and Clinical Aspects*. Printed in the United States of America.

endogenous system might help us understand the way in which exogenously administered analgesics exert their effects on mother and fetus.

Enkephalins, endorphins, and dynorphins are peptides released by the human body (Snyder, 1977). Lipotropin is co-released with ACTH after cleavage from proopiomelanocortin (POMC) in the anterior pituitary and is partially cleaved to gamma lipotropin, methionine-enkephalin, leucine-enkephalin, and β-endorphin. Other sites in which POMC is found are the hypothalamus, placenta, and adrenal glands.

Maternal β-endorphin is a large molecule that does not cross the blood-brain barrier. Beta-endorphin secretion in plasma increases during the pain of labor and during anxiety and correlates with the patient's perception of pain intensity (Steinbroeck et al., 1982; Fettes et al., 1984). Plasma levels of β-endorphin level are lower in pregnant women than in nonpregnant women (Hoffmann et al., 1984). With the beginning of contractions, the β-endorphin level in the hypophysis rises and acts as a central analgesic (Oliver et al., 1977). Proof of this central analgesic action comes from two studies. In obstetric patients, intrathecal administration of β-endorphin caused profound anesthesia (Oyama et al., 1980). In rats, there is a progressive increase in the pain threshold throughout pregnancy, probably because of a progressive increase of endogenous opioids in the substantia gelatinosa, which can be blocked by naltrexone administration (Ginzler et al., 1980). Sandman et al. (1995) reported an intriguing observation. They showed that the normal pattern of corelease of β-endorphin and ACTH measured 10 weeks before delivery was dissociated in subjects later asking for epidural anesthesia during birth. This uncoupling may result from modified control of POMC expression during pregnancy or from unique proteolytic expression of POMC, and thus may alter pain tolerance during delivery (Sandman et al., 1995).

Studies of the effects of analgesia during labor and delivery on the levels of β-endorphin have yielded conflicting results. In one study, epidural analgesia was shown to lower maternal β-endorphin (Abboud et al., 1983), whereas in another study no correlation between plasma endorphins in maternal and umbilical veins during epidural analgesia was found (Joupilla et al., 1983). A further study compared the difference in neuroendocrine stress response in severe pre-eclamptic women who had a cesarean section either under general anesthesia or epidural analgesia. It was shown that under general anesthesia ACTH and β-endorphin levels increased from baseline levels, whereas under epidural analgesia the levels of these hormones decreased or remained unchanged. The anesthetic technique did not alter the concentrations of stress hormones in the neonate (Ramanthan et al., 1991).

During labor, the β-endorphin plasma concentration in the fetus rises. The concentration in the umbilical vein is higher than that in the artery, probably because of the production of β-endorphin in the placenta (Nakay et al., 1978; Goebelsman et al., 1984). Beta-endorphin has a molecular weight of 3,500 and is unlikely to cross from mother to fetus (Rust et al., 1980). Most of the β-endorphin is produced by the hypophysis of the fetus (Facchinetti et al., 1982; Goebelsman et al., 1984). Premature delivery or fetal distress causes the β-endorphin levels in the fetus to rise (Distler et al., 1988; Distler, 1989; Shaaban et al., 1982). The other stress axis, the sympathomedullary system, is also known to store and release opioids, particularly enkephalins. These are unstable compounds that are rapidly hydrolyzed by specific enkephalinase enzymes (Bovill, 1991), making clinical studies difficult. In animals, it has been demonstrated that Met-enkehalin is co-released with catecholamines (Livett et al., 1981; Moore et al., 1993).

Exogenous Opioids

Pharmacology of Systemic Opioids

Only a few systemic opioids have been used as analgesics in labor and delivery.

Morphine has too many undesirable effects to be of further use in modern obstetric practice. Its hypotensive effects on the mother and its slow onset of action make titration difficult. Infants are highly susceptible to the respiratory depressant effect of intravenous administration of morphine.

Meperidine (pethidine) is a narcotic frequently used in obstetrics. Usual doses are 50–100 mg intramuscularly and 25–50 mg intravenously. The peak analgesic action occurs 40–50 minutes after an intramuscular administration and 5–10 minutes when given intravenously. The duration of action is three to four hours (Shnider and Levinson, 1994). When given intravenously, maternal and fetal blood concentrations rise rapidly after 90 seconds (Crawford and Rudowsky, 1965). Maternally administered meperidine may produce neonatal respiratory depression, as evidenced by delay in sustained respiration, decreased Apgar scores (Shnider and Moya, 1964), lower oxygen saturation (Taylor et al., 1955), decreased minute ventilation (Roberts et al., 1957), respiratory acidosis (Koch et al., 1968), and abnormal neurobehavior after birth (Brackbill et al., 1974). Fetal exposure to meperidine is highest two to three hours after intramuscular administration of the drug to the mother (Savonna-Ventura et al., 1991). The concentration of normeperidine, an active metabolite of meperidine, rises steadily in fetal blood. Fetal changes attributed to meperidine persist for 72 hours after birth. The use of meperidine in complicated pregnancies was studied by Rhien et al. (1995). They compared a group of 214 infants whose mothers received meperidine with 401 infants whose mothers did not receive meperidine. All these deliveries (the control and treatment groups) were complicated with meconium-stained amniotic fluid. This study failed to identify additional neonatal risks if meperidine was used.

Other opioids are not widely used and are rarely studied for their systemic use in women in labor. However, it is important to understand the pharmacology of, for example, fentanyl and sufentanil administered intravenously. These drugs are widely used for epidural and spinal administration, and accidental intravenous injection is possible.

Fentanyl was administered intravenously as a labor analgesic. Doses of 50–100 μg per hour as needed (PRN) were given to women in labor. A total mean dose of

142 μg was given (range 50–600 μg). No major side effects were seen, apart from mild sedation. Umbilical blood fentanyl concentration never exceeded 0.4 ng/ml (Rayburn et al., 1988). In a study in which fentanyl was compared with meperidine, moderate to severe pain was recorded in both groups during active labor. No mothers in the fentanyl group suffered side effects, compared with 20% in the meperidine group. In the meperidine group, 13% of the babies received naloxone at birth compared to 2% in the fentanyl group (Rayburn et al., 1989). In gravid ewes, Craft et al. (1983) showed the rapid rise and decline of fetal fentanyl blood concentrations (appearance after 1 minute and peak at 5 minutes) after maternal IV injection of 50–100 μg fentanyl. In humans, the ratio of umbilical vein concentration to maternal artery concentration (UV/MA) is 0.31 (Estaphanous et al., 1984).

Sufentanil was never popular for systemic administration for labor pain relief because of its potency. Therefore, intravenous sufentanil in pregnant humans was never studied. In pregnant sheep, Vertommen et al. (1995) showed that after a maternal injection of 50 μg sufentanil a mean peak level of sufentanil was detected in maternal plasma at 1 minute (1.28 ng/ml). A mean peak plasma level of 0.037 ng/ml in the fetus was attained 3 minutes after injection. Fetal sufentanil levels decreased in parallel with maternal levels, as evidenced by a constant maternal-fetal ratio of 5:5 for 15–60 minutes after the injection of sufentanil.

A few studies with butorphanol and nalbuphine, two agonist-antagonist narcotic analgesics, showed no advantages over other narcotics.

Tramadol is a centrally acting analgesic agent belonging to the group of weak opioids (Arend et al., 1978). It is reported that in therapeutic doses, fewer side effects will occur, especially less respiratory depression than with other opioids (Cossman et al., 1988). Bitch et al. (1980) reported that 50 mg tramadol administered intramuscularly was effective in relieving labor pain in more than 60% of subjects; analgesia began about 10 minutes after injection and lasted for as long as 45 minutes. Viegas et al. (1993) compared intramuscular tramadol 50 mg and 100 mg with intramuscular meperidine 75 mg for relief of labor pain. They found that pain relief was similar with meperidine and 100 mg tramadol, but that the meperidine group suffered more side effects. However, further research is needed for tramadol to gain acceptance as the drug of choice for intramuscular application in women in labor.

Pharmacology of Spinal Opioids

The discovery of opioid receptors in the substantia gelatinosa of the spinal cord opened the possibility of giving opioids intrathecally in the direct vicinity of these opioid receptors and of interrupting local nocioceptive transmission (Behar et al., 1979). The amount of administered opioids could be reduced and relief of pain was achieved earlier without systemic respiratory depression of mother and child (Irestedt, 1993). However, several disadvantages associated with intrathecal opioids have now been reported, limiting their use.

Several studies describe the administration of intrathecal morphine during parturition (Scott et al., 1980; Baraka et al., 1981; Abboud et al., 1984; Leighton et al., 1989). Morphine, a highly ionized, water-soluble opioid, produced analgesia of long duration but slow onset. The slow onset of action, plus a high incidence of side effects, such as nausea, vomiting, pruritus, and the potential for delayed respiratory depression, limits the usefulness of intrathecal morphine for labor analgesia. Intrathecal injection of a more lipid-soluble opioid leads to rapid relief of labor pain with fewer side effects, but the duration of analgesia is relatively short (Leicht et al., 1990; Honet et al., 1992). Intrathecal fentanyl 25 μg has a rapid onset of analgesia but lasts only 60–90 minutes (Zakowsky et al., 1991). In a retrospective study of a group of patients who received intrathecal fentanyl 25–30 μg plus 0.25–0.3 mg morphine and 6–8 mg lidocaine, Rust et al. (1994) reported excellent pain relief without respiratory depression. However, a significant proportion of patients experienced pruritus and urinary retention.

From a theoretical standpoint, sufentanil would be an ideal drug for intrathecal use. Its high lipophilicity should limit the rostral spread of this opioid in the cerebrospinal fluid and speed its onset of action. When D'Angelo et al. (1994) compared 10 μg intrathecal sufentanil with 12 mg bupivacaine administered epidurally, they found a rapid-onset analgesia with intrathecal sufentanil. However, they found the same incidence of hypotension in both groups and a rapid cephalic spread of the intrathecal sufentanil. These observations were confirmed by Cohen et al. (1993) and Grieco et al. (1993), who also showed a short mean duration of action (123 minutes). When 2.5 mg intrathecal bupivacaine was added to 10 μg intrathecal sufentanil, it significantly prolonged labor analgesia (from 114 minutes in the sufentanil group to 148 minutes in the combined sufentanil/bupivacaine group) without adverse maternal or fetal side effects (Campbell et al., 1995). A different approach to prolong the effects of lipophilic intrathecal opioids, by adding epinephrine, failed in one study to demonstrate any extension of analgesia (Camann et al., 1993), whereas in another study the effect was significantly prolonged (Campbell et al., 1997). Another possibility for prolonging the effects of intrathecal analgesia is the use of in-dwelling small-gauge spinal catheters. In a study by Honet et al. (1992), the analgesic efficacy of intermittent injections of intrathecal fentanyl (10 μg), meperidine (10 mg), or sufentanil (5 μg) during the first stage of labor was compared. They concluded that intermitted intrathecal injections of fentanyl, meperidine, or sufentanil can provide adequate analgesia during first-stage labor. Meperidine appears to provide more reliable analgesia as the first stage of labor progresses. However, variable decelerations of the fetal heart rate occurred more frequently in the fentanyl and the meperidine groups. Other side effects included nausea and mild pruritus. The safety of spinal catheters is also a concern.

To combine the fast onset of intrathecal opioids with the possibility of titration to meet the needs of the individual patient, the combined spinal-epidural technique (CSE) has gained popularity in obstetric analgesia. The same drugs and dosages can be used as described above. Norris et al. (1994) collected data on 388 women who received epidural anesthesia and 536 women who received a CSE anesthesia. It was shown that complications with both techniques are few. Hypotension complicates about 10% of cases of intrathecal opioid or epidural local anesthetic technique. Intentionally puncturing the dura with a small-gauge pencil-point needle during the induction of CSE labor analgesia does not increase the risk of postpartum headache. However, other studies indicated a risk of nausea and vomiting of 44–50% (Caldwell et al., 1994; Herspolsheimer and Schretenthaler, 1994), a risk of pruritus of 81–94% (Vercauteren, 1996), and a higher incidence of postdural puncture headache (Kartawiadi et al., 1996). Heyman et al. (1996) suggested that, due to the possibility of additional side effects, informed consent should be obtained prior to performing this technique (see also Vercauteren, 1996).

We conclude that the sole use of intrathecal opioids for labor analgesia has too many disadvantages to be recommended. More research on in-dwelling intraspinal catheters and CSE techniques is required before these approaches can replace epidural use of combinations of opioids and local anesthetics.

Pharmacology of Epidural Opioids

Since its introduction, epidural analgesia has been proved the safest and most effective method for pain relief during labor and delivery. Incremental addition of opioids in labor improves the safety and efficiency of epidural analgesia. Morphine, fentanyl, and sufentanil are the most frequently studied opioids for epidural use.

Morphine is not the drug of choice for epidural use because its onset of action is only 20–45 minutes after administration (Hughes et al., 1984). It causes a high incidence of maternal side effects such as nausea (53%), urinary retention (43%), and somnolence (43%) (Abboud et al., 1984). Morphine is hydrophilic and might cause late respiratory depression, which is dangerous when the patient is not adequately monitored. Because of these side effects, interests have turned to the more lipophilic opioids such as fentanyl and sufentanil.

In several studies, epidural fentanyl in combination with low doses of bupivacaine improved the quality of analgesia and reduced the severity of motor blockade and the incidence of hypotension (Cohen et al., 1987; Cellano et al., 1988). However, many side effects are reported after the use of epidural fentanyl. In the mother, 100 μg epidural fentanyl may cause late respiratory depression (Brockway et al., 1987; Wang et al., 1992). Neonates can also suffer from respiratory depression. In a study by Noble et al. (1991), two neonates had to be given naloxone after the mother received epidural fentanyl, and in a study by Carrie et al. (1981), one neonate had to be intubated. However, these results were contradicted in a study by Preston et al. (1987), in which Apgar scores, neurobehavior, and adaptive capacity scores (NACS) were normal and neonatal blood levels at delivery were below the level expected to cause respiratory depression. Similar conclusions were drawn in a study of pregnant ewes by Craft et al. (1984), in which the placental passage and uterine effects after epidural fentanyl were investigated. The investigators showed that an epidural injection of 50 μg fentanyl has little effect on maternal or fetal cardiovascular and acid base status, uterine tone, and uterine blood flow. They also demonstrated only minimal placental passage of fentanyl to the fetus.

Continuous epidural infusions containing a combination of low concentrations of local anesthetics and narcotic have become increasingly popular for labor analgesia. Bader et al. (1995) examined the potential for fetal drug accumulation after a continuous (up to 15 hours) epidural infusion of 0.125% bupivacaine with 2 μg/ml fentanyl. They concluded that the concentrations of both drugs remained low and that none of the neonates showed any significant accumulation of drug or adverse effects as demonstrated by umbilical blood gases and neurobehavioral scores.

The most recent addition to our therapeutic arsenal for epidural analgesia is sufentanil. The analgesic effect of sufentanil was investigated in several studies. The addition to sufentanil to bupivacaine 0.25% did not improve the quality of analgesia, but the duration was prolonged (Jorrot et al., 1989). Van Steenberghe et al. (1987) combined 7.5 μg and 15 μg sufentanil with bupivacaine 0.125% plus epinephrine during labor in 107 women and found superior analgesia with faster onset and longer duration compared with local anesthetic alone. The hourly bupivacaine requirement was significantly reduced, and "top-up" injections were required less frequently. They also found that the addition of sufentanil allowed relief of any residual pain resulting from an incomplete sensory block. Although the 1-minute Apgar scores were significantly lower in the group that received 15 μg sufentanil 5 minutes after birth, there were no differences among the three groups (Van Steenberghe et al., 1987). Vertommen et al. (1991), in a study of 695 women, showed that the addition of sufentanil to bupivacaine 0.125% not only improved analgesia but also reduced the incidence of instrumental deliveries. The addition of up to 30 μg sufentanil did not cause neonatal respiratory depression (see also Van Aken et al., 1994). The conclusion that the chances of neonatal respiratory depression are small was confirmed by other studies. Using the chronic maternal-fetal sheep model, Vertommen et al. (1995) found that after the epidural administration of 50 μg sufentanil, the maternal blood sufentanil concentration was 0.059 ng/ml. No fetal blood sufentanil could be detected. Palot et al. (1992) compared the placental transfer of fentanyl and sufentanil after continuous epidural administration in women in labor and found that placental transfer of fentanyl was significantly higher than the transfer of sufentanil. Loftus et al. (1995) contradicted these results and found that the fetal/maternal ratio was higher for sufentanil than for fentanyl. However, because of its greater potency, less epidural sufentanil is needed, so that lower maternal concentrations and lower fetal concentrations were shown (Loftus et al., 1995). When continuous infusion containing a combination of bupivacaine and sufentanil was investigated, Cohen et al. (1996) found that an epidural opioid infusion (fentanyl 2 μg/ml compared with sufentanil 1 μg/ml) with very low doses of bupivacaine (0.015%) achieved an overall high level of patient satisfaction in both groups without serious maternal or neonatal side effects. At the fentanyl to sufentanil ratio used here, patients receiving sufentanil had lower pain scores, and substantially fewer patients required bupivacaine rescue (Cohen et al., 1996).

One potential disadvantage of epidural opioids is their effect on gastric emptying (Geddes et al., 1991; Wright et al., 1992; Ewah et al., 1993). Geddes et al. (1991) added fentanyl 100 μg to epidural bupivacaine 0.5% after cesarean section and demonstrated a statistically significant delay in gastric emptying after surgery, as did Ewah et al. (1993) and Wright et al. (1992). However, addition of smaller doses of opioids do not delay gastric emptying. Zimmerman et al. (1996) demonstrated that a bolus of 50 μg epidural fentanyl followed by an infusion delivering fentanyl at 20 μg/hour does not delay gastric emptying in women in labor two hours after epidural analgesia is initiated. Other side effects from epidural opioids are pruritus (1.3%) and nausea and vomiting (1.0%) (Norris et al., 1994). Thus, addition of small doses of opioids for epidural use result in fewer side effects compared with the systemic and spinal use of opioids.

It has been shown that epidural anesthesia might prolong labor. In a study by Newton et al. (1995), continuous epidural analgesia with bupivacaine and fentanyl did not result in a change in myometrial contractility in the first hour after the initiation of analgesia. However, despite more oxytocin therapy, the rate of cervical dilatation was significantly lower in the epidural group than in the nonepidural group. Operative deliveries were more common in patients with epidural analgesia (Newton et al., 1995). In contrast, Philipsen and Jensen (1989) could not show adverse outcomes associated with epidural analgesia, and Chestnut et al. (1994) showed that there was no prolongation of the first stage of labor. However, in all of these studies it is difficult to compare the groups with and without epidural catheters.

When there is a prolongation of the first stage of labor, the causes are speculative. The small amount of bupivacaine in maternal blood may have an adverse effect on the propagation and strength of myometrial contractions, or perhaps patients with epidural analgesia are not able to move around, thus reducing uterine efficiency (Newton et al., 1995). Finally, uterine activity induced by exogenous oxytocin may be less effective than endogenous oxytocin (Newton et al., 1995).

In the second stage of labor, epidural analgesia attenuates the normal rise in maternal oxytocin through inhibition of the Ferguson reflex (Goodfellow et al., 1985). The resultant decrease in uterine activity can contribute to an increased incidence in instrumental delivery. Thus, the role of opioids in the duration of first and second stages remains unclear.

Postoperative Analgesia

Opioids in obstetrics are used not only in the delivery room but also for the prevention of postoperative pain. The best way to treat postoperative pain is by patient-controlled analgesia (PCA). PCA provides better pain relief and is preferred by patients to nurse-administered PRN opioids after cesarean section. PCA can be given intravenously (PCIA) or via an epidural route (PCEA). Peach et al. (1994) compared the two routes of administration, using meperidine, in a randomized double-blind, cross-over study and showed that PCEA with meperidine produces high-quality pain relief with few side effects and has significant advantages over PCIA meperidine. The optimal initial dose of meperidine is 25 mg, which has a fast onset of action and a relatively long duration of action (Ngan Kee et al., 1996). However, concerns exists about the accumulation of normeperidine in maternal plasma and breastmilk.

Morphine, fentanyl, and sufentanil have also been administered epidurally for postcesarean delivery analgesia as bolus injections (Rosen et al., 1988) and by continuous infusions (Fisher et al., 1988). Both fentanyl and sufentanil (with and without bupivacaine) were compared with morphine in this population of patients (Fisher et al., 1988; Rosen et al., 1988) and were found to cause a lower incidence of opioid-induced side effects. The addition of epinephrine (Leicht et al., 1990) to fentanyl or sufentanil has been reported to reduce opioid requirements and perhaps improve the quality of analgesia (Cohen et al., 1993). Cohen et al. (1993) compared a group of patients who received epidural fentanyl 2 μg/ml, bupivacaine 0.01%, and epinephrine 0.5 μg/ml with patients who received epidural sufentanil 0.8 μg/ml, bupivacaine 0.01%, and epinephrine 0.5 μg/ml. They concluded that both epidural regimens offer satisfactory analgesia with mild side effects and are associated with high overall satisfaction scores. Vomiting during the infusion was more common with sufentanil, as was dizziness after the termination of the infusion. They concluded that epidural sufentanil offers no advantages over epidural fentanyl.

Epidurally administered hydromorphone provides a duration of postoperative analgesia comparable to epidural morphine with significantly fewer side effects in nonobstetric patients. However, Halpern et al. (1996) compared 0.6 mg hydromorphone epidurally with 3 mg morphine epidurally in postcesarean section patients and found no difference in the analgesic effectiveness or side effects of those compounds.

A promising development for postoperative analgesia is the sustained-release formulation of opioids. In a study by Kim et al. (1996), a lipid-based sustained-release formulation of morphine (DTC401) was studied in rats to ascertain if it could provide sustained analgesia without causing supraspinal effects. They concluded that a single dose of DCT401 administered epidurally results in a prolonged duration of analgesia 3- to 19-fold longer than that produced by morphine sulphate alone. The formulation did not demonstrate supraspinal toxic effects until a dose of 2,000 μg was given. The markedly lower CSF and serum peak concentrations of morphine after DCT401, compared with morphine alone, limits the lack of undesirable side effects (Kim et al., 1996).

We can conclude that the drug of choice for PCEA use remains controversial.

REFERENCES

Abboud, K., Shnider, S.M., and Daily, A. (1984). Intrathecal administration of hyperbaric morphine for the relief of pain in labour. *Br. J. Anaesth.* **56,** 1351–1359.

Abboud, T.K., Sarkis, F., Hung, T.T., Khoo, S.S., Varakian, L., and Henriksen, L. (1983). Effects of epidural anesthesia during labour on maternal plasma β-endorphin levels. *Anesthesiology.* **59,** 1–5.

Arend, L., von Arnim, B., and Nijsen, J. (1978). Tramadol and pentazocin in a double blind crossover comparison. *Arzneim.-Forsch/Drug Res.* **28** (1a), 199–208.

Bader, A., Fragneto, R., Terui, K., Arthur, G.R., Loferski, B., and Datta, S. (1995). Maternal and neonatal Fentanyl and bupivacaine concentrations after epidural infusions during labor. *Anesth. Analg.* **81,** 829–832.

Baraka, A., Noueihid, R.D., and Haji, S. (1981). Intrathecal injection of morphine for obstetric analgesia. *Anesthesiology.* **54,** 136–140.

Behar, M., Magora, F., Olshwang, D., and Davidson, J.T. (1979). Epidural morphine in treatment of pain. *Lancet.* **1,** 527–528.

Bitch, M., Emmrich, J., and Hary, J. (1980). Obstetric analgesia with tramadol. *Fortschr. Med.* **16,** 632–634.

Bovill, J.G. (1991). Opioids. In Dundee, J.W., Clarke, R.S.J., and McCaughy, W. (eds.), *Clinical anesthetic pharmacology.* Boston: Lichnow & Co., 203–230.

Brackbill, Y., Kane, J., and Maniello, R.L. (1974). Obstetric meperidine usage and assessment of neonatal status. *Anesthesiology.* **40,** 116–120.

Brockway, M.S., Noble, D.W., Sharwood-Smith, G.H., and McClure, J.H. (1990). Profound respiratory depression after extradural fentanyl. *Br. J. Anaesth.* **64,** 243–245.

Caldwell, L.E., Rosen, M.A., and Shnider, S.M. (1994). Subarachnoid morphine and fentanyl for labor analgesia: Efficacy and adverse effects. *Reg. Anesth.* **19,** 2–8.

Camann, W.R., Mintzer, B.H., Denney, R.A., and Datta, S. (1993). Intrathecal sufentanil for labor analgesia effects of added epinephrine. *Anesthesiology.* **78,** 870–874.

Campbell, D.C., Banner, R., Crone, L.A., Gore, D., Hickman, W., and Yip, R.W. (1977). Addition of epinephrine to intrathecal bupivacaine and sufentanil for ambulation labor. *Anesthesiology.* **86,** 525–531.

Campbell, D.C., Camann, W.R., and Datta, S. (1995). The addition of bupivacaine to intrathecal sufentanil for labor analgesia. *Anesth. Analg.* **81,** 305–309.

Carrie, L.E.S., O'Sullivan, G.M., and Seegobin, R. (1981). FORUM epidural fentanyl in labour. *Anaesthesia.* **36,** 965–999.

Cellano, D., and Capogna, G. (1988). Epidural fentanyl plus bupivacaine 0,125 per cent for labour: Analgesic effects. *Can. J. Anaesth.* **35,** 375–378.

Chestnut, D.H., Vincent, D.R., Jr., McGrath, J.M., Choi, W.W., and Bates, J.N. (1994). Does early administration of epidural analgesia affect obstetric outcome in nulliparous women who are receiving intravenous oxytocin? *Anesthesiology.* **80,** 1193–1200.

Cohen, S., Amar, D., Pantuck, C.B., Pantuck, E.J., Goodman, E.J., Widrow, J.S., Kansas, R.J., and Brady, J.A. (1993). Postcesarean delivery epidural patient-controlled analgesia. *Anesthesiology.* **78,** 486–491.

Cohen, S.E., Tan, S., Albright, G.A., and Halpern, J. (1987). Epidural fentanyl/bupivacaine mixtures for obstetric analgesia. *Anesthesiology.* **67,** 403–407.

Cohen, S., Ama, D., Pantuck, C.B., Pantuck, E.J., Goodman, E.J., and Leung, D.H. (1996). Epidural analgesia for labour and delivery: Fentanyl or sufentanil? *Can. J. Anaesth.* **43,** 341–364.

Cossmann, M., and Wilsman, K.M. (1988). Application of tramadol injection (TRAMAL) in acute pain: Open trial to assess the acute effect and safety after a single parental administration. *Therapeut. News.* **130** (36), 633–636.

Craft, J.R., Coaldrake, L.A., Bolan, J.C., Mondino, M., Mazel, P., and Gilman, R.M. (1983). Placental passage and uterine effects of fentanyl. *Anesth. Analg.* **62,** 894–898.

Craft, J.B., Robichaux, A.G., Kim, H., Thorpe, D.H., Mazel, P., Woolf, W.A., and Stolte, A. (1984). The maternal and fetal cardiovascular effects of epidural fentanyl in the sheep model. *Am. J. Obstet. Gynecol.* **148,** 1098–1104.

Crawford, J.S., and Rudofsky, S. (1965). The placental transmission of pethidine. *Br. J. Anaesth.* **37,** 929–933.

D'Angelo, R., Anderson, M.T., Philip, J., and Eisenach, J.C. (1994). Intrathecal sufentanil compared to epidural bupivacaine for labor analgesia. *Anesthesiology.* **80,** 1209–1215.

Distler, W. (1989). Schmerzmodulation unter der Geburt durch endogene Opiate. *Gynäkologe.* **22,** 100–103.

Distler, W., Schwenzer, T.H., Umbach, G., and Graf, M. (1988). β-Endorphin bei Frühgeburten und reifen Neugeborenen nach vaginaler und abdominaler Entbindung. *Geburtshilfe Frauenheilkd.* **48,** 140–142.

Esthaphenous, F.G. (1984). *Opioids in anesthesia.* Boston: Butterworth, 104–108.

Ewah, B., Yau, K., and King, M. (1993). Effect of epidural opioids on gastric emptying in labour. *Int. J. Obstet. Anesth.* **2,** 125–128.

Facchinetti, F., Bagnoli, F., Bracci, R., and Genazzani, A.R. (1982). Plasma opioids in the first hours of life. *Pediatr. Res.* **16,** 95–98.

Fettes, I., Fox, J., Kuzniak, S., Shime, J., and Gare, D. (1984). Plasma levels of immunoreactive beta-endorphin and adrenocorticotropic hormone during labor and delivery. *Obstetr. Gynecol.* **64,** 382–384.

Fisher, R.L., Lubenow, T.R., Liceaga, A., McCarthy, R.J., and Ivankoviek, A.D. (1988). Comparison of continuous epidural infusion of fentanyl-bupivacaine and morphine-bupivacaine in management of postoperative pain. *Anesth. Analg.* **67,** 559–563.

Geddes, S.M., Thorburn, J., and Logan, R.W. (1991). Gastric emptying following cesarean section and the effect of epidural fentanyl. *Anesthesia.* **46,** 1016–1018.

Ginzler, A.R. (1980). Endorphin-mediated increases in pain threshold during pregnancy. *Science.* **210,** 193–195.

Goebelsman, U., Abboud, T.K., Hoffman, D.I., and Hung, T.T. (1984). β-endorphin in pregnancy. *Eur. J. Obstet. Gynecol. Reprod. Biol.* **17,** 77–81.

Goodfellow, C.F., Hull, M.G.R., Swaab, D.F., Dogterom, J., and Buys, R.M. (1985). Oxytocin deficiency at delivery with epidural analgesia. *Br. J. Obstet. Gynaecol.* **95,** 1246–1250.

Grieco, W., Norris, M., Leighton, B.L., Arkoosh, V.A., Huffnagle, H., Honet, J.A., and Costello, D. (1993). Intrathecal sufentanil analgesia: The effects of adding morphine or epinephrine. *Anesth. Analg.* **77,** 1149–1154.

Halpern, S.H., Arellano, R., Preston, R., Carstoniu, J., O'Leary, G., Roger, S., and Sandler, A. (1996). Epidural morphine vs. hydromorphone in post-cesarean section patients. *Can. J. Anaesth.* **43,** 595–598.

Herspolsheimer, A., and Schretenthaler, J. (1994). The use of intrapartum intrathecal narcotic analgesia in a community based hospital. *Obstet. Gynecol.* **84,** 931–963.

Heyman, H.J. (1995). Complications of combined spinal-epidural technique for labor analgesia: Complicating the informed consent process? *Anesth. Analg.* **80,** 854–855.

Hoffman, D.I., Abboud, T.K., Haase, H.R., Hung, T.T., and Goebelsman, U. (1984). Plasma β-endorphin concentrations prior to and during pregnancy, in labor and after delivery. *Am. J. Obstet. Gynecol.* **150,** 492–496.

Honet, J.E., Arkoosh, V.A., Norris, M.C., Huffnagle, J., Silverman, N.S., and Leighton, B.L.

(1992). Comparison among intrathecal fentanyl, meperidine, and sufentanil for labor analgesia. *Anesth. Analg.* **75,** 734–739.

Hughes, S.C., Rosen, M.A., Shnider, S.M., Abboud, T.K., Stefani, S.J., and Norton, M. (1984). Maternal and neonatal effects of epidural morphine for labor and delivery. *Anesth. Analg.* **63,** 318–324.

Irestedt, L. (1993). The effects of analgesia and anaesthesia on fetal and neonatal stress response. In Reynolds, F. (ed.), *Effects on the baby of maternal analgesia and anaesthesia.* London: W.B. Saunders, 148–162.

Jorrot, J.C., Lirzin, J.D., Daillard, P., Jacquinot, P., and Conseiller, C. (1989). A combination of sufentanil and 0.25% bupivacaine administered epidurally for ostetrical analgesia: Comparison with fentanyl and placebo. *Ann. FR. Anesth. Reanim.* **8** (4), 321–325.

Joupilla, R., Joupilla, P., Karlqvist, K., Kaukoranta, P., Leppaluota, J., and Vuolteenako, O. (1983). Maternal and umbilical venous plasma immunoreactive β-endorphin levels during labor with and without epidural analgesia. *Am. J. Obstet. Gyn.* **147,** 799–802.

Kartawiadi, S.L., Vercauteren, M.P., Van Steenberghe, A.L., and Adriaensen, H.A. (1996). Spinal analgesia during labor with low-dose bupivacaine, sufentanil, and epinephrine. *Reg. Anesth.* **21,** 191–196.

Kim, T., Muranda, A., Gruber, A., and Kim, S. (1996). Sustained-release morphine for epidural analgesia in rats. *Anesthesiology.* **85,** 331–338.

Koch, G., and Wandel, H. (1968). Effect of meperidine on the postnatal adjustment of respiration and acid-base balance. *Acta Obstet. Gynecol. Scand.* **47,** 27–37.

Leicht, C.H., Evans, D.E., and Durkin, W.J. (1990). Intrathecal sufentanil for labor analgesia: Results of a pilot study. *Anesthesiology.* **73,** A980.

Leicht, C.H., Kelleher, A.J., Robinson, D.E., and Dickerson, S.E. (1990). Prolongation of postoperative epidural sufentanil analgesia with epinephrine. *Anesth. Analg.* **70,** 323–325.

Leighton, B.L., DeSimone, C.A., Norris, M.C., and Ben-David, B. (1989). Intrathecal narcotics for labor revisited: The combination of fentanyl and morphine intrathecally provides rapid onset of profound, prolonged analgesia. *Anesth. Analg.* **69,** 122–125.

Livett, B.C., Dean, D.M., Whelan, L.G., Udenfiend, S., and Rossier, J. (1981). Co-release of encephalins and catecholamines from cultured adrenal chromaffin cells. *Nature.* **289,** 317–319.

Loftus, J.R., Hill, H., and Cohen, S.E. (1995). Placental transfer and neonatal effects of epidural sufentanil and fentanyl administration with bupivacaine during labor. *Anesthesiology.* **83,** 300–308.

Moore, J. (1993). The effects of analgesia and anaesthesia on the maternal stress response. In Reynolds, F. (ed.), *Effects on the baby of maternal analgesia and anaesthesia.* London: W.B. Saunders, 148–162.

Nakay, Y., Nakao, K., Oki, S., and Imura, H. (1978). Presence of immunoreactive β-lipotropin and β-endorphin in human placenta. *Life Sciences.* **23,** 213–218.

Newton, E.R., Schroeder, B.C., Knape, K.G., and Bennet, B.L. (1995). Epidural analgesia and uterine function. *Obstet. Gynecol.* **85,** 749–755.

Ngan Kee, W.D., Lam, K.K., Chen, P.P., and Gin, T. (1996). Epidural meperidine after cesarean section: A dose response study. *Anesthesiology.* **85,** 289–294.

Noble, D.W., Morrison, L.M., Brockway, M.S., and McClure, J.H. (1991). Adrenaline, fentanyl, or adrenaline and fentanyl as adjuncts to bupivacaine for extradural anesthesia in elective cesarean section. *Br. J. Anaesth.* **66,** 645–650.

Norris, M.C., Grieco, W.M., Borkowski, M., Leighton, B.L., Arkoosh, V., Huffnagle, H.J., and Huffnagle, S. (1994). Complications of labor analgesia: Epidural versus combined spinal epidural techniques. *Anesth. Analg.* **79,** 529–537.

Oliver, C., Mical, R.S., and Porter, J.C. (1977). Hypothalamic-pituitary vasculature: Evidence for retrograde blood flow in the pituitary stalk. *Endocrinology.* **101,** 598–604.

Oyama, T., Matsuki, A., Taneichi, T., Ling, N., and Guillemin, A. (1980). β-Endorphin in obstetric analgesia. *Am. J. Obstet. Gynecol.* **137,** 613–616.

Palot, M., Visseaux, H., Botmans, C., Levson, J.C., and Lemoing, J.P. (1992). Placental transfer and neonatal distribution of fentanyl, alfentanil, and sufentanil after continuous epidural administration for labor. *Anesthesiology.* **77,** A991.

Peach, M.J., Moore, J.S., and Evans, S.F. (1994). Meperidine for patient-controlled analgesia after cesarean section: Intravenous versus epidural administration. *Anesthesiology.* **80,** 1268–1276.

Philipsen, T., and Jensen, N.H. (1989). Epidural block for parenteral meperidine as analgesic in labor: A randomised study concerning progress in labor and instrumental deliveries. *Eur. J. Obstet. Gynecol. Reprod. Biol.* **30,** 27–33.

Preston, M.D., Rosen, M., Daniels, M., Glosten, B., Shnider, S., Ross, B., Dailey, P., and Hughes, S. (1987). Epidural fentanyl with lidocaine for cesarean section (abstract). *Anesthesiology.* **67,** A442.

Ramanthan, J., Coleman, P., and Sibai, B. (1991). Anesthetic modification of hemodynamic and neuroendocrine stress responses to cesarean delivery in women with severe preeclampsia. *Anesth. Analg.* **73,** 772–779.

Rayburn, W., Rathke, A., Leuschen, M.P., Chleborad, J., and Werdner, W. (1989). Fentanyl citrate analgesia during labor. *Am. J. Obstet. Gynecol.* **161,** 202–206.

Rayburn, W., Smith, C.V., Parriott, J.E., and Woods, R.E. (1989). Randomized comparison of meperidine and fentanyl during labor. *Obstet. Gynecol.* **74,** 604–607.

Rhien, A., Rhien, F., Wiedemann, B., and Distler, W. (1995). Pethidine-anwendung bei Geburten mit mekoniumhaltigem Fruchtwasser: Einfluß auf fetal outcome und respiratorische Störungen. *Z. Geburtsch. Neonatol.* **199,** 103–106.

Roberts, H., Kane, K.M., and Percival, N. (1957). Effects of some analgesic drugs used in childbirth. *Lancet.* **1,** 128–130.

Rosen, M.A., Dailey, P.A., Hughes, S.C., Leight, C.H., Shnider, S.M., Jackson, C.E., Baker, B.W., Cheek, D.B., and Connor, D.E. (1988). Epidural sufentanil for postoperative analgesia after cesarean section. *Anesthesiology.* **68,** 448–454.

Rust, M., Csontos, K., Mahr, W., Hollt, V., Zilker, T., Hegemann, M., and Teschemacher, H. (1980). Zum Verhalten von β-Endorphin in Perinatalperiode. *Geburtshilfe Frauenheilkd.* **40,** 769–777.

Rust, L.A., Waring, R.W., Hall, G.L., and Nelson, E.I. (1994). Intrathecal narcotics for obstetric analgesia in a community hospital. *Am. J. Obstet. Gynecol.* **170,** 1643–1648.

Sandman, C.A., Wadhwa, P.D., Chicz-DeMet, A., Porto, M., and Garite, T.J. (1995). Third trimester POMC disregulation predicts use of anesthesia at vaginal delivery. *Peptides.* 187–190.

Savonna-Ventura, C., Sammut, M., and Sammut, C. (1991). Meperidine blood concentrations at time of birth. *Int. J. Gynecol. Obstet.* **36,** 103–107.

Scott, P.V., Bowen, F.E., Cartwright, P., Rao, B.C., Deely, D., Wotherspoon, H.J., and Gumrein, J.M. (1981). Intrathecal morphine as a sole analgesic during labour. *Anesthesiology.* **54,** 136–140.

Shaaban, M.M., Hung, T.T., Hoffman, D.I., Lobo, R.A., and Goebelsman, K. (1982). β-

Endorphin and β-lipotropin concentrations in umbilical cord blood. *Am. J. Obstet. Gynecol.* **144,** 560.

Shnider, S.M., and Levinson, G. (1994). Anesthesia for obstetrics. In *Miller, R.D. (ed.),* Anesthesia. 2031–2076.

Shnider, S.M., and Moya, F. (1964). Effects of meperidine on the newborn infant. *Am. J. Obstet. Gynecol.* **89,** 1009–1011.

Snyder, S.H. (1977). Opiate receptors in the brain. *N. Engl. J. Med.* **296,** 266–271.

Steinbrook, R.A., Carr, D.B., Datta, S., Naulty, J.S., Lee, C., and Fisher, J. (1982). Dissociation of plasma cerebrospinal fluid beta-endorphin-like immunoactivity levels during pregnancy and parturation. *Anesth. Analg.* **61,** 893–897.

Taylor, E.S., von Fumetti, H.H., and Essig, L.L. (1955). The effects of demerol and trichorethylene on arterial oxygen saturation in the newborn. *Am. J. Obstet. Gynecol.* **69,** 348.

Van Aken, H., Kick, O., and Weißauer, W. (1994). Geburtschilfliche Periduralanästhesie mit Sufentanil. *Anaesthesist.* **43,** 667–670.

Van Steenberghe, A., Debroux, H.C., and Noorduin, L.H. (1987). Extradural bupivacaine with sufentanil for vaginal delivery. *Br. J. Anaesth.* **59,** 1518–1522.

Vercauteren, M. (1996). Epidural analgesia for labor pain: (Still) the method of choice. *Acta Anesthesiol. Belg.* **47,** 163–169.

Vertommen, J.D., Marcus, M.A.E., and Van Aken, H. (1995). The effects of intravenous and epidural sufentanil in the chronic maternal-fetal sheep preparation. *Anesth. Analg.* **80,** 71–75.

Vertommen, J.D., Vandermeulen, E., Van Aken, H., Vaes, L., Soetens, M., van Steenberghe, A., Mourisse, P., Willaret, J., Noorduin, H., Devlieger, H., and Van Assche, A. (1991). The effects of the addition of sufentanil to 0.125% bupivacaine on the quality of analgesia during labor and on the incidence of instrumental deliveries. *Anesthesiology.* **74,** 809–814.

Viegas, O.A.C., Khaw, B., and Ratnam, S.S. (1993). Tramadol in labour pain in primiparous patients. A prospective comparative clinical trial. *Eur. J. Obstet. Gynecol. Reprod. Biol.* **49,** 131–135.

Wang, C.Y. (1992). Respiratory depression after extradural fentanyl. *Br. J. Anaesth.* **69,** 544.

Wright, P.M.C., Allen, R.W., Moore, J., and Donelly, J. P. (1992). Gastric emptying during lumbar extradural analgesia in labour: Effect of fentanyl supplementation. *Br. J. Anesth.* **68,** 248–251.

Zakowsky, M.I., Goldstein, M.J., Ramanathan, S., and Turndorf, H. (1991). Intrathecal fentanyl for labor analgesia. *Anesthesiology.* **75,** A840.

Zimmerman, D.L., Breen, T.W., and Fick, G. (1996). Adding fentanyl 0,0002% to epidural bupivacaine 0,125% does not delay gastric emptying in laboring parturients. *Anesth. Analg.* **82,** 612–616.

Index

Note: page numbers printed in **boldface** type refer to tables or figures